CATEGORY - OBS & Gy.

THE MANAGEMENT OF THE MENOPAUSE

ANNUAL REVIEW 1998

THE MANAGEMENT OF THE MENOPAUSE
ANNUAL REVIEW 1998

Edited by
John Studd

Chelsea & Westminster Hospital, London, UK

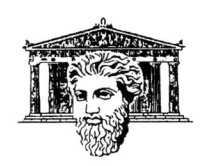

The Parthenon Publishing Group
International Publishers in Medicine, Science & Technology

NEW YORK   LONDON

Published in the USA by
The Parthenon Publishing Group Inc.
One Blue Hill Plaza, PO Box 1564,
Pearl River, New York 10965, USA

Published in the UK and Europe by
The Parthenon Publishing Group Ltd.
Casterton Hall, Carnforth,
Lancs. LA6 2LA, UK

ISSN 1460-1397

British Library Cataloguing-in-Publication Data
The management of the Menopause: annual review 1998
 1. Menopause—Periodicals
 I. Studd, John W. W.
 618.1'75'005

ISBN 1-85070-022-2

Copyright © 1998 The Parthenon Publishing Group Limited

No part of this publication may be reproduced, in any form, without permission from the publishers except for the quotation of brief passages for the purpose of review.

Typeset by AMA Graphics Ltd., Preston, UK
Printed and bound by Butler & Tanner Ltd., Frome and London, UK

Contents

	List of principal contributors	ix
	Introduction J. Studd	xiii
1	The menopausal transition H. Teede and H. G. Burger	1
2	Depression and the menopausal transition A. Collins	13
3	Estrogens and skin M. P. Brincat and R. Galea	19
4	The effect of estrogens on wound healing M. Calvin, J. Rymer, S. R. Young and M. Dyson	27
5	The effect of estrogen deficiency on the bladder A. Hextall and L. Cardozo	39
6	Sexuality and the menopause A. Graziottin	49
7	Arthritis, estrogens and menopause F. M. Cicuttini and T. D. Spector	59
8	Contraception for women over forty A. E. Gebbie	67
9	Epidemiology of phytoestrogens and cancer M. S. Morton and K. Griffiths	81
10	Ovum donation for premature menopause H. I. Abdalla and A. K. S. Kan	93
11	New delivery systems for hormone replacement therapy I. S. Fraser and Y. Wang	101

12	Endometrial risks with hormone replacement therapy *J. H. Pickar*	111
13	The clinical problem of treating osteoporosis with estrogens *E. F. Eriksen and M. Kassem*	121
14	Timing of postmenopausal estrogen for optimal bone mineral density *D. L. Schneider and D. J. Morton*	135
15	Value of bone markers in osteoporosis and related diseases *M. Bonde and C. Christiansen*	143
16	Nutritional support for osteoporosis *A. Carey and B. Carey*	159
17	Estrogens and neurotransmitters *A. R. Genazzani, C. Salvestroni, A. Spinetti, P. Monteleone and F. Petraglia*	169
18	Estrogens and cerebral blood flow *W. L. McCullough and K. F. Gangar*	177
19	Estrogens and prevention of Alzheimer's disease *V. W. Henderson*	183
20	Hormone replacement therapy and breast cancer mortality *L. Bergkvist*	193
21	Estrogens after breast cancer *S. L. Nand, J. A. Eden and B. G. Wren*	199
22	The cardioprotective effects of estrogens *F. Grodstein and M. J. Stampfer*	211
23	Estrogen therapy after coronary artery thrombosis *J. M. Sullivan*	221
24	Hormone replacement therapy and diabetes mellitus *A. A. Oladipo, I. F. Godsland and J. C. Stevenson*	231
25	Treatment of progestogen intolerance *N. Panay and J. Studd*	241
26	Hormone replacement therapy after hysterectomy *J. Studd and G. Khastgir*	257

27	Efficacy of combined estrogen–androgen preparations in the postmenopause *B. B. Sherwin*	271
28	Andropause *A. Vermeulen and V. A. Giagulli*	279
	Index	297

List of principal contributors

H. I. Abdalla
Fertility and Endocrinology Centre
The Lister Hospital
Chelsea Bridge Road
London SW1W 8RH
UK

L. Bergkvist
Department of Surgery
Centrallasarett
S721 89 Västerås
Sweden

M. Bonde
Osteometer BioTech A/S
Herlev Hovedgade 207
DK-2730 Herlev
Denmark

M. P. Brincat
Faculty of Medicine and Surgery
Department of Obstetrics and Gynecology
University of Malta
St. Luke's Hospital Medical School
Gwardamangia
Malta

M. Calvin
Tissue Repair Research Unit
Department of Anatomy and Cell Biology
Guy's Hospital
London SE1 9RT
UK

A. Carey
Department of Obstetrics and Gynaecology
Chelsea & Westminster Hospital
Fulham Road
London SW10 9NH
UK

F. M. Cicuttini
Department of Epidemiology and Preventive Medicine
Alfred Hospital
Prahran
Victoria 3181
Australia

A. Collins
Department of Clinical Neuroscience
Karolinska Hospital
S171 76 Stockholm
Sweden

E. F. Eriksen
University Department of Endocrinology
Aarhus Amtssygehus
DK-8000 Aarhus C
Denmark

I. S. Fraser
Department of Obstetrics and Gynaecology
University of Sydney
NSW 2006
Australia

A. E. Gebbie
Community Gynaecology
Family Planning and Well Woman Services
18 Dean Terrace
Edinburgh EH4 1NL
UK

A. R. Genazzani
Department of Obstetrics and Gynecology
University of Pisa
Via Roma 67
56100 Pisa
Italy

A. Graziottin
Via San Secondo 19
10128 Turin
Italy

V. W. Henderson
Department of Neurology (PMB-B104)
University of Southern California School of
   Medicine
1420 San Pablo Street
Los Angeles, CA 90033
USA

A. Hextall
38 Barnfield Avenue
Kingston upon Thames
Surrey KT2 5RE
UK

G. Khastgir
Department of Obstetrics and Gynaecology
Chelsea & Westminster Hospital
Fulham Road
London SW10 9NH
UK

W. L. McCullough
Department of Obstetrics and Gynaecology
St. Mary's Hospital
Milton Road
Portsmouth PO3 6AD
UK

M. S. Morton
University of Wales College of Medicine
Tenovus Cancer Research Centre
Tenovus Building
Heath Park
Cardiff CF4 4XX
UK

S. L. Nand
School of Obstetrics and Gynaecology
Royal Hospital for Women
Barker Street
Randwick
NSW 2031
Australia

N. Panay
Academic Department of Obstetrics and
   Gynaecology
Chelsea & Westminster Hospital
Fulham Road
London SW10 9NH
UK

J. H. Pickar
Clinical Research
Wyeth-Ayerst Research
PO Box 8299
Philadelphia, PA 19101-8299
USA

D. L. Schneider
Department of Medicine
University of California
San Diego
9500 Gilman Drive
La Jolla
CA 92093-0638
USA

B. B. Sherwin
Department of Psychology
McGill University
Stewart Biology Building
1205 Dr Penfield Ave
Montreal, Quebec
Canada H3A 1B1

M. J. Stampfer
Department of Medicine
Harvard Medical School
181 Longwood Avenue
Boston
MA 02115
USA

J. C. Stevenson
Wynn Department of Metabolic Medicine
Division of Medicine
Imperial College School of Medicine
21 Wellington Road
London NW8 9SQ
UK

J. Studd
Department of Obstetrics and Gynaecology
Chelsea & Westminster Hospital
Fulham Road
London SW10 9NH
UK

J. M. Sullivan
The University of Tennessee Memphis
College of Medicine
Department of Medicine
Division of Cardiovascular Diseases
951 Court Avenue, Room 353D
Memphis, TN 38163
USA

H. Teede
Prince Henry's Institute of Medical Research
PO Box 5152
Clayton
Victoria 3168
Australia

A. Vermeulen
Department of Internal Medicine
Section of Endocrinology
University Hospital
De Pintelaan 185
9000 Gent
Belgium

Introduction

The explosion of interest and publications concerning the menopause and osteoporosis is most welcome as this will encourage the correct, safe treatment of so many women with these common problems. I think it is necessary to have an annual update which should attempt to bring together the most advanced thinking from the experts in this field. I am delighted that Parthenon Publishing has been so encouraging in this venture and has produced, with great skill, *The Management of the Menopause: Annual Review 1998*.

The secret of an annual review is to ask about 50 people to write chapters on the assumption that 25 chapters will turn up some time near the finishing post. The rest can be updated and with others form the bulk of the next edition. This explains why a few notable workers are not featured in this present volume and why certain important subjects such as SERMS or Contraindications to estrogen therapy will find their way into *Annual Review 1999*. Already, invitations have been sent to the team for this volume but I must invite any who are interested to write to me and submit ideas and titles which they may wish to contribute.

I have to admit that I am very pleased with this edition as I see it in proof form. I am committed to producing this each year and, with your help, I expect it to improve year by year and become an essential part of the literature of this fascinating area of medicine.

John Studd, DSc, MD, FRCOG
Chelsea & Westminster Hospital
London, UK

1
The menopausal transition

H. Teede and H. G. Burger

The long-term implications of estrogen deficiency in postmenopausal women have received much attention over the past decade. The impact on the cardiovascular system, the skeletal system and, more recently, the central nervous system remains the subject of ongoing research. In recent years, that field has expanded to include the years prior to the menopause. To clarify existing terminology, the menopause is defined by the World Health Organization[1] as the permanent cessation of menstruation resulting from the loss of ovarian follicular activity. The perimenopause is the phase extending from the onset of symptoms of the ensuing menopause to 1 year after the final menstrual period. The menopausal transition refers to that time of the perimenopause prior to the final menstrual period, essentially encompassing a phase of transition from fertile, ovulatory cycles with well-characterized hormone profiles to the postmenopause, with low estrogen and progesterone, and high gonadotropin levels. Longitudinal studies have characterized the menopausal transition with a median age of onset of 45.5–47.5 years and an average duration of 4 years[2,3]. The incidence of dysfunctional uterine bleeding and hysterectomy are maximal during the menopausal transition, and the incidence of symptoms is similar to that in postmenopausal women[2]. During these years, women seek medical consultation more frequently than pre- or postmenopausal women. In this setting, current knowledge of the menopausal transition, including the physiological changes, clinical features and management, is reviewed.

REPRODUCTIVE HORMONAL DYNAMICS: NORMAL PHYSIOLOGY

An initial review of the function of the hypothalamic–pituitary–ovarian axis during the mid-reproductive years is warranted to provide a background for subsequent observations throughout the transition. The pituitary is regulated by pulsatile secretion of gonadotropin releasing hormone (GnRH) from the hypothalamus. In turn, the pituitary produces gonadotropins: luteinizing hormone (LH) and follicle stimulating hormone (FSH). Gonadotropins are responsible for the regulation of ovarian function and are subject to predominantly negative feedback by the sex steroids estrogen and progesterone. Regulation of FSH is more complex as it is subject to an additional negative feedback system mediated by the inhibins, and pituitary secretion of FSH has an autonomous component as well as being GnRH-dependent.

Inhibin is a dimeric glycoprotein produced in the granulosa cells of the ovary, as reviewed by Burger[4]. There are two distinct subtypes, A and B, with a common α subunit and one of two β chains. The β subunits demonstrate functional, structural and molecular differences to render the two subtypes distinct hormones with different physiological roles[5]. Inhibin A is produced mainly by the granulosa cells of the dominant follicle in the follicular phase and by the corpus luteum during the luteal phase. Inhibin B (Figure 1) is probably a product of the cohort of growing antral follicles in the early to

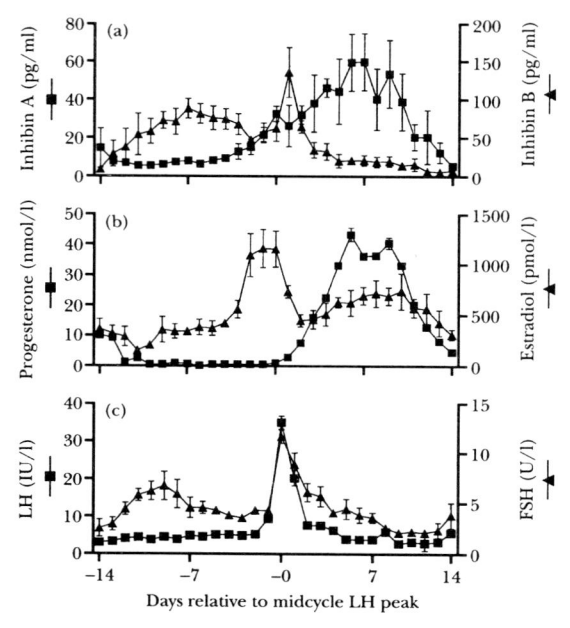

Figure 1 Plasma concentrations of (a) inhibin A and inhibin B, (b) estradiol and progesterone and (c) luteinizing hormone (LH) and follicle stimulating hormone (FSH) during female menstrual cycle: data displayed with respect to day of midcycle LH peak. Adapted from reference 5, with permission

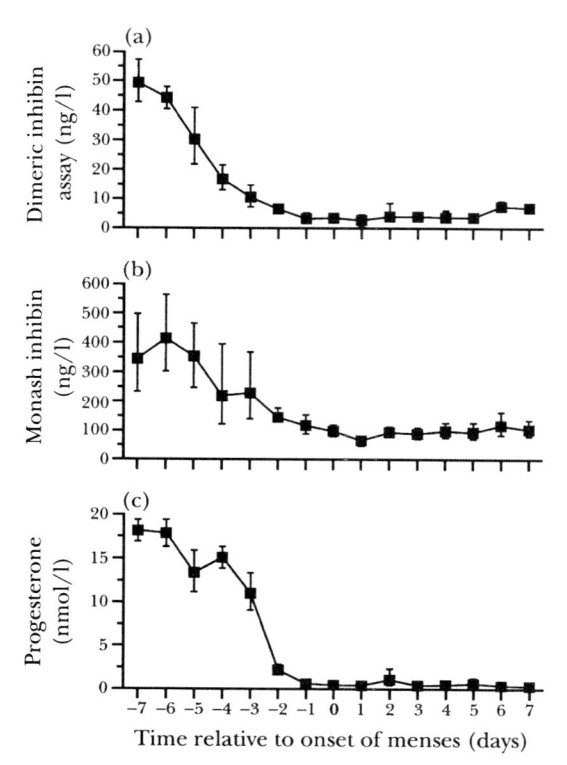

Figure 2 Geometric mean concentrations (± 67% confidence interval) of (a) dimeric inhibin compared with (b) Monash inhibin and (c) progesterone during luteal–follicular transition: first day of menstruation represents day zero. Adapted from reference 6, with permission

mid-follicular phase, and falls to low levels in the luteal phase[5,6]. The function of the inhibins includes paracrine regulation of the gonads and closed-loop negative feedback on FSH at the level of the pituitary with levels inversely correlated with FSH[7,8]. Administration of FSH has also been shown to stimulate inhibin production[9]. Activins, discovered during the purification of inhibin, are formed from the dimerization of two inhibin B subunits. Activins primarily act in paracrine regulatory functions in the ovary and in the pituitary, where activin B is responsible for the autonomous component of FSH secretion[10]. Most studies of the physiology of inhibin have employed a heterologous radio-immunoassay developed in Melbourne and called the 'Monash assay'. It is non-selective, detecting inhibins A and B and inactive free α subunits[4]. Subsequent work has demonstrated that the Monash assay parallels the patterns seen with inhibin A (Figure 2). Recent assays have been developed based on two-site detection of both active dimeric inhibins A and B, and their physiology in the menstrual cycle has been documented[5,6].

REPRODUCTIVE HORMONAL DYNAMICS IN MENOPAUSAL TRANSITION

The physiology of the hormonal milieu during the menopausal transition is still being clarified. Current understanding encompasses the exponential decline of oocyte numbers as menopause approaches[11], with fluctuating ovarian hormone production and altered feedback regulation on the pituitary as a result of approaching ovarian failure. The significant role of inhibin has been appreciated in recent years. Reyes and colleagues[12] studied ovulating women in the age range 20–50 years. Follicle

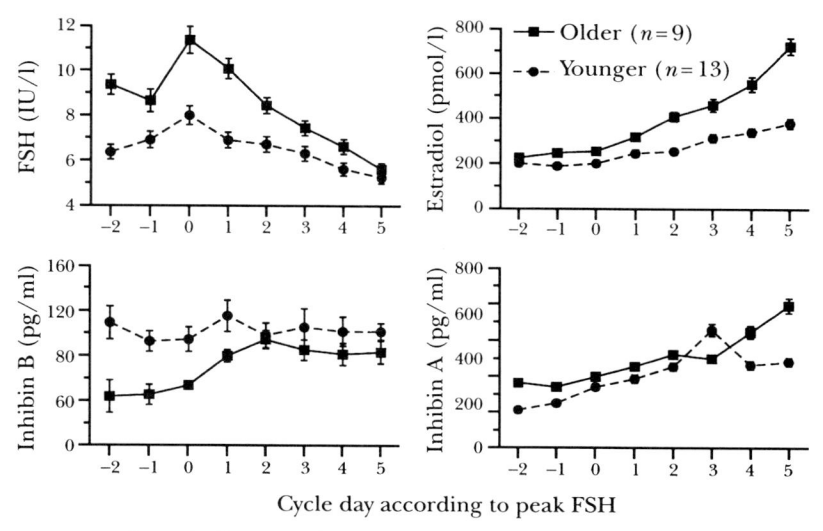

Figure 3 Mean concentrations (± SEM) of follicle stimulating hormone (FSH), estradiol, inhibin B and inhibin A plotted relative to day of maximal FSH peak comparing younger and older cycling women. Adapted from reference 19, with permission

stimulating hormone was noted to increase with age; however, estradiol did not decline prior to menopause. Lee and co-workers[13] had a similar finding with a rising FSH but no decline in levels of estradiol. It became obvious that other factors were responsible for the observed rise in FSH and this dilemma was touched on in the 1970s when these observations on estrogen and FSH were first noted. Sherman and Korenman[14] proposed that reductions in an 'inhibin-like substance' similar to that found in men, could be the primary stimulus for FSH elevation. While longitudinal studies were still to be completed, further evidence to support this theory of declining inhibin prior to the menopause was sought with most studies using the non-specific Monash assay. Evidence for a reduced inhibin reserve with age[15] is supported by studies on women undergoing *in vitro* fertilization. Hughes and associates[16] demonstrated that inhibin responses to gonadotropin hyperstimulation were significantly lower in women over 35 years compared with those of younger women, whereas the estradiol responses were similar in all groups. Cross-sectional studies demonstrated declining inhibin with increasing age and elevated FSH[7,17,18]. The longitudinal phase of the Melbourne Midlife Women's Health Study is currently being analyzed; however, inhibin fell prior to the menopause[17]. The fall in immunoreactive inhibin levels was associated with a rise in FSH and preceded a fall in estrogen levels. A recent study has provided evidence (Figure 3) that it is a fall in inhibin B in the follicular phase of the cycle that particularly accounts for the age-associated rise in FSH, with estradiol levels being slightly higher in the older women[19].

The fall in inhibin levels correlates with physiological changes occurring in the ovary as follicle numbers (the source of inhibin production) decline dramatically. Autopsy studies[20], oophorectomy studies[11] and mathematical models[21] have all indicated that the rate of follicular depletion increases during the menopausal transition, with a greater percentage of follicles becoming atretic at any one time. Accelerated follicular development of recruited follicles is also observed[19]. At this time, the primary event, which stimulates this process of accelerated follicular depletion, is not understood and remains a topic of ongoing research. Vihko[22] found that levels of FSH receptors on ovarian follicles are reduced in the years preceding the menopause, and suggested that there is a disturbance of follicular maturation and function prior to exhaustion of follicles. Likewise, an increasing percentage of cycles are anovulatory as women approach the menopause[23,24]. Consistent with this, the level of progesterone declines as the menopause approaches[25].

Follicular development has also been demonstrated to be erratic[26,27] with consequent variability in estrogen levels. Several cases of elevated estrogen production in the setting of multiple developing follicles have been documented in the perimenopause. Metcalf and colleagues[28], in a longitudinal study of 31 women, documented that in 14 women, on 32 separate occasions, elevated FSH with high estrogen levels occurred. Fitzgerald and co-workers[29] noted perimenopausal women had the most variability in ovarian steroid profiles, but found the mean serum estrogen levels were no different from those of younger women. Santoro and colleagues[25] recently studied daily urine profiles in a longitudinal study of women aged 47–50 years. Overall, the perimenopausal women had a greater estrone conjugate excretion than did mid-reproductive-aged women. Variability was again evident, with episodes of marked hyperestrogenism and elevated FSH levels documented in many of the women studied. Brown[27] demonstrated this many years ago; unfortunately, little recognition was given to these findings because they were thought to be incompatible with the conventional thinking of slowly progressive decline in estrogen in this setting. In fact, Brown analyzed urinary steroid profiles in 85 'climacteric' women. Figure 4 exemplifies the patterns documented in one of these women from age 42 to 48 years. Estrogen levels fluctuated, with periods of hyperestrogenism, consistent with multiple follicles developing at any one time. Follicle stimulating hormone levels tested in the 47th year also demonstrated classic fluctuations. Pregnanediol levels declined with obvious increases in anovulatory cycles. These fluctuating hormone profiles would explain the presence of variable symptoms, including those of estrogen excess and the high incidence of dysfunctional uterine bleeding. Interestingly, an increase in the rate of follicle development with elevated FSH and estrogen has been reviewed by Baird[30] in adolescents with anovulatory dysfunctional uterine bleeding.

The concept of altered hypothalamic–pituitary sensitivity during the perimenopause is also important to consider. It has been demonstrated that hormone replacement therapy (HRT) does not suppress gonadotropin production completely, and also that estrogen suppression of the hypothalamic–pituitary axis is not as reliable in the setting of the menopausal transition. Van Look and associates[31] performed a longitudinal study on women with dysfunctional uterine bleeding in the perimenopause and on regularly menstruating control subjects. Serial steroid and gonadotropin levels were analyzed under basal conditions and during dynamic testing. Results were compared with those of premenopausal controls. In contrast with results from controls, exogenous estradiol did not have any consistent suppressive effect on gonadotropins in these women. This, along with the documentation of elevated estrogens in the presence of elevated gonadotropins, indicates that feedback is altered. Metcalf and colleagues aptly stated 'the only conclusion which can be made with confidence concerning pituitary–ovarian function in individual perimenopausal women is that it is unsafe to generalize'[28].

Ovarian interstitial cells under LH stimulation produce androgens, with adrenal androgens being the other primary source. Androgen profiles remain controversial even in postmenopausal women and, in the transitional period, the literature on androgens demonstrates many inconsistencies. Bancroft and Caewood[32] recently studied sex steroid profiles in women aged 40–60 years in a cross-sectional study. The study concluded that androgen profiles are inherently complex with no clear patterns related to the menopause emerging after multivariate analysis. Lifestyle factors including smoking and nutrition showed significant impact[32]. Burger and co-workers[17] demonstrated a decline of 1.7% per year in serum testosterone in women in the transition. However, after correction for age and body mass index (BMI), testosterone was higher in women as they approached the menopause. Generally,

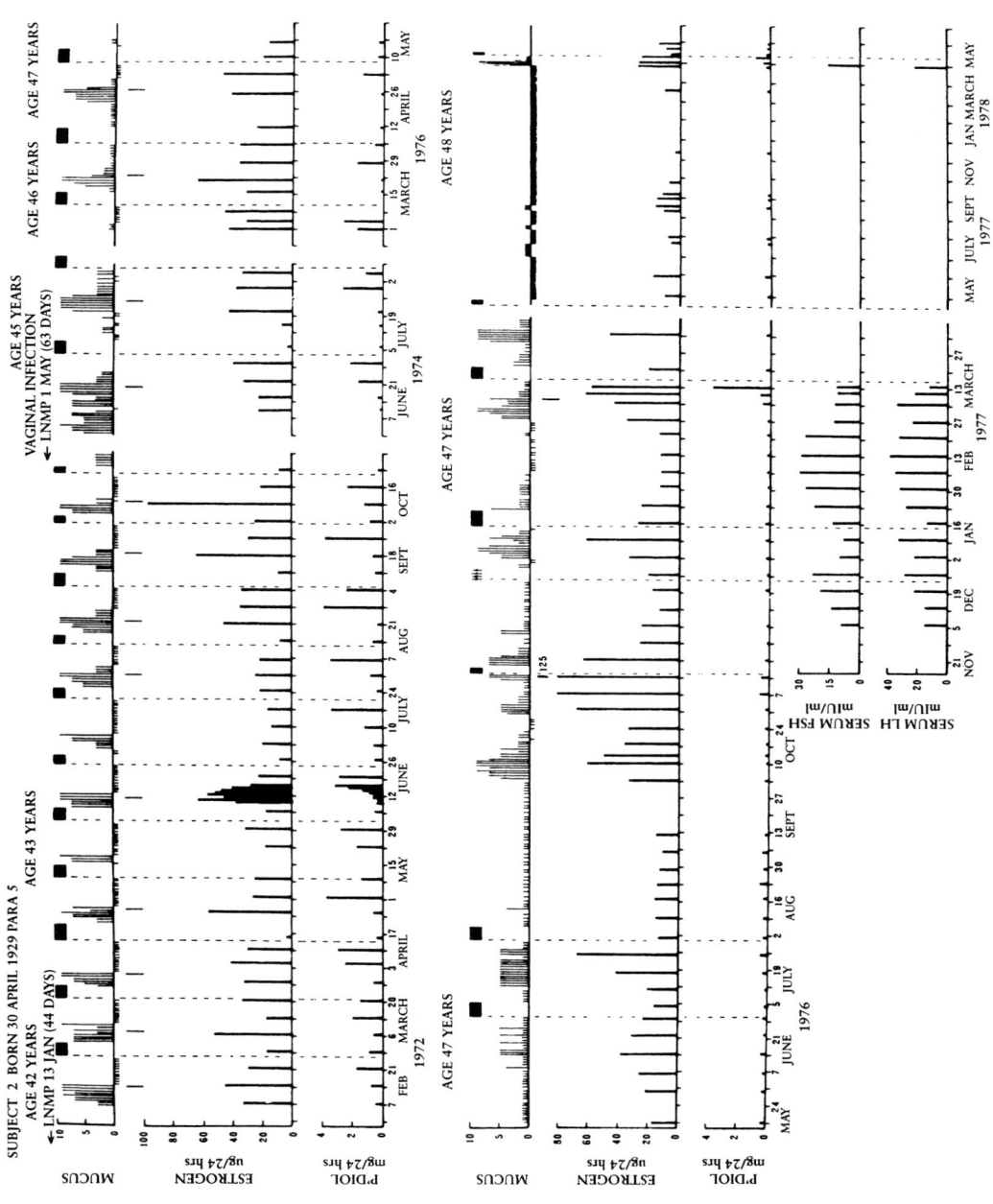

Figure 4 Weekly urinary estrogen and pregnanediol (progesterone metabolite) values, mucus scores and menstrual bleeding (documented by black blocked areas) over 6 years in a woman in menopausal transition aged 42–48 years: serum follicle stimulating hormone (FSH) and luteinizing hormone (LH) values were measured in the 47th year. Adapted from reference 27, with permission

there appear to be no significant changes in androgen levels across the transition. It is possible that the levels may fall many years prior to the menopausal transition[33].

Based on the foregoing discussion, the primary endocrine event with reproductive aging may be a fall in inhibin B, allowing FSH to rise which, in turn, leads to accelerated follicle development and increased estrogen secretion in older women until the follicle pool has been exhausted.

CLINICAL FEATURES OF THE MENOPAUSAL TRANSITION

Symptoms

Women in the perimenopausal years are more likely to seek medical consultation than their pre- or postmenopausal counterparts[2]. In this setting, clinicians would benefit from an optimal understanding of symptoms experienced during these years. A number of studies have demonstrated that factors including culture, education and socioeconomic environment all influence individual experiences of the menopause. The nature of symptoms attributable to physiological hormonal changes *per se* remains controversial, despite extensive study in industrialized nations. Longitudinal, population-based studies have described several distinct clusters of symptoms that demonstrate different characteristics[34]. This is exemplified by vasomotor symptoms that demonstrate the most instability during the transition, no doubt influenced by fluctuating hormone profiles. Clusters of dysphoric mood and neuromuscular symptoms, however, appear more stable and are believed to reflect psychosocial events and not simply hormonal changes *per se*.

Although specific symptoms are not unique to the transitional period, there are several features that warrant discussion. While genitourinary symptoms are not prominent prior to the menopause, vasomotor symptoms including hot flushes and night sweats, disturbances of sexuality and psychological symptoms are all markedly increased[34,35]. Studies have noted symptoms to be maximal during the transition and the immediate postmenopausal period (Figure 5). Negative psychological symptoms were at their highest incidence while a sense of well-being was at its lowest in several studies comparing symptoms in pre-, peri- and postmenopausal women[37]. In case studies and cross-sectional studies, symptoms of estrogen excess and deficiency were described often in the same individual over time. Breast tenderness, menorrhagia, migraine, nausea, shorter cycle length and a shorter follicular phase were described[25,27,31]. These were thought at the time to be incompatible with conventional concepts of gradually declining estrogen. More recently, as studies on hormone profiles confirmed considerable inter- and intraindividual variation, with transient periods of estrogen excess in the setting of

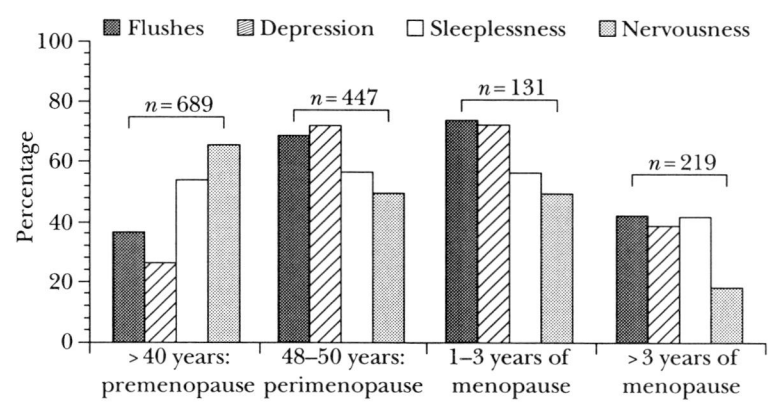

Figure 5 Incidence of symptoms in women from age 40 to several years postmenopause. Adapted from reference 36, with permission

elevated FSH, these symptoms were clarified. Given that estrogen levels are often well preserved, even elevated on occasion, the understanding of vasomotor symptoms becomes more complex. This is exemplified by the fact that women who receive estrogen implants experience flushes when estrogen levels are in the high normal range but levels are decreasing[38]. Consistent with this, women have documented cyclical patterns to their flushes[26], and it may be that flushes are occurring in response to fluctuations rather than simply low levels of estrogen. In contrast with this, evidence also exists correlating estrogen levels with flush frequency in a longitudinal study of women in the transition[39] (Figure 6). There remains a great deal to understand about the etiology of vasomotor disturbances.

Women may experience significant symptoms related to hormonal fluctuations as described above. They also have to contend with menstrual disturbances with irregular and heavy cycles. Fitzgerald and colleagues described age-related changes in the reproductive cycle[29]. Cycles are, in general, shorter with a shorter follicular phase during later years. Cycle length eventually increases and irregular cycles occur. Dysfunctional uterine bleeding, with persistent elevation of unopposed estrogens[40], occurs most frequently in perimenopausal women, who have the greatest maximal thickness of endometrium[29] and have the highest incidence of hysterectomy. Interestingly, after studying ovarian secretion of estrogen in women with dysfunctional uterine bleeding, it was suggested in 1974 by Fraser and Baird[40] that it occurs secondary to inappropriate estrogen secretion resulting from multiple follicles developing, owing to abnormal gonadotropin release. Ironically, this would well describe the hormone profile we have confirmed some 24 years later.

Bone turnover

A rapid phase of bone turnover is well documented in the early postmenopausal period and contributes significantly to osteoporosis in later life. Recently, several studies have focused on bone turnover in the menopausal transition. Interpreting studies on bone turnover, like much of the research during this phase of reproductive life, presents difficulties. Specific issues include lack of uniformity on definitions of the respective phases of later reproductive life as well as difficulty in analyzing changes specific to each reproductive phase. Despite this, evidence is emerging for alterations in bone turnover prior to the menopause. Guthrie and associates[41] studied bone mineral density (BMD), hormone profiles and bone turnover markers in a cross-sectional study in the menopausal transition as a component of the Melbourne Midlife Women's Health Study. Age was the primary determinant of femoral neck changes in BMD; however, lumbar spine density was influenced by menopausal status as well as age[41]. Interestingly, decline in bone density was noted prior to the decline in estrogen levels, but was accompanied by an increase in mean FSH levels. Guthrie and associates hypothesized that factors other than estrogen may be influencing bone turnover. Nilas and Christiansen[42] also reported radial bone loss in women in the transitional period associated with increased FSH, but not reduced estrogen levels. A study by Steinberg and

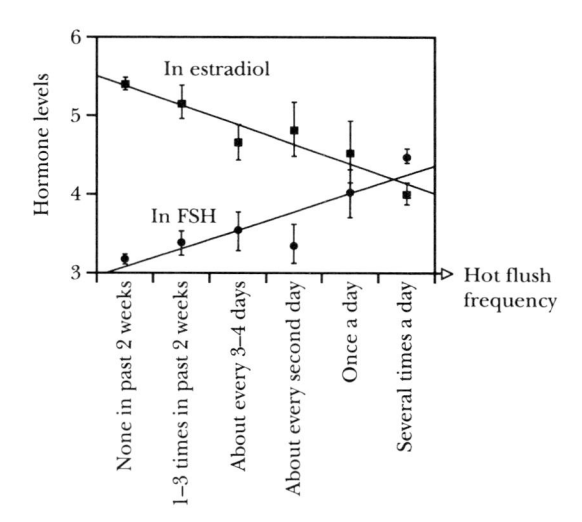

Figure 6 Relationship between frequency of hot flush reporting and mean (± SEM) of log transformed values of follicle stimulating hormone (FSH) and estradiol in women in the Melbourne Midlife Women's Health Study. Adapted from reference 39, with permission

co-workers[43] has demonstrated cross-sectional changes in BMD in the perimenopause. Once again, FSH was inversely correlated with BMD; however, estrogen and testosterone levels did correlate with lower BMD in this study. Johnston and colleagues[44] noted that BMD was lower in women prior to the cessation of menses, and estrone levels were again correlated with BMD. Slemenda and co-workers[45] undertook a longitudinal study over 3 years and demonstrated that women in the later phase of the menopausal transition had elevated FSH and reduced radial BMD; however, those in the early transitional phase with irregular cycles and normal FSH did not demonstrate reduced BMD.

Clearly, the opportunity to improve peak bone mass has passed in women reaching the menopausal transition. Prevention of further bone loss is ideal to prevent later osteoporotic fracture. The preventive effects of exercise on bone turnover in the perimenopause have been studied. Goto and associates[46] concentrated on the protective effects of exercise in 26 women, aged 39–65 years, in a longitudinal study over 5 years. Peri- and postmenopausal women both demonstrated bone loss in the hip and lumbar spine despite regular exercise. Pharmacological intervention for women with low bone density in the transition is still to be clarified. An interesting study by Shargil[47] demonstrated that women taking oral contraceptives for 3 years over the transitional period had higher BMD compared with that of controls. A study by Draper and Roland[48] focused on the willingness of perimenopausal women to consider hormone replacement therapy for osteoporosis prevention. Seventy per cent of respondents to a questionnaire considered osteoporosis to be an important indication for HRT. Given the emerging evidence that bone turnover increases, BMD falls and oral contraceptive therapy is protective preceding menopause, it may well be timely to consider osteoporosis and skeletal health earlier than conventionally thought, especially in women with a high risk of osteoporotic fracture.

Cardiovascular risk factors

Structural vascular disease is the culmination of years of exposure to many complex interacting factors. The acute effects of estrogen deficiency would not be expected to result in an increased incidence of vascular disease in the short term. This is reflected in the epidemiology of vascular disease in women, with those over 60 years primarily affected. Therefore, the relevant issues relating to the vascular system in the menopausal transition are related to risk-factor management. Jensen and colleagues[49] and others have noted adverse changes in risk profiles between pre- and postmenopausal women. Few studies have addressed the issue of cardiovascular risk across the menopausal transition. Matthews and co-workers[50] focused on changes throughout the years surrounding the menopause; however, definitions in this study differed from those employed here, resulting in difficulty separating observed changes into pre- and postmenopausal timing. No substantial changes were noted in lipid profiles except for a small change in triglyceride levels. An interesting

Table 1 Plasma lipid concentrations in 100 perimenopausal women taking the oral contraceptive pill (OCP) and 100 controls over 3 years. Adapted from reference 47, with permission

Months of study	Total cholesterol (mg/100 ml) OCP	Controls	Triglycerides (mg/100 ml) OCP	Controls	LDL cholesterol (mg/100 ml) OCP	Controls	HDL cholesterol (mg/100 ml) OCP	Controls
On admission	260 ± 5	260 ± 10	130 ± 12	130 ± 10	120 ± 8	115 ± 15	37 ± 5	35 ± 6
6	255 ± 13	263 ± 10	110 ± 8	125 ± 4	98 ± 6	120 ± 10	45 ± 6	33 ± 4
12	246 ± 8	260 ± 17	78 ± 10	132 ± 9	80 ± 11	140 ± 8	50 ± 3	30 ± 6
24	230 ± 10	288 ± 9	76 ± 7	170 ± 19	58 ± 7	156 ± 6	56 ± 6	27 ± 5
36	230 ± 9	200 ± 15	70 ± 10	210 ± 13	60 ± 10	168 ± 12	55 ± 6	29 ± 5

LDL, low density lipoprotein; HDL, high density lipoprotein

study by Shargil[47] looked at the effects of 3 years of treatment with triphasic low-dose oral contraceptives in 100 women and 100 controls aged 40–50 years. The perimenopausal women on the oral contraceptive preparation demonstrated an improvement in lipid profile compared with that of controls (Table 1). Estrogen supplementation in the setting of estrogen deficiency in postmenopausal women has been well documented to improve vascular risk factors and reduce the incidence of cardiovascular disease. Darling and associates[51] noted that estrogens and conventional lipid lowering agents (in low dose) are both effective in improving lipid profiles. Further studies are needed in this area to document the timing of onset of adverse changes in vascular risk factors as women approach the menopause.

MANAGEMENT

In the setting of variable hormone profiles and symptoms, how should a physician approach the assessment and management of women approaching the menopause? The complexity of the physiology dictates that the solutions may not be simple. Studies in perimenopausal women have noted the variations in FSH, inhibin and estrogen levels to be transient and, therefore, unreliable in diagnosing approaching menopause or predicting the stage of any given woman in the menopausal transition[9,52]. However, if FSH is to be used, for example, in women who have had a hysterectomy, early follicular phase samples have been shown to be the most reliable[52]. Serum estrogen levels add another complication, as cycle phase and relationship with ovulation are extremely difficult to estimate at this time, yet are essential to interpret serum estrogens.

A more rational approach would appear to be the acquisition of individual longitudinal symptom data on women who present with perimenopausal complaints. The importance of daily menstrual pattern documentation was emphasized by Treloar[3]. The Melbourne Midlife Women's Health Study demonstrated that hormone profiles correlate well with symptoms and cycle features[17]. Offering individuals a diary for the recording of menstrual disturbances and symptoms can be a useful exercise in self-education for women and a useful assessment tool for clinicians.

The primary symptoms in the menopausal transition relate to dysfunctional uterine bleeding, irregularity of cycles and hot flushes, together with insomnia and emotional symptoms which are prevalent during this period. Education, support and advice on lifestyle issues are essential in the approach to management. Dietary intervention has received considerable attention in the community at large as well as in the medical field. Phytoestrogens or plant-based agents with estrogenic activity may offer benefit to women at this time of life[53]. At present, few studies on menopausal symptom relief have been completed, with existing studies showing conflicting results. While phytoestrogens may indeed offer women a non-pharmacological alternative with an appealing side-effect profile in the future, further research is required not only into symptom prevention but also into the estrogenic actions of these compounds on other target organs including bone and the cardiovascular system.

Pharmacological alternatives include conventional hormone replacement therapy, a low-dose oral contraceptive pill or progesterone therapy alone. Progesterone is useful in the management of irregular menses and menorrhagia, and has also been documented in two separate randomized, placebo-controlled trials to reduce hot flushes[54,55]. Although progesterone may induce side-effects, it is often well tolerated in this age group[56]. The use of conventional HRT to induce cycle regularity, reduce hormone fluctuations and reduce symptoms is more difficult than in the predictable estrogen deficiency state of the postmenopausal woman. While HRT may be appropriate in the later stages of the transition with hormone profiles more akin to those of postmenopausal women, women in the earlier stages of the transition with more erratic hormone profiles are likely to encounter difficulties. As discussed above, evidence exists for altered hypothalamic–pituitary sensitivity during the transition, which is important to consider when making therapeutic decisions. Low-dose oral contraceptive pills provide a viable alternative as they offer the advantage of suppressing hypothalamic–pituitary function, therefore suppressing turbulent endogenous hormonal activity. Upton[57] reviewed the safety of the oral contraceptive pill in this age group with the conclusion that low-dose preparations are safe in non-smoking, non-hypertensive women up to the age of 50 years. The increased risk of cerebrovascular accidents in women on low-dose oral contraceptives is primarily expressed in smokers and women who are hypertensive[58]. The issue of when to change from oral contraception to HRT is difficult. Castracane and colleagues[59] addressed this issue of when fertility and estrogen production have declined sufficiently to allow safe transition to HRT. In premenopausal women, compared to peri- and postmenopausal women, rebound levels of estradiol and FSH were measured following withdrawal of the oral contraceptive pill. Levels of FSH and estradiol did not behave consistently, highlighting the difficulties in interpreting the results of hormone profiles over these years. At the present time, it remains a clinical dilemma when to safely cease contraception and not expose patients to the risk of pregnancy.

CONCLUSION

The physiology of the menopausal transition is still being clarified. Existing data show that it is a time of exponential decline in oocyte number with turbulent hormone profiles with reduced inhibin reserve, fluctuating estrogen and generally rising FSH levels. In this setting, the ideal assessment is individual, longitudinal and symptom-based, best achieved by the use of a perimenopause diary rather than isolated hormone levels. Therapeutic options are complex, as the underlying hormonal milieu and associated symptoms are variable. The low-dose oral contraceptive pill improves lipid profiles, and reduces bone loss as well as preventing symptoms, regulating menses and providing contraception: thus, especially in the early transitional years, it may be the best treatment alternative.

References

1. World Health Organization. *Research on the Menopause in the 1990s*. Report of a WHO Scientific Group. Geneva: WHO, 1996
2. McKinlay SM, Brambilla DJ, Posner JG. The normal menopause transition. *Maturitas* 1992; 14:103–15
3. Treloar AE. Menstrual cyclicity and the premenopause. *Maturitas* 1981;3:249–64
4. Burger HG. Clinical utility of inhibin measurements. *J Clin Endocrinol Metab* 1993;76:1391–6
5. Groome NP, Illingworth PJ, O'Brien M, et al. Measurement of dimeric inhibin B throughout the human menstrual cycle. *J Clin Endocrinol Metab* 1996;81:1401–5
6. Groome NP, Illingworth PJ, O'Brien M, et al. Detection of dimeric inhibin throughout the human menstrual cycle by two-site enzyme immunoassay. *Clin Endocrinol* 1994;40:717–23
7. Burger HG. Evidence for a negative feedback role of inhibin in FSH regulation in women. *Hum Reprod* 1993;8(Suppl 2):129–32
8. MacNaughton J, Banagh M, McCloud P, et al. Age-related changes in follicular stimulating hormone, luteinising hormone, estradiol and immunoreactive inhibin in women of reproductive age. *Clin Endocrinol* 1992;36:339–45
9. Hee JP, MacNaughton J, Banagh M, et al. FSH induces dose-dependent stimulation of immunoreactive inhibin secretion during the follicular phase of the human menstrual cycle. *J Clin Endocrinol Metab* 1993;76:1340–3
10. Corrigan AZ, Bilezikjian LM, Carroll RS, et al. Evidence for an autonomous role of activin B within rat anterior pituitary culture. *Endocrinology* 1991;128:1682–4
11. Richardson SJ, Senikas V, Nelson JF. Follicular depletion during the menopausal transition: evidence for accelerated loss and ultimate exhaustion. *J Clin Endocrinol Metab* 1987;65:1231
12. Reyes FI, Winter JS, Faiman C. Pituitary ovarian relationships preceding the menopause. I. A cross-sectional study of serum follicle-stimulating hormone, luteinizing hormone, prolactin, estradiol and progesterone levels. *Am J Obstet Gynecol* 1977;129:557–64

13. Lee SJ, Lenton EA, Sexton L et al. The effect of age on the cyclical patterns of plasma LH, FSH, estradiol and progesterone in women with regular menstrual cycles. *Hum Reprod* 1988;3:851–5
14. Sherman BM, Korenman SG. Hormonal characteristics of the human menstrual cycle throughout reproductive life. *J Clin Invest* 1975;55:699–706
15. Pellicer A, Simon C, Mari M, et al. Effects of aging on the human ovary: the secretion of immunoreactive α-inhibin and progesterone. *Fertil Steril* 1994;61:663–8
16. Hughes EG, Robertson DM, Handelsman DJ, et al. Inhibin and estradiol responses to ovarian hyperstimulation: effects of age and predictive value for *in vitro* fertilization outcome. *J Clin Endocrinol Metab* 1990;70:358–64
17. Burger HG, Dudley EC, Hopper JL, et al. The endocrinology of the menopausal transition: a cross-sectional study of a population-based sample. *J Clin Endocrinol Metab* 1995;80:3537–45
18. Lenton EA, Kretser DM, Woodward AJ, et al. Inhibin concentrations throughout the menstrual cycles of normal, infertile and older women compared with those during spontaneous conception cycles. *J Clin Endocrinol Metab* 1991;73:1180–90
19. Klein NA, Illingworth PJ, Groome NP, et al. Decreased inhibin B secretion is associated with the monotropic rise of FSH in older, ovulatory women: a study of serum and follicular fluid levels of dimeric inhibin A and B in spontaneous menstrual cycles. *J Clin Endocrinol Metab* 1996;81:2742–5
20. Block E. Quantitative morphological investigations of the follicular system in women. Variations in different ages. *Acta Anat* 1952;14:108–23
21. Faddy MJ, Gosden RG, Gougeon A, et al. Accelerated disappearance of ovarian follicles in mid-life: implications for forecasting menopause. *Hum Reprod* 1992;7:1342–6
22. Vihko KK. Gonadotrophins and ovarian gonadotrophin receptors during the perimenopause transition period. *Maturitas* 1996; (Suppl 23):S19–22
23. Doring GK. The incidence of anovulatory cycles in women. *J Reprod Fertil* 1969 (Suppl 6):77–81
24. Metcalf MG. Incidence of ovulatory cycles in women approaching the menopause. *J Biosoc Sci* 1979;11:39–48
25. Santoro N, Brown JR, Adel T, et al. Characterization of reproductive hormonal dynamics in the perimenopause. *J Clin Endocrinol Metab* 1996;81:1495–501
26. Metcalf MG, Donal RA. Fluctuating ovarian function in a perimenopausal woman. *NZ Med J* 1979;89:45–7
27. Brown JB, Harrisson P, Smith MA, Burger HG. *Correlations between Mucus Symptoms and the Hormonal Markers of Fertility throughout Reproductive Life*. Ovulation Method Research Centre of Australia, 1981
28. Metcalf MG, Donald RA, Livesey JH. Pituitary–ovarian function in normal women during the menopausal transition. *Clin Endocrinol* 1981;14:245–55
29. Fitzgerald CT, Self MW, Killick SR, et al. Age related changes in the female reproductive cycle. *Br J Obstet Gynecol* 1994;101:229–33
30. Baird DT. Anovulatory dysfunctional uterine bleeding in adolescence. In Flamigni C, Verturolil S, Givens JR, eds. *Adolescence in Females*. Chicago: Year Book Medical Publishers, 1985:273–85
31. Van Look PF, Lothian H, Hunter WM, et al. Hypothalamic–pituitary–ovarian function in perimenopausal women. *Clin Endocrinol* 1977;7:13–31
32. Bancroft J, Caewood EH. Androgens and the menopause; a study of 40–60 year old women. *Clin Endocrinol* 1996;45:577–87
33. Zumoff B, Strain GW, Miller LK et al. Twenty-four hour mean plasma testosterone concentration declines with age in normal premenopausal women. *J Clin Endocrinol Metab* 1995;80:1429–30
34. Mitchell ES, Woods NF. Symptom experiences of mid-life women: observations from the Seattle midlife women's health study. *Maturitas* 1996;25:1–10
35. Dennerstein L, Smith AM, Morse CA, et al. Menopausal symptomatology: the experience of Australian women. *Med J Aust* 1993;159:232–6
36. Upton GV. The contraceptive and hormonal requirements of the premenopausal woman: the years from 40–50. *Int J Fertil* 1986;30:44–55
37. Hunter M, Battersby R, Whitehead M. Relationships between psychological symptoms, somatic complaints and menopausal status. *Maturitas* 1986;8:217–28
38. Gangar KF, Cust MP, Whitehead MI. Symptoms of oestrogen deficiency associated with supraphysiological plasma oestradiol concentrations in women with oestradiol implant. *Br Med J* 1993;299:601–2
39. Guthrie JR, Dennersein L, Hopper JL, et al. Hot flushes, menstrual status, and hormone levels in a population-based sample of midlife women. *Obstet Gynecol* 1996;88:437–42
40. Fraser IS, Baird DT. Blood production and ovarian secretion rates of estradiol-17β and estrone in women with dysfunctional uterine bleeding. *J Clin Endocrinol Metab* 1974;39:564–9
41. Guthrie JR, Ebling PR, Hopper LJ, et al. Bone mineral density and hormone levels in

menopausal Australian women. *Gynecol Endocrinol* 1996;10:199–205
42. Nilas L, Christiansen C. Bone mass and its relationship to age and the menopause. *J Clin Endocrinol Metab* 1987;65:697–702
43. Steinberg RK, Freni-Titulaer W, Depuey EG, *et al.* Sex steroids and bone density in premenopausal and perimenopausal women. *J Clin Endocrinol Metab* 1989;69:533–9
44. Johnston CC Jr, Hui SL, Witt RM, *et al.* Early menopausal changes in bone mass and sex steroids. *J Clin Endocrinol Metab* 1985;61:905–11
45. Slemenda C, Hui SL, Longcope C, *et al.* Sex steroids and bone mass. A study of changes about the time of menopause. *J Clin Invest* 1987;80:1261–9
46. Goto S, Shigeta H, Hyakutake S, *et al.* Comparison between menopausal-related changes in bone mineral density of the lumbar spine and the proximal femur in Japanese female athletes. *Calcif Tissue Int* 1996;59:461–5
47. Shargil AA. Hormone replacement therapy in perimenopausal women with a triphasic contraceptive compound: a three-year prospective study. *Int J Fertil* 1985;30(1):15–28
48. Draper J, Roland M. Perimenopausal women's views on taking hormone replacement therapy to prevent osteoporosis. *Br Med J* 1990;300:786–8
49. Jensen J, Nilas L, Christiansen C. Influence of menopause on serum lipids and lipoproteins. *Maturitas* 1990;12:321–31
50. Matthews KA, Wing RR, Kuller LH. Influence of the perimenopause on cardiovascular risk factors and symptoms of middle-aged healthy women. *Arch Intern Med* 154:1994;2349–55
51. Darling GM, Johns JA, McCloud PI, *et al.* Estrogen and progestin compared with simvastatin for hypercholesterolemia in postmenopausal women. *N Engl J Med* 1997;337:595–601
52. Burger HG. Diagnostic role of follicle-stimulating hormone (FSH) measurements during the menopausal transition – an analysis of FSH, estradiol and inhibin. *Eur J Endocrinol* 1994;130:38–42
53. Wahlqvist M, Dalais F. Phytoestrogens: emerging multifaceted plant compounds. *Med J Aust* 1997;167:119–20
54. Kirkham C, Hahn PM, Van Vugt DA, *et al.* A randomized, double-blind, placebo-controlled, cross-over trial to assess the side effects of medroxyprogesterone acetate in hormone replacement therapy. *Obstet Gynecol* 1991;78:93–7
55. Prior JC, Alojado N, Vigna Y, *et al.* Estrogen and progestin are equally effective in symptom control post-ovariectomy – a one-year, double-blind, randomized trial in premenopausal women. *Endocr Soc Abstr* 1994;12H:411
56. Prior JC, Alojado N, McKay DW, *et al.* No adverse effects of medroxyprogesterone treatment without estrogen in postmenopausal women: double-blind, placebo-controlled, cross-over trial. *Obstet Gynecol* 1994;83:24–8
57. Upton GV. Contraception for the perimenopausal patient. *Obstet Gynecol Clin North Am* 1987;14:207–27
58. Petitti DB, Sidney S, Bernstein A, *et al.* Stroke in users of low dose oral contraceptives. *N Engl J Med* 1996;335:8–15
59. Castracane DV, Gimpel T, Goldzieher JW. When is it safe to switch from oral contraceptives to hormonal replacement therapy? *Contraception* 1995;52:371–6

2
Depression and the menopausal transition

A. Collins

INTRODUCTION

There continues to be considerable controversy as to whether mood change and psychological symptoms are linked to menopausal status or whether psychosocial factors play a more important role for the development of these symptoms. There is also controversy regarding the incidence of depression at menopause and whether the hormonal changes are, in fact, associated with an increased risk of negative mood change among women. The surge in prescription of hormone replacement therapy (HRT) for women in recent years has highlighted the question of whether hormones have a positive effect on mood and psychological functioning and whether they enhance the quality of life of menopausal women.

PSYCHOPATHOLOGY

At the turn of the century, Kraepelin[1] introduced the term 'involutional melancholia', a condition that was characterized by anxiety and confusion with a poor prognosis. Werner and colleagues[2] considered this to be an extreme form of menopausal syndrome. In these early discussions of the menopause as a cause of melancholia, there was no clear distinction between menopause and involution. These ideas did not receive scientific support but continued to influence a number of clinicians. As late as 1979, Weissman[3] concluded that there was no evidence to support the theory of involutional melancholia and the term has since been removed from psychiatric textbooks.

Earlier psychoanalytic writers held a predominantly negative view of menopausal women. The women who had invested the most in motherhood and child-rearing were assumed to grieve the loss of reproductive capacity the most. Deutsch, in her book *The Psychology of Women*[4], referred to the loss of reproductive capacity as 'partial death'. According to psychoanalytic interpretation, the menopause was considered a time of disappointment and mortification as well as decline in sexual attractiveness. More recent research has addressed the issue of loss of reproductive ability and the 'empty nest'. Women are believed to become depressed because their children are leaving home. However, Neugarten[5] failed to find evidence for the view that the empty nest period is a time of crisis. She remarked that women become more reflective and more willing to satisfy egoistic impulses during transition to the menopause. Barnett and Baruch[6] concluded that there was no evidence that the empty nest presented a problem to the majority of women.

HORMONES AND MOOD IN POSTMENOPAUSAL WOMEN

Researchers have assumed that there is an association between depressed mood and declining estrogen levels influenced partly by reports of depression in the postpartum period and in the late luteal phase of the cycle as part of the premenstrual syndrome, both conditions being characterized by relative estrogen deficiency[7]. Also, findings from basic neuroscience have provided information on brain chemistry and how the sex steroid may influence brain structure and function. Estrogen has also been shown to have important neuroprotective properties. Circulating estrogen levels influence the structure and biochemistry of the brain by altering the concentration and availability of neurotransmitter amines, including serotonin. Estrogen has been shown to enhance both transport and availability of serotonin in the brain. Furthermore, estrogen receptors are found in the hypothalamus, pituitary and limbic forebrain[8,9]. Therefore, limbic system function, which largely subserves emotion, can be influenced by circulating estrogen. These mechanisms explain how estrogen may affect mood during the menopausal transition in a certain proportion of women[10]. A few clinical studies have indicated that estrogen replacement improves mood and increases a sense of wellbeing in menopausal women[11–13]. Sherwin[10] has shown that estrogen in combination with androgen is effective in treating depression in women who have undergone hysterectomy with oophorectomy. Sherwin also found that estrogen in doses conventionally used in HRT treatment had mood enhancing effects in non-depressed women; however, these doses were not effective in women with more severe depressive symptoms[14]. On the other hand, others have criticized the clinical treatment studies on methodological grounds, and contend that there is not enough evidence to show that hormone replacement has an effect on depression other than that of a placebo effect and relief from vasomotor symptoms[15–17].

IS THERE A MENOPAUSAL SYNDROME?

Earlier research assumed the presence of a menopausal syndrome including both vasomotor and psychological symptoms such as depressed mood. A range of other symptoms that have been associated with the menopause include forgetfulness, fatigue, concentration problems, irritability, depressed mood, decrease in sexual desire, mood swings, anxiety and sleep-related problems. These are all diffuse symptoms which may occur at any age and in both sexes. Such symptoms also occur in certain major psychiatric disorders, particularly anxiety and depression. The question is, whether these symptoms are widely experienced by menopausal women or confined to a minority who seek help. A large number of clinical studies have attempted to establish a relationship between these symptoms and menopausal status. Many of these studies have been criticized on methodological grounds, for example relying on selected populations such as clinic attenders or using inadequate measures of symptoms. Hay and colleagues[18] pointed out that a considerable percentage of women attending menopause clinics were found to be depressed at the time of the clinic attendance. Their study showed that there was a peak of depression in clinic attenders in the 4 years before and after the last menstrual period. Morse and co-workers[19] reported that the help-seeking woman at menopause is very different in her behavior and personality and suffers from more frequent symptoms than women of the same age range who do not attend clinics.

Population-based studies have shown that about 20% of perimenopausal women have depressed mood as a central problem. According to Holte[20], dysphoric mood is related to menopausal status and the biological changes associated with the menopause, whereas Kaufert and colleagues[21] emphasized that changes in social roles and family are more important in determining mood changes in women than changes in hormonal levels.

Results from the epidemiological studies indicate that there is an increase in minor somatic and psychological complaints at the time of the menopause. About 75–80% of women experience vasomotor symptoms. However, results concerning psychological symptoms and depression are much more controversial. Results from an Australian survey[22] showed that there was no increase of depressed mood in the menopausal age range. Hallstrom[23], in a Swedish study, found no fluctuation in the prevalence of psychiatric disorder but reported that women who presented with irregular periods and who could be considered perimenopausal had a higher frequency of psychological symptoms. Ballinger, in a review[24], concluded that results from general population surveys did not indicate a major effect of the menopause on a variety of common psychiatric symptoms.

It is not clear that the menopause is associated with an increased incidence of depression[25]. Instead, it seems that the highest incidence of depression occurs in the 30–45-year age range. This study also found that previous medically treated depression was associated with early menopause. A recent review using meta-analytical techniques concludes that there is no substantial evidence to support the view that natural menopause causes depression[26]. Hunter[27], in a critical editorial, also expressed serious concerns regarding the view that the menopause causes depression, and emphasized that depressed mood is most likely related to adverse psychosocial factors and previous episodes of depression. McKinlay and associates[28] showed that only surgical but not natural menopause was associated with depressed mood.

PSYCHOSOCIAL FACTORS AFFECTING MOOD CHANGE AND SYMPTOMS

The menopause occurs in the context of midlife for women, and may be seen to represent a phase of increased vulnerability. The interaction of psychological and biological factors is probably important in determining women's reactions to the hormonal changes. Women's earlier experiences, their personality, earlier coping style and acquired behavioral patterns influence their way of reacting to the hormonal changes. Middle age is considered to be a period of increased role change and occurrence of stressful life events, particularly those called exit events. Such events include children moving out, elderly parents developing illnesses and requiring assistance or dying, partners or close friends aging or developing disease, separation and divorce.

More recent research emphasizes women's social roles, role conflicts and life stress as important variables contributing to mood state and well-being. Social and family factors were found to be more important in the etiology of psychological symptoms such as depression than were changing hormonal levels. McKinlay and associates[28] found that the major influences on the risk of developing depression were health problems, somatic symptoms and causes of worry such as husband or children. Very similar results were reported by Kaufert and colleagues[21], who found that the risk of depression was increased by poor general health and by current interpersonal stresses. Avis and co-workers, in a re-analysis of their longitudinal data[29], found that there was, in fact, a transient increase in depression parallel to the drop in estrogen levels, but this could be attributed mainly to the presence of vasomotor symptoms and a negative attitude to the menopause.

Methodological problems associated with research in this area include criteria for menopausal status, inadequate sampling and the use of small clinical trials. The criteria for menopause are not always reported, and McKinlay and associates[30] have emphasized the importance of defining menopausal status by providing strict criteria for each stage. Holte[31] has addressed the importance of using population-based samples as opposed to small clinical samples as well as the use of standardized instruments for measuring symptoms. He also pointed out that dysphoric mood is not the same as clinical depression, and most of the scales used are not adapted to measuring the kind of depressed mood that women may experience at menopause.

Currently, there are at least three ongoing population-based longitudinal studies which examine biological as well as psychological measures using standardized rating scales. The results to date concerning mood changes are very similar. Woods and Mitchell[32] reported from the Seattle Women's Health Study that somatic health, definition of femininity and a positive attitude to the menopause, not menopausal status, were the best predictors of positive mood at menopause. Dennerstein[33] reported from the Melbourne Women's Health Study that negative affect was mainly explained by a negative attitude to the menopause, but menopausal status and the presence of vasomotor symptoms also contributed to negative mood states. This would indicate that the declining estrogen levels are somehow associated with negative mood. Our own results from a longitudinal study of Swedish women[34] support the Australian results, and showed that a negative attitude to aging and the menopause, life stress and worry about ailing parents as well as vasomotor symptoms and menopausal status were significant predictors of depressed mood. Women who had recently undergone a hysterectomy with bilateral oophorectomy were significantly more depressed than other women. It seems that psychosocial factors, attitude to the menopause and somatic symptoms are the strongest predictors of mood change at menopause. To some extent, biological factors may also be associated with dysphoric mood at menopause.

FACTORS THAT SERVE AS BUFFERS

Social support serves as a buffer against menopausal symptoms. Van Keep[35] reported that women with many friends and high social support had less frequent symptoms. Holte[17] found that Norwegian women with a good social network and an income of their own had less frequent psychosocial symptoms. Employment and an income served as buffers against vasomotor symptoms. Results from different studies show that women with less education, monotonous work and little control over their work tend to suffer from more severe symptoms. Barnett and Baruch[36] have stressed that earlier research has emphasized women's traditional roles as homemakers and wives without considering women's work role as being central. The majority of women are employed outside the home. Job satisfaction is an important contributor to mental health during all phases of the life span. In our longitudinal study, we have focused on women's work role during transition to menopause. The results showed that women who were more involved in their work had a better health profile, a lower systolic blood pressure and lower body weight compared to women who perceived their work role as less important.

Personality traits, behavioral patterns and sex roles can also influence women's experience of the menopausal years. Polit and Larocco[37] found a strong association between personality traits and psychological symptoms during the menopause. Women with more severe symptoms had lower self-esteem, were more emotionally dependent and had a more negative attitude to the menopause. In a Swedish study[38], we found that women with a more traditional sex role experienced more frequent vasomotor symptoms than other women. Moreover, there was a relationship between psychological symptoms and anxiety-proneness as well as external locus of control, i.e. the feeling that external factors are determining important events in one's life.

Expectations and learned behavioral patterns probably play an important part in coping with the changes occurring at menopause. Neugarten[5] showed that younger women frequently had a more negative attitude to the menopause than those women who already were postmenopausal. According to Myra Hunter[39], attitude to the menopause, earlier periods of depressed mood and lower socioeconomic status as well as unemployment, were the main predictors of depressed mood in women at menopause.

CONCLUSION

The results reviewed above show that psychosocial factors and attitude to the menopause play an important part in the way women cope with the stresses of the menopause. Newer research has shown that a woman's entire life situation including her past experiences, her present social network and involvement in work are important for her mood state and well-being. Negative stereotypes and society's view of older women also have important implications for how women view themselves. The hormonal changes occurring at menopause and their influence may be enough to trigger emotional reactions such as depression[40]. Basic neuro-scientific research has provided evidence that estrogen plays an important role in brain chemistry and function which may have implications for mood, psychological functioning and aging. The menopausal transition can be seen as a period of increased vulnerability and possible symptom formation including depressed mood. It can also be seen as a period of psychological development entailing turmoil and crisis, but with a potential for personal growth and increased maturity and a stronger sense of identity. For those women who develop depression, it is important to examine recent life events, personality factors and predispositions, earlier ways of coping with stress, social network and work role. Counseling women within such a framework may prove to be effective. It is vital to look for different dimensions when diagnosing mood changes and to individualize treatment. It is also important to look for signs of increased vulnerability to hormonal fluctuation such as earlier premenstrual symptoms, negative reactions to oral contraceptives or a history of postpartum 'blues'. Two of the recent longitudinal studies have indicated an association between menopausal status and mood ratings demonstrating a need for further research, to disentangle the relationship between depressed mood, menopausal status and hormone levels.

It should be remembered that vasomotor symptoms and sleep disturbances may contribute to depressed mood and, in helping women to choose a treatment that will alleviate these symptoms, be it hormone replacement, alternative treatments or lifestyle changes, it may prove to be beneficial also in improving well-being and mood. Women should be encouraged to make autonomous choices about treatment and they should be given adequate information about different treatment options. Attitude to older women should also be changed and women's competence should be recognized. More information and education is needed to dispel myths and negative stereotypes which may affect mood.

In summary, psychosocial factors, life events and attitude to the menopause play an important part in influencing women's mood and well-being at the time of the menopause. It is suggested that an integration of disciplines into an interactive approach to the menopause be advocated, one that recognizes the interplay between the individual woman and her psychosocial environment. Menopausal symptoms including depressed mood are then seen as a result of an increased vulnerability to the hormonal changes taking place in interaction with critical psychosocial factors and attitude to the menopause.

References

1. Kraepelin E. Lecture 1 – Introduction: melancholia. In Johnson T, ed. *Lectures in Clinical Psychiatry*. New York: MacMillan, 1906
2. Werner AA, Johns GA, Hoctor EF. Involutional melancholia. Probable etiology and treatment. *J Am Med Assoc* 1934;103:13–16
3. Weissman MM. The myth of involutional melancholia. *J Am Med Assoc* 1979;242:742–4
4. Deutsch H. The climacterium. In Deutsch H, ed. *The Psychology of Women*. New York: Green & Stratton, 1945
5. Neugarten B, Kraines J. Menopausal symptoms in women of various ages. *Psychosom Med* 1965;27:266–73
6. Barnett R, Baruch G. Women in the middle years: a critique and research theory. *Psychol Women Q* 1978;3:187–97
7. Arpels J. The female brain hypoestrogenic continuum from the premenstrual syndrome to menopause. *J Reprod Med* 1996;41:633–9
8. McEwen BS. Estrogens and structural and functional plasticity of neurons. Implications for memory, aging and neurodegenerative processes. *Ciba Foundation Symp* 1995 191:52–66
9. McEwen BC, Alves SE, Bulloch K, *et al*. Ovarian steroids and the brain: implications for cognition and aging. *Neurology* 1997;48(Suppl. 7):S8–15
10. Sherwin B. Hormones, mood and cognitive functioning in post-menopausal women. *Obstet Gynecol* 1996;87(Suppl):20S–6S
11. Ditkoff EC, Gary WG, Cristo M, *et al*. Estrogen improves psychological functioning in asympto-

matic postmenopausal women. *Obstet Gynecol* 1991;78:991–5
12. Barrett-Connor E, Kritz-Silverstein D. Estrogen replacement and cognitive function in older women. *J Am Med Assoc* 1993;269:2637–41
13. Studd J. Depression and the menopause: estrogens improve symptoms in some middle aged women. *Br Med J* 1997;314:977–8
14. Sherwin B. The impact of different doses of estrogen and progestin on mood and sexual behavior in postmenopausal women. *J Endocrinol Metab* 1991;72:336–43
15. Coope J. Hormonal and nonhormonal interventions for menopausal symptoms. *Maturitas* 1996;23:159–68
16. Hunter M. Emotional wellbeing, sexual behavior and hormone replacement therapy. *Maturitas* 1990;12:299–314
17. Holte A. The search for a climacteric mood disorder: methodological problems and recent results. In Wijma K, von Schoultz B, eds. *Reproductive Life: Advances in Research in Psychosomatic Obstetrics and Gynecology*. Carnforth, UK: Parthenon Publishing, 1992:352–8
18. Hay AG, Bancroft J, Johnstone EC. Affective symptoms in women attending a menopause clinic. *Br J Psychiatry* 1994;164:513–16
19. Morse C, Smith A, Dennerstein L, *et al*. The treatment-seeking woman at menopause. *Maturitas* 1994;18:161–73
20. Holte A. Influence of natural menopause on health complaints: a prospective study of healthy Norwegian women. *Maturitas* 1992;14:127–41
21. Kaufert P, Gilbert P, Tate R. The Manitoba project: a re-examination of the link between menopause and depression. *Maturitas* 1992;14:143–55
22. Woods NF, Mitchell ES. Pathways to depressed mood for midlife women. *Res Nurs Health* 1997;20:119–29
23. Hallstrøm T. *Mental Disorder and Sexuality in the Climacteric*. Copenhagen: Scandinavian University Books, 1973
24. Ballinger CB. Psychiatric aspects of the menopause. *Br J Psychiatry* 1990;156:773–87
25. Harlow B, Cramer D, Annis K. Association of medically treated depression and age at menopause. *Am J Epidemiol* 1995;141:1170–6
26. Nicol-Smith L. Causality, menopause and depression: a critical review of the literature. *Br Med J* 1996;313:1129–32
27. Hunter M. Depression and the menopause. *Br Med J* 1996;313:1217–18
28. McKinlay J, McKinlay S, Brambilla D. The relative contribution of endocrine and social circumstances to depression in mid-aged women. *J Health and Soc Behav* 1987;28:345–63
29. Avis NE, Brambilla D, McKinlay S, *et al*. A longitudinal analysis of the association between menopause and depression. *Ann Epidemiol* 1994;4:214–20
30. McKinlay S, Brambilla DJ, Posner JG. The normal menopausal transition. *Maturitas* 1992;14:103–15
31. Holte A. Influences of natural menopause on health complaints: a prospective study of healthy Norwegian women. *Maturitas* 1992;14:127–41
32. Woods NF, Mitchell ES. Patterns of depressed mood in midlife women: observations from the Seattle Women's Health Study. *Res Nurs Health* 1996;19:111–23
33. Dennerstein L. Wellbeing and the menopausal transition. *J Psychosom Obstet Gynecol* 1997;18:95–101
34. Collins A, Landrgen BM. Psychosocial factors associated with the use of hormonal replacement therapy in a longitudinal follow-up of Swedish women. *Maturitas* 1997;28:1–9
35. Van Keep P, Kellerhans J. The impact of sociocultural factors on symptom formation. *Psychother Psychosom* 1974;23:251–63
36. Barnett R, Baruch G. Gender, social role and distress. In Barnett R, Baruch G, eds. *Gender and Stress*. New York: Free Press, 1987:122–43
37. Polit D, LaRocco S. Social and psychological correlates of menopausal symptoms. *Psychosom Med* 1980;42:335–42
38. Collins A, Landgren BM. Experience of symptoms, estrogen use and reproductive health during transition to menopause. *Maturitas* 1995;25:101–11
39. Hunter M. Psychosocial aspects of the climacteric. In Studd J, Whitehead M, eds. *The Menopause*. Oxford: Blackwell, 1988:55–64
40. Dennerstein L. Psychiatric aspects of the climacteric. In Studd J, Whitehead M, eds. *The Menopause*. Oxford: Blackwell, 1988:43–54

3
Estrogens and skin

M. P. Brincat and R. Galea

INTRODUCTION

The skin is one of the largest organs in the body containing a sizeable proportion of total body collagen. This organ is composed of a population of cells of diverse embryonic origin which, under normal conditions, exist side by side in complete harmony, forming a complex mosaic.

ANATOMICAL CONSIDERATIONS

Skin is composed of two main layers. A thin outer layer, the epidermis, is composed of keratinocytes (keratin-producing cells) of ectodermal origin intermingled with melanin-producing cells, the melanocytes, which arise from a specialized embryonic ectodermal tissue, the neural crest. The other layer is the dermis, a stroma that forms the main bulk of the skin and is intimately bound with the overlaying epidermis; finger-like processes or dermal papillae project upwards into corresponding recesses in the epidermis. In contrast to the epidermis, the dermis is predominantly fibrous and contains blood vessels. It is of mesodermal origin like all connective tissue (including bone). It also contains several structures derived from the embryonic ectoderm, e.g. sweat glands and hair follicles. The fibers present in the dermis consist of two main types of fibrous protein, collagen (97.5%) and elastin (2.5%)[1]. Collagen constitutes approximately one-third of the total mass of the body and 20% of total protein. It is a major constituent of all connective tissues, some 88% of which is found in the dermis and in bones, the amount of collagen being almost equally shared. Collagen fibers are responsible for the main mass and resilience of the dermis. This collagen is disposed mainly in a parallel arrangement to the skin surface. The elastin fibers, on the other hand, form a subepidermal network and are only thinly distributed. Collagen is produced by fibroblasts. These cells contain abundant endoplasmic reticulum where secreted proteins such as collagen are synthesised from the main types of collagen found in connective tissues, types I, II, III, V and XI.

The dermis and the epidermis are nourished by blood vessels that pass upwards from the subcutaneous layer. In the dermis, they form relatively small channels (arterioles) which pass towards the undersurface of the epidermis forming a rich capillary network in the dermal papillae. It is these vessels that are responsible for the menopausal flush, the most characteristic symptom of the menopause, affecting some 75% of all women in their first menopausal year[2] and still affecting 25% of them 5 years later[3]. Connective tissue consists of an extracellular matrix and cellular elements. The extracellular matrix is composed of two classes of macromolecules, the collagens and the polysaccharide glycosaminoglycans (GAGs). The chains of GAGs allow rapid diffusion of water molecules and are responsible for the turgor in the compressive forces. Collagen fibrils, on the other hand, resist stretching of the tissues. By weight, GAGs amount to less than 5% of the fibrous protein, the rest being composed largely of collagen with some elastin[4]. Although the bulk of the body collagen is remarkably stable, a fraction of the collagen in all tissues is continuously degraded and replaced, even in old age. Such a change in overall collagen metabolism can be approximately followed by assaying the excretion of peptide-bound hydroxyproline in urine[5], as excretion of these substances is largely caused by collagen degradation[6]. Changes in collagen metabolism can also be followed by urinary assay of collagen pyridinium cross-links. Collagen changes with age, in quality, type and amount. Growth of connective tissue involves collagen biosynthesis, and this is reflected in an increased tissue level of intracellular post-translational enzymes. Both the rates of translation and the levels of these enzymes decrease with age[7]. Our study of collagen markers indicated that, after the menopause, the rate of collagen breakdown (osteoclastic activity) increased dramatically when compared to a faster rate of collagen production (osteoblastic activity). With estrogen replacement therapy, this situation was reversed with osteoblastic activity and evidence of collagen formation, hence, reduced. However, this was greatly affected by the larger decrease in collagen breakdown which led to an overall positive balance, thereby explaining the increase in bone mass and possibly also the increase in dermal skin thickness in women on estrogen replacement[8] (Figure 1).

MENOPAUSE, SKIN AND BONE

The menopause is a major event in the life of a woman. This hypoestrogenic state gives rise to profound effects on all organs containing connective tissue. Albright and colleagues, as early as 1940[9], speculated that postmenopausal osteoporosis was part of a generalized connective tissue disorder, having observed that the skin of women with this disorder was noticeably thin. McConkey and associates[10] showed that transparent skin on the back of the hand was most common in women over 60 years of age and the prevalence of osteoporosis in women with transparent skin was 83% versus 12.5% in women with opaque skin. In fact, postmeno-

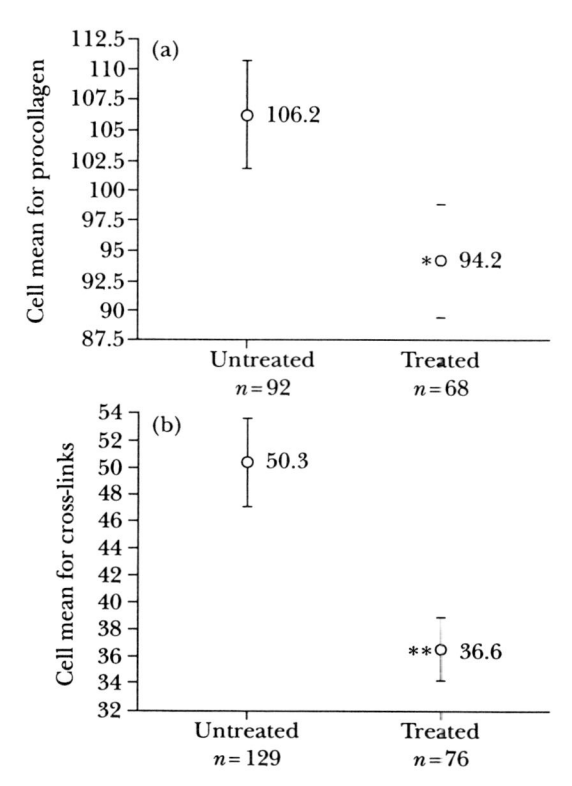

Figure 1 Plots of mean procollagen (a) and cross-links (b) in untreated patients and in patients on hormone replacement therapy. There was 11.3% change in bone formation and 27.2% change in bone resorption in treated compared to untreated patients. *$p < 0.05$; **$p < 0.005$

pausally, there is a decline in skin thickness and skin collagen, causing skin deterioration as evidenced by dry, wrinkled, flaky and easily bruised skin. There is also a decline in the bone mass. These two organs, containing some 30% of all the connective tissues in the body, show a deterioration which can be prevented and even reversed with appropriate and adequate estrogen replacement[11–14].

Atrophy of the dermis after the menopause is due to a decrease in the dermal skin collagen content of the dermis. The amounts of hydroxyproline and glycosylated hydroxylysine[15,16] in type I collagen and of immature and reducible cross-links decrease with age[17]. To what extent these changes are fundamental to the aging process is still unknown. This decrease is not only arrested but reversed by hormone replacement therapy[18]. Estrogens have, in fact, been shown to enhance the dermal contents of water, GAGs and collagen. Both estrogen and androgen receptors have been identified on dermal fibroblasts[19]. In a study to identify specific estrogen-sensitive structures[20], normal human skin was examined for the binding of the estrogen receptor D5 antibody which is associated with p29, a 29-kDa protein found in the cytoplasm of normal estrogen-sensitive cells. Strong and specific staining was seen in the epidermis, with a gradient showing the most intense staining in the granular layer. Similar positive staining was seen in the hair follicles and sebaceous glands. Variable staining was seen in the eccrine glands and vessels. These findings demonstrate p29 to be present in these structures and, hence, that estrogens may exert a specific effect on these tissues.

Estrogens could increase the rate of collagen production[21] by altering the degree of polymerization of GAGs. Estrogens increase the hydroscopic qualities[22], probably though enhanced synthesis of dermal hyaluronic acid[23]. Collagenous fibrils were found to be less fragmented in the dermis of women treated with estrogens[24].

Most studies have measured the thickness of the dermis, as this is the layer which is mainly connective tissue. Subcutaneous tissue is an added variable, and results from studies using Harpenden's calipers, which also include subcutaneous fat, have been conflicting[25,26]. Ultrasound can nowadays be used to measure skin thickness. Ultrasound examination has been used by dermatologists when assessing dermal malignancies. Good reproducibility has been obtained by using high-frequency (20 MHz) ultrasound to determine the thickness of the skin excluding the subcutaneous tissue. The dermal skin thickness itself, composed as it is of connective tissue including the predominant protein, collagen as well as elastin (small amounts) and glycoaminoglycans, also has more than one variable that is affected by estrogen replacement and the menopause. In rat work, for example[21], castrated rats that were given estrogens had a 70% increase in their glycosaminoglycans content in 2 weeks. Similar increases in women would lead to skin thickness increases of far more than that which would be expected from a collagen content increase alone.

EFFECTS OF SEX STEROIDS ON SKIN COLLAGEN CONTENT

In animals, estrogens appear to alter the vascularization of the skin[27], and a change in the connective tissue of the dermis occurs as is reflected by increased mucopolysaccharide incorporation, hydroxyproline turnover and alterations in ground substance. In addition to increased dermal turnover of hyaluronic acid, the dermal water content is enhanced with estradiol therapy[23]. Rauramo and Punnonen[28] observed that oral estrogen therapy in castrated women caused thickening of the epidermis for 3 months which persisted for 6.

Punnonen[29], using two different strengths of estrogens in castrated women, showed a statistically significant thickening of the epidermis after 3 months with both strengths, but this thickness persisted only with the lower dose. One-third of patients on the higher dose started showing significant thinning of the epidermis, possibly because the dosage and treatment was too strong and, therefore, was exerting a corticosteroid-like effect.

Comparing a group of patients who had been on estradiol and testosterone implants from 2 to 10 years to a group of untreated postmenopausal women, it was shown that the treated group had a highly significant greater skin collagen content than the untreated group. Optimum skin collagen was obtained after 2 years of an optimum estrogen regimen that was calculated. Too high or too low levels of estradiol gave lower levels of collagen[30]. The same conclusions were also reported in relation to the epidermis[31].

The decline in skin collagen content after the menopause occurs at a much more rapid rate in the initial postmenopausal years than in the later years. Some 30% of skin collagen is lost in the first 5 years after the menopause[30] with an average decline of 2.1% per postmenopausal year over a period of 20 years. The increase in skin collagen content after 6 months of sex hormone therapy depends on the collagen content at the start of treatment[30]. In women with a low skin collagen content, estrogens are initially of therapeutic and later of prophylactic value, while in those with mild loss of collagen content in the early menopausal years, estrogens are of prophylactic value only. Thus, a deficiency in skin collagen can be corrected but not over-corrected.

Skin collagen content has been shown to have a strong correlation with dermal skin thickness[30]. Using 100-mg subcutaneous estradiol implants, significant increases in skin thickness and metacarpal index occurred over a 1-year period. Most of the increase occurred in the first 6 months.

Brincat and Castelo-Barcia and their associates[32-34] have shown that, following the menopause, skin collagen content and skin thickness are increased in women on hormone replacement therapy (HRT) compared to age-matched women on no treatment (Figure 2). Prospective studies have shown that skin thickness, skin collagen and bone mass increase in postmenopausal women who start estrogen replacement (HRT). The mechanical properties of the skin have been shown to be improved with HRT[35] and to reach premenopausal levels. In this study, the mechanical properties of the skin were defined by extensibility and elasticity measurements using a computerized device.

Computerized measurements of skin deformability and viscoelasticity revealed differences between women on estrogen therapy, postmenopausal women on no treatment and non-menopausal controls. This parallels the changes noted elsewhere with skin collagen. A sharp increase in skin extensibility was shown during the perimenopause in untreated women. Estrogen replacement therapy appeared to limit the age-related increase in cutaneous extensibility, thereby exerting a preventive effect on skin slackness. No effect of HRT was found on other parameters of skin viscoelasticity. Hormone replacement therapy has a beneficial effect on some mechanical properties of skin and, thus, may slow the progress of intrinsic cutaneous aging[35].

Brincat and colleagues[36-38] found significant correlations between the skin (dermal) collagen, skin thickness (measured radiologically) and metacarpal index, both in postmenopausal women who had been on HRT and in untreated postmenopausal women. The common factor is the connective tissue present at all three sites. These findings were irrespective of the woman's age, number of years since the menopause, original skin thickness or metacarpal index.

IMPLICATIONS IN OTHER SITUATIONS: FUTURE WORK

Skin thickness change has many potential implications regarding other tissues. One study that is currently underway seems to show that estrogen replacement therapy in postmenopausal women on long-term corticosteroids may lead to an increase in skin thickness over a period of 6 months[39].

Likewise, changes in the wall thickness of the carotid media have been shown to occur in a closely related fashion in a cross-sectional study comparing postmenopausal controls to women on oral HRT and women with estradiol implants. The mean thickness of the media was greater in women on oral HRT and still greater in women with implants[40,41] (Figure 3). As the media in the carotid is almost entirely composed of connective tissue, this situation is similar to that of skin thickness. Indeed, a paper presented

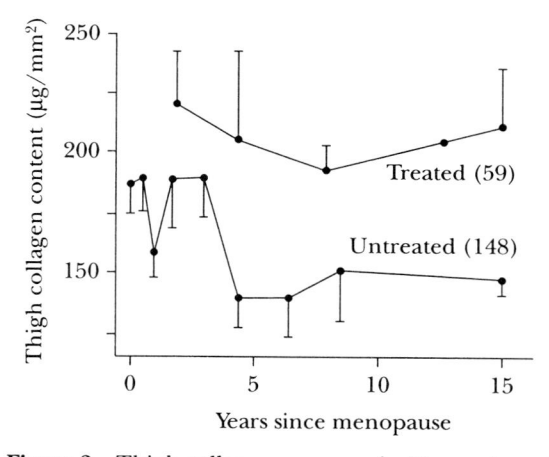

Figure 2 Thigh collagen compared with number of years since menopause

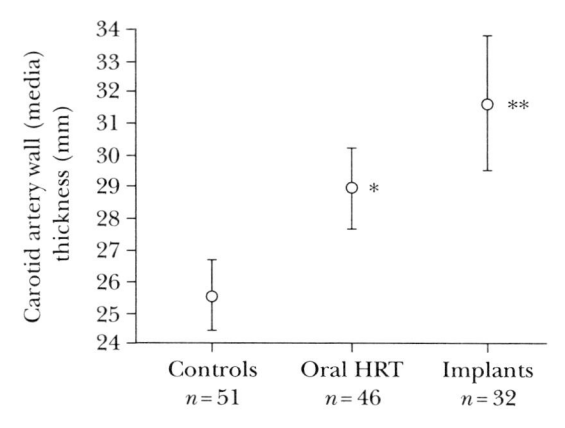

Figure 3 Plot of carotid artery wall (media) (mean ± SE) thickness in postmenopausal women on no treatment, on oral hormone replacement therapy (HRT) and with estradiol implant. Controls vs. oral HRT, $*p < 0.05$; controls vs. implants, $**p < 0.005$; oral HRT vs. implants, NS

indicated a correlation between skin thickness and the carotid artery media[42].

Attempts to identify the correct value of skin thickness measurement that could be used as a screening for postmenopausal osteoporosis have been underway for some time[42]. Skin thickness does seem to have a role in screening for osteoporosis. Of course, the entire field of adequate prediction of fractures, whether by skin thickness, bone density or any other method, is fraught with huge difficulties owing to the fact that there are so many variable contributions to the issues of when and where an individual will fracture. Even relatively expensive tests such as bone density measurements seem to be not much better than skin thickness measures in predicting fractures so, as a screening test, the faster and considerably cheaper skin thickness assessment by high frequency ultrasound or radiological methods is still an attractive proposition. Bone densitometry assessments would then be utilized as a second tier of screening or possibly even relegated to a purely diagnostic role, and a role in assessing response to therapy.

CONCLUSIONS

It is an old adage that skin is a manifestation of inner health, but its own health is also important in the self-esteem of the individual, with its quality, elasticity, translucency and hydration having important cosmetic implications.

The hypoestrogenic state prevailing in the menopause has a profound effect on the skin that is not simply age-related but, as with bone loss, leads to rapid deterioration which can be prevented and even reversed with appropriate and adequate estrogen replacement. These effects have been demonstrated in the epidermis, dermis, collagen content of the dermis, glycosaminoglycan content of the dermis and skin thickness. The mechanical properties of the skin after the menopause have been shown to benefit from HRT. Skin and bone each contain some 40% of the total body collagen. Collagen marker studies have shown that the bone changes associated with the menopause are connective tissue changes. This connective tissue deficiency in bone is mirrored in the individual's skin changes, although the correlation is not exact.

The deleterious effects of the menopause on connective tissue in skin, like those in bone, can be reversed by HRT, in part or totally, in most women.

References

1. Bailey AJ, Etherington DJ. Metabolism of collagen and elastin. In Florkin M, Neuberger A, Van Dienen LLM, eds. *Comprehensive Biochemistry*. London: Elsevier Scientific, 1980;5:408–31
2. McKinlay SM, Jeffreys M. The menopausal syndrome. *Br J Prev Med Soc Med* 1974;28:108–15
3. Thompson B, Hart SA, Durno D. Menopausal age and symptomatology in a general practice. *J Biosoc Sci* 1973;5:71–2
4. Alberts B, Bray D, Laws J, et al. Cell–cell adhesion and the extracellular matrix. In Alberts B, et al., eds. *Molecular Biology of the Cell*. New York: Garland Publishing Inc, 1983;12:673–715

5. Kivirikko KI. Urinary excretion of hydroxyproline in health and disease. *Int Rev Connect Tissue Res* 1973;5:93–163
6. Krane SM, Kontrwitz FG, Byrne M, et al. Urinary excretion of hydroxylysine and its glycosides as an index of collagen degradation. *J Clin Invest* 1977;59:819–27
7. Amen H, Crara J, Ryhanent, et al. Assay of proto collagen lysyl hydroxylase activity in the skin of human subjects and changes in the activities with age. *Clin Chim Acta* 1973;47:289–94
8. Brincat M, Galea R, Muscat Baron Y, et al. Changes in bone collagen markers and in bone density in hormone treated and untreated postmenopausal women. *Maturitas* 1997;27:171–7
9. Albright F, Bloomberg E, Smith PH. Postmenopausal osteoporosis. *Trans Assoc Amer Phys* 1940;55:298–305
10. McConkey B, Fraser GR, Bligh AS, et al. Transparent skin and osteoporosis. *Lancet* 1963;1:693–5
11. Punnonen R, Vilska S, Rauramo L. Skinfold thickness and long-term post-menopausal hormone therapy. *Maturitas* 1984;5:259–62
12. Dunn LB, Damesyn M, Moore AA, et al. Does estrogen prevent skin aging? Results from the First National Health and Nutrition Examination Survey (NHANESI). *Arch Dermatol* 1997;133:339–42
13. Schmidt JB, Binder M, Demschik G, et al. Treatment of skin aging with topical estrogens. *Int J Dermatol* 1996;35:669–74
14. Maheux R, Naud F, Rioux M, et al. A randomized, double-blind, placebo-controlled study on the effect of conjugated estrogens on skin thickness. *Am J Obstet Gynecol* 1994;170:642–9
15. Barnes MJ, Constable BJ, Morton LF, et al. Age-related variations in hydoxylation of lysine and proline on collagen. *Biochem J* 1974;139:461–8
16. Murai A, Miyahara T, Shiozawa S. Age-related variations in glycosylation of hydroxyproline in human and rat skin collagens. *Biochim Biophys Acta* 1975;404:345–8
17. Ristch J, Kivirikko KI. Intracellular enzymes of collagen biosynthesis in rat liver as a function of age and in hepatic injury induced by dimethylnitrosamine: changes in prolyl hydroxylase, lysyl hydroxylase, collagen galactosyltransferase and collagen glucosyltransferase activities. *Biochem J* 1976;158:361–7
18. Hall DA, Reed FB, Noki G, et al. The relative effects of age and corticosteroid therapy on the collagen profiles of dermis from subjects with rheumatoid arthritis. *Age Ageing* 1974;3:15–22
19. Stumpf WE, Sur M, Joshi SE. Estrogen target cells in the skin. *Experimentia* 1976;30:196
20. Jemec GB, Wojnarowska F. The distribution of p29 protein in normal human skin. *Br J Dermatol* 1987;117:217–24
21. Boucek RJ, Noble NL, Woessner JF Jr. Properties of fibroblasts. In Page IH, ed. *Connective Tissue Thrombosis and Atherosclerosis*. New York: Academic Press, 1959:193–211
22. Danforth DN, Vies A, Breen M, et al. The effect of pregnancy and labour on the human cervix: changes in collagen, glycoproteins and glucosaminoglycans. *Am J Obstet Gynecol* 1974;120:641–51
23. Grosman N, Hindberg E, Schen J. The effect of oestrogenic treatment on the acid mucopolysaccharide pattern in skin of mice. *Acta Pharmacol Toxicol* 1971;30:458–64
24. Goldzieher MA. The effects of oestrogens on the senile skin. *J Gerontol* 1946;1:196
25. Varila E, Rantala I, Ikarinem A, et al. The effect of topical oestriol on skin collagen of postmenopausal women. *Br J Obstet Gynaecol* 1995;102:985–9
26. Tan CY, Stratham B, Marks R, et al. Skin thickness measurements by pulsed ultrasound: its reproducibility, validation and variability. *Br J Dermatol* 1994;96:1392–4
27. Goodrich SM, Wood JE. The effect of oestradiol 17β on peripheral venous distensibility and velocity of venous blood flow. *Am J Obstet Gynecol* 1966;96:407–12
28. Rauramo L, Punnonen R. Wirking einer oralen estrogentherapie mit oestriolsuccinat auf die haut hastierter. *Fraunen Haut Gerchluts Kr* 1969;44:463–70
29. Punnonen R. Effect of castration and peroral therapy on skin. *Acta Obstet Gynaecol Scand* 1973;21 (Suppl):1–4
30. Brincat M, Moniz CF, Studd JWW, et al. Sex hormones and skin collagen content in postmenopausal women. *Br Med J* 1983;287:1337
31. Shahrad P, Marks RA. Pharmacological effect of oestrone on human epidermis. *Br J Dermatol* 1977;97:383–6
32. Brincat M, Moniz CF, Studd JWW, et al. Long-term effects of the menopause and sex hormones on skin thickness. *Br J Obstet Gynaecol* 1985;92:256–9
33. Brincat M, Moniz CF, Studd JWW, et al. Sex hormones and skin collagen content in postmenopausal women. *Br Med J* 1983;287:1337–8
34. Castelo-Barcia C, Pons F, Gratacos E, et al. Relationship between skin collagen and bone changes during ageing. *Maturitas* 1994;18:199–206
35. Pierard GE, Letawe C, Dowlati A, et al. Effect of hormone replacement therapy for menopause

on the mechanical properties of skin. *J Am Geriatr Soc* 1995;43:662–5
36. Brincat M, Studd JWW, Moniz CF, *et al.* Skin thickness and skin collagen mimic an index of osteoporosis in the postmenopausal woman. In Christiansen C, *et al.*, eds. *Osteoporosis. Proceedings of the Copenhagen International Symposium on Osteoporosis*, Vol. 1. 1984:353–5
37. Brincat M, Studd JWW, Moniz CF, *et al.* Skin thickness measurement. A simple screening method for determining patients at risk of postmenopausal osteoporosis. In Christiansen C, *et al.*, eds. *Osteoporosis. Proceedings of the Copenhagen International Symposium on Osteoporosis*, Vol. 1. 1984:323–6
38. Brincat M, Moniz CJ, Kabalan S, *et al.* Decline in skin collagen content and metacarpal index after the menopause and its prevention with sex hormone replacement. *Br J Obstet Gynaecol* 1987; 94:126–9
39. Muscat Baron Y, Brincat M, Galea R. Bone density and skin thickness changes in postmenopausal women on long term steroid therapy. In Wren BG, ed. *Progress in the Management of the Menopause.* Carnforth, UK: Parthenon Publishing, 1997: 179–82
40. Muscat Baron Y, Brincat M, Galea R. Carotid artery wall thickness in women treated with hormone replacement therapy. *Maturitas* 1997;27: 47–53
41. Muscat Baron Y, Brincat M, Galea R. Carotid artery wall thickness changes in estrogen treated and untreated postmenopausal women. *Obstet Gynecol* 1998; in press
42. Brincat M, Galea R, Muscat Baron Y. A screening model for osteoporosis using dermal skin thickness and bone densitometry. In Wren BG, ed. *Progress in the Management of the Menopause.* Carnforth, UK: Parthenon Publishing, 1997: 175–8

4
The effect of estrogens on wound healing

M. Calvin, J. Rymer, S. R. Young and M. Dyson

INTRODUCTION

With the declining trends in birth rate and increases in longevity in the western world, postmenopausal women are representing a greater percentage of the population and there are increasing medical concerns for their health. During the past few decades, several studies have documented the deleterious impact of the menopause on bone mass[1,2] and cardiovascular disease, and the reduction of risk in these areas by hormone replacement therapy (HRT)[3]. This may be attributed to the fact that these degenerative disorders are responsible for many fatalities in people over 50 years of age. However, the possible effects of the postmenopausal deficiency in ovarian hormones on skin are less well documented, despite skin being the largest organ of the body and the primary barrier against microbial invasion, dehydration and mechanical, chemical, osmotic, thermal and photic damage.

After the menopause, women start to complain of dry, flaky skin and easy bruising. These symptoms are often reversible with HRT, usually within the first 6 months of administration[4]. It is evident, therefore, that the sex hormones and, in particular, estrogens play an important part in the maintenance of skin quality in women and, thus, may also play a pivotal role in the healing of skin post-injury. This is of paramount clinical importance both in terms of financial cost and human suffering, as many of the chronic wounds such as venous ulcers, pressure sores[5] and burns[6] afflict the elderly population, of whom postmenopausal women comprise the majority.

The demonstration of estrogen receptors in various cells in human skin[7–9] and in cells such as macrophages[10], fibroblasts[11] and endothelial cells[12] that play vital roles in the healing process, suggests a direct effect of estrogens on both intact and wounded skin. However, there is a paucity of information regarding the effects of estrogens on these targets. There have been a number of studies on epidermal[13] and dermal thickness[14], skin mitotic figures[15], elastic properties[16] and collagen content of skin[17]; however, collectively, the results have been inconclusive. Furthermore, few and contradictory observations have been reported on the influence of estrogens on wound healing in extragenital tissues.

The aim of this chapter is to provide a survey of the literature that is available regarding the physiological effect of estrogens on the various phases of cutaneous repair described by Clark[18]: (1) inflammation, (2) new tissue formation (proliferation) and (3) matrix formation and remodeling, although many of the studies were performed in the 1960s and 1970s before much of our current knowledge on wound repair was acquired. Research carried out on the effects of estrogens, both in terms of their deficiency and replacement, on the process of tissue repair in various animal models is described and discussed, together with the very limited work undertaken in humans.

Some of the earliest work was investigated in gingival tissue in the field of periodontology, prompted by the clinical symptoms of chronic gingival inflammation in pregnant women[19,20]. The studies that followed examined, in laboratory animals, the influence of female sex hormones on healing using subcutaneous implantation of cellulose sponges, stainless steel and Teflon® cylinders, the production of sterile abscesses etc., in addition to cutaneous wounds.

In recent years, there has been negligible work on the effects of estrogens on tissue repair, emphasizing the need for further experimentation in this area. However, some of the more up-to-date research on the influence of estrogens on the individual cell types, for example, neutrophils, macrophages, fibroblasts and components of the extracellular matrix, such as collagen, that play a fundamental role in the healing wound, is included.

EFFECTS OF ESTROGENS ON THE INFLAMMATORY PHASE OF WOUND REPAIR

The inflammatory phase of repair is marked by platelet accumulation, coagulation, an increased permeability of the vessels adjacent to the wound and leukocyte migration into the wound bed. Studies investigating the effects of estrogens on these processes are addressed.

One of the earliest experiments[21] examined the influence of excessive amounts of estradiol dipropionate on the walls of turpentine abscesses produced subcutaneously in male and female rats. The investigators found that, in the animals receiving estradiol, the walls of the abscesses were thin, very poorly demarcated from the surrounding edematous tissue, and almost completely void of granulation tissue and fibroblastic response, consisting almost entirely of polymorphonuclear leukocytes (PMNLs), suggesting a lack of progression in healing from the early inflammatory phase of repair.

Rigdon and Chrisman[22], who examined local areas of inflammation in the skin of rabbits, found that intramuscular injections of estradiol benzoate did not influence the inflammatory phase of healing in terms of vascular permeability, measured by the leakage of injected trypan blue, nor the emigration of PMNLs from the vessels into the wound site. However, both these studies involved the administration of physiologically excessive amounts of estradiol, and there seems to be an optimum physiological estrogen dose for their beneficial effects to be demonstrated on epidermal thickness and collagen content in intact skin[23–25]; this may also apply to the process of healing, resulting in detrimental effects if the estrogen dose is too high.

Following the clinical observations of chronic gingival inflammation in pregnant women[19,20] and those using hormonal contraceptives[26], there have been a number of studies on the effects of estrogens and progesterone on the inflammatory process in gingival tissue. Lindhe and colleagues[27] reported that pregnant rats, and non-pregnant rats treated with a combination of estrogen and progesterone, showed an increased permeability of the gingival vasculature to intravenously injected trypan blue; an enhanced inflammatory response was further substantiated from the findings of increased exudate in pregnant women[28] and hormone-treated dogs[29].

Subsequent to these findings, Nyman and his colleagues carried out a series of investigations[30–34] studying the effects of estrogens and progesterone on granulation tissue outside the oral cavity, including that developing at the site of wounds to the skin. This was some of the first work carried out on the effects of estrogens on cutaneous healing. In one of these experiments, Nyman and colleagues[33], investigating vascular permeability in the inflammatory phase of healing in wounded ovariectomized rabbits treated with daily intramuscular injections of estradiol benzoate and progesterone, demonstrated a significantly lower amount of exudate in the estradiol- and progesterone-treated rabbits than in the controls up to, but not on, day 4 post-injury. These results are in accordance with those of Hugoson and Lindhe[29], who reported that, after gingival wounding, progesterone- and stilbestrol-treated female dogs exhibited a significantly lower exudation than controls. The observation by Nyman and colleagues[33] of differences in vascular exudation between the groups up to, but not on day 4, suggests that the influence of the hormones on vascular permeability in wounded areas is limited to the first few days (i.e. the inflammatory phase) of the healing process. It is possible that it was the estradiol component of the hormonal administration that suppressed exudation, as treatment with progesterone alone was found to enhance vascular exudation during the inflammatory phase of healing in the ovariectomized rabbits.

In a large study involving 300 ovariectomized rats, Lundgren[35] analyzed the influence of daily estradiol benzoate intramuscular injections on the amount of exudation and inflammatory cell migration following the subcutaneous implantation of Teflon cylinders in the backs of the animals. The authors found that, compared to the control group, the degree of exudate accumulation in the cylinder was markedly decreased in the estrogen-treated rats up to 1 week after implantation and there was a smaller number of PMNLs within the cylinder for 21 days.

Contrary to the results observed by Lundgren[35], Pallin and co-workers[36], who examined granulation tissue formation in cellulose sponges implanted subcutaneously in the backs of 98 ovariectomized rats, found that daily intramuscular injections of estrogen resulted in similar histological findings to those for the control group in terms of infiltration of PMNLs and monocytes.

Some of the more recent research, although not specifically on the effects of estrogens on the inflammatory phase of tissue repair following the creation of a wound or inflammatory area, has investigated the influence of these hormones on some of the properties of the cells and vasculature that are involved in this phase of healing.

Gouveia and associates[37] found that conjugated estrogens inhibited the vascular permeability of virgin rat uterine horns in inflammatory conditions. The findings are in accordance with those of Murthy and colleagues[38], who found that high doses of estrogen decreased the inflammatory exudate present in cutaneous rat wounds, suggesting that estrogens may influence vascular permeability and the resulting degree of inflammatory exudate accumulation.

The demonstration of estrogen receptors in human megakaryocytes[39] and a relationship between an increase in thrombus formation and increased levels of estrogens from the oral contraceptive pill[40] and, to a lesser extent, HRT[41] suggest that platelet aggregation during the inflammatory phase of wound healing may be affected by estrogens. This theory is supported by a study by Rosenblum and co-workers[42], who have reported that treatment with estradiol implants enhances platelet aggregation in mice at the site of microvascular injury in the pial arterioles of the brain, compared to placebo-treated controls.

Contrary to the above findings, Aune and colleagues[43] found significant reductions in the formation of thromboxane B2 in 32 postmenopausal women treated with HRT for 12 months. From these findings, the authors concluded that HRT reduces the cellular activation of blood platelets, which may account for some of the beneficial effects in reducing the risk of cardiovascular disease, although it is not known whether estrogens would have the same effect on platelets in the wound environment.

Neutrophils are the first cells to arrive at the wound site in substantial numbers during the inflammatory phase of repair, and they play an important role in the phagocytosis of pathogenic bacteria and debris[44]. Micromolar concentrations of estrogens have been found to enhance the oxidative metabolism of activated human PMNLs possibly by an increase in their myeloperoxidase activity[45], suggesting that either postmenopausal estrogen deficiency or replacement with hormonal therapy may have an effect on the phagocytic activity of PMNLs in the inflammatory phase of wound healing, via an action on the myeloperoxidase enzyme system. These findings were supported by Magnusson and Einarsson[46], who demonstrated a significant increase in phagocytic capacity of PMNLs *in vivo* in ovariectomized sows after a 6 week treatment period with physiological levels of 17β-estradiol.

Josefsson and colleagues[47] reported that physiological and pharmacological doses of estradiol significantly suppressed the inflammatory response in ovariectomized mice, after intradermal injection of cholera toxin to induce local inflammation. The authors concluded that the estradiol significantly suppressed the bone marrow production of leukocytes and affected the distribution of PMNLs in peripheral blood. Recently, Ito and co-workers[48], in accordance with similar findings by Miyagi and associates[49], demonstrated that physiological concentrations of 17β-estradiol in humans significantly reduced the chemotaxis of PMNLs. Pre-incubation with estrogen receptor antagonists eliminated the inhibitory effect, suggesting a receptor-dependent mechanism.

Monocytes and the macrophages they differentiate into, also play crucial roles in the healing wound, not only by eliminating deleterious materials by phagocytosis in the inflammatory phase, but also by generating chemotactic and growth factors critical to the co-ordination of granulation tissue formation in the proliferative phase of repair. The demonstration of estrogen receptors in both the human monocytic leukemia cell line J111 and rat peritoneal macrophages by Gulshan and colleagues[10] suggests that estrogens may have a direct effect on this cell type. Indeed, one of our recent studies investigating the effects of ovarian hormone deficiency on the infiltration of neutrophils and monocytes into the wound bed post-injury, in a rat model, supports this[50]. Following the creation of full-thickness excised lesions at either 2 weeks or 4 months post-ovariectomy, the 48 ovariectomized rats showed markedly reduced numbers of PMNLs, monocytes and macrophages in the wound bed on days 3 and 5 post-injury but, by day 10, these cells were frequently more numerous in the ovariectomized groups than in the sham-ovariectomized controls, where the numbers had reduced as occurs typically in the proliferative and remodeling phases of healing. This suggests that the inflammatory phase of repair may be delayed as well as depressed, and that this may be related to a detrimental effect of estrogen and/or progesterone deficiency on the early stages of healing.

A significantly reduced number of mature tissue macrophages was noted in the ovariectomized groups compared to the controls on days 3, 5, 10 and 22 post-injury in the tissue wounded at either 2 weeks or 4 months post-ovariectomy. As the total monocyte and macrophage number was shown to be higher in the ovariectomized groups than in the control groups by 10 days post-injury, it is possible that the reduced levels of ovarian hormones resulting from ovariectomy had an effect on the ability of the monocyte or immature macrophage to differentiate into its mature form[50].

EFFECTS OF ESTROGENS ON THE PROLIFERATIVE PHASE OF WOUND REPAIR

The proliferative phase of repair is characterized by: (1) re-epithelialization restoring the cutaneous barrier; (2) angiogenesis, the neovasculature supplying much of the nutrition required for healing; (3) fibroplasia, during which the matrix of the granulation tissue and scar tissue is formed; and (4) wound contraction, reducing wound size and, thus, the need for scar tissue. Studies investigating the effects of estrogens on these processes are addressed.

Taylor and colleagues[51] investigated the effects of daily estradiol dipropionate injections on the healing of sutured full-thickness cutaneous wounds in male rats, and found that fibroblastic infiltration and proliferation was not altered by the administration of estradiol. In contrast, Murthy and associates[38], examining the effects of subcutaneous estrogen injections following cutaneous wounding in male and female rats, reported a significantly reduced fibroblastic response and retarded collagen synthesis and maturity in the estrogen-treated groups.

The influence of estrogens on granulation tissue formation, provoked by the subcutaneous insertion of a plastic ring in the back of female rats, was examined by Jorgensen and Schmidt[52]. The authors found no significant differences in the dry weight of granulation tissue, nor in the content of hydroxyproline taken to indicate collagen content, in the estradiol-treated group compared to the controls. These results are in conflict with those of Portugal and colleagues[53], who observed an inhibited fibroblast reaction in the walls of turpentine-provoked abscesses following the combined administration of testosterone and estradiol, and those of Robertson and Sanborn[54], who, having provoked carrageenin granulomas in guinea-pigs, showed that injection of stilbestrol resulted in increased fibroblast infiltration and collagen production. Possible explanations for these discrepancies may be the utilization of different techniques to stimulate granulation tissue formation and the administration of different forms and doses of the estrogen with or without the addition of other hormones, such as testosterone.

In a study involving 300 ovariectomized rats, Lundgren[35], analyzing the influence of daily intramuscular injections of estradiol benzoate on the amount of granulation tissue formed following the subcutaneous implantation of Teflon cylinders in the backs of the animals, found that the estrogen-treated rats developed a significantly smaller amount of granulation tissue than the controls. These findings are in accordance with those of Nyman[32], Lundgren[55] and Pallin and associates[56], who have reported a markedly reduced amount of granulation tissue following the administration of estrogen in ovariectomized rabbits and rats.

The various studies of the effects of estrogens on vascularity, blood flow etc. during the proliferative phase of healing also appear to show contradictory results. Lindhe and colleagues[57] found that estrogens had no effect on vascular proliferation following mechanical injury to the pinnae of ovariectomized rabbits. Nyman and co-workers[31] evaluated the vascularity of granulation tissue by microangiography following the creation of full-thickness cutaneous wounds in 40 ovariectomized rabbits. The authors reported that daily intramuscular injections of estradiol for 4 weeks did not influence the number of vessels in the wounded tissue, supporting the observations by Lindhe and colleagues[57].

In contrast, Lundgren[55], also using microangiographical techniques, observed a significant suppression in vascularization in an estrogen-treated group of ovariectomized rats, compared to controls. Discrepancies between the results of the two studies can probably be explained by the use of different species of experimental animal and the administration of estrogens for differing durations, in addition to the utilization of different contrast mediums which may affect the degree of visualization of the vascular system.

Blood flow (determined by Xe^{133} clearance) was analyzed within granulation tissue formed in subcutaneously implanted stainless steel wire mesh cylinders in 15 estradiol- and progesterone-treated ovariectomized rabbits[34]; no observations were made as to the effects of estrogen-only administration. In both the hormone-treated and control groups there was a gradual increase in blood flow of the granulation tissue from day 7 after implantation to day 21, indicating an improvement of the microcirculation in parallel with the nutritional needs of the proliferating cells. This finding is in agreement with that of Nyman[32], who showed an increase from day 7 to day 21 in the oxygen tension of wound fluid of rabbits treated with a similar combination of hormones. However, the clearance data showed no difference in blood flow between the groups in the course of granulation tissue formation during the proliferative phase of repair.

Some of the more recent research, although not dealing specifically with the effects of estrogens on the proliferative phase of tissue repair, does demonstrate the influence of these hormones on some of the properties of the cells and vasculature that are involved in the process.

The demonstration of high-affinity estrogen receptors in monocytes and macrophages[10] suggests that estrogens may have a direct effect on these cell types, which play a vital role in regulating the co-ordination of granulation tissue development. A study by Hu and associates[58] showed that ovariectomy led to reduced synthesis of interleukin-1 (IL-1) by rat peritoneal macrophages, but estradiol replacement therapy administered to the rats increased synthesis. These findings suggest that estradiol may indirectly affect the proliferative phase of wound healing as IL-1 is thought to be involved in the formation of granulation tissue possibly by stimulating hyaluronic acid synthesis[59] and collagen deposition[60].

Shanker and colleagues[61] demonstrated that estrogen modulates platelet-derived growth factor-A (PDGF-A) gene expression by monocytes/macrophages and, thus, may indirectly influence the proliferative phase, as PDGF is mitogenic and chemotactic for fibroblasts[62], plays a role in angiogenesis by the attraction of cells that stimulate angiogenic factors[63] and is thought to stimulate wound contraction[64]. Thus, estrogen deficiency adversely affecting the synthesis of PDGF could be a possible explanation for the significantly slower rate of cutaneous wound contraction in ovariectomized rats compared to sham-ovariectomized controls, demonstrated in one of our recent studies[65]. In the rats wounded at 4 months post-ovariectomy, the ovariectomized rat wounds were approximately 30% larger than the controls on days 3 and 5 post-injury, whereas no significant difference was observed between the sham-ovariectomized and ovariectomized groups wounded at 2 weeks post-ovariectomy, indicating that the effects of ovarian hormone deficiency on this process are delayed. These findings suggest that the effects of ovariectomy on wound contraction are not only dependent on the plasma levels of estrogens but also on the duration of the deficiency.

Fibroblasts synthesize the matrix at the wound site in addition to facilitating wound contraction and releasing angiogenic factors which influence new blood vessel formation, emphasizing the important role that this cell plays in the proliferative phase of healing. Levine and co-workers[66] and Luo and associates[67] both claimed that estradiol did not affect fibroblast proliferation in fetal and adult human prostates although further investigations are required to establish whether this is true of the wound environment. Sato and colleagues[68] observed that treatment with 17β-estradiol decreased the level of procollagenase and prostromelysin produced by cultured rabbit uterine fibroblasts, but increased the production of tissue inhibitor of metalloproteinases (TIMP) by these cells, suggesting that collagenolysis is negatively regulated by 17β-estradiol. Collagenolysis is an important phenomenon in both the overlapping proliferative and remodeling phases of tissue repair as, with synthesis, it regulates the amount of collagen in the granulation tissue and ultimately in the scar; thus, 17β-estradiol may influence this process of wound healing indirectly by regulating the proteases involved in collagen degradation.

The presence of estrogen receptors in the nuclei of cultured human aortic and umbilical vein endothelial cells[12] suggests that estrogens may influence the process of angiogenesis in the proliferative phase of wound repair via a direct effect on endothelial cells. Morales and co-workers[69] found that the addition of 17β-estradiol increased the attachment of endothelial cells to laminin, collagen types I and IV and fibronectin, demonstrating that estradiol enhances endothelial cell activities important in neovascularization, and suggesting a promoting influence of estrogens on angiogenesis and, thus, an effect on the proliferative phase of healing.

EFFECTS OF ESTROGENS ON MATRIX FORMATION AND REMODELING

During the remodeling phase of repair, the skin responds to injury with a dynamic continuation of collagen synthesis and degradation, and the once highly vascular granulation tissue matures into less vascular scar tissue. Studies investigating the effects of estrogens on this process, particularly on the tensile strength of scar tissue, are addressed.

Taylor and colleagues[51], testing the tensile strength of full-thickness cutaneous wounds in 60 male rats, found that there was no significant difference between the estradiol-treated and control groups from day 2 to day 7 post-wounding, i.e. there was a steady increase in wound strength as it progressed from the inflammatory into the proliferative phase of repair. These findings were supported by studies performed by Nyman and associates[30], assessing the tensile strength of incised cutaneous wounds in 34 ovariectomized rabbits, and by Pallin and co-workers[56], examining the tensile strength of granulation tissue after the insertion of subcutaneous cellulose sponges in ovariectomized rats. Both investigations demonstrated that daily intramuscular injections of estradiol benzoate in the animals had no influence on the tensile strength measurements compared to controls.

Jorgensen and Schmidt[52] studied the effects of estradiol on the tensile strength of cutaneous linear wounds but observed results conflicting with those above. The authors claimed that administration of estradiol injections to female rats significantly increased the tensile strength of the wounds on the 10th day post-wounding compared to the control group. The discrepancies may be due to the use by Jorgensen and Schmidt[52] of different animals for the control and test wounds, the administration of high pharmacological doses of estradiol and experimentation on rats with intact ovaries, as opposed to physiological doses administered to ovariectomized rabbits, whereby each animal acted as its own control, which was the methodology employed by Nyman and colleagues[30].

The findings of Jorgensen and Schmidt[52] are in accordance with a more recent study investigating the effects of estrogens on the healing of the rat genital tract[70], which showed that the administration of estradiol implants increased the tensile strength of anastomosed uterine horns during the first 14 days of healing but, thereafter, no significant differences between the estradiol and control groups were found. If a similar pattern of healing is true for cutaneous wounds, this supports our observations of no significant difference in the breaking strength of wounded tissue between ovariectomized rats and sham-ovariectomized controls at 22 days post-injury[71]. Estrogen deficiency following ovariectomy may have resulted in a reduced breaking strength within the first 2 weeks post-injury, which was not demonstrated by day 22 when the breaking strength of the tissue was assessed by Calvin[71].

In contrast to the findings of all the studies presented above, Murthy and colleagues[38] observed a marked reduction in tensile strength between the 7th and 15th day post-wounding in estrogen-treated rats compared with controls. The authors suggested that estrogen administration resulted in a delayed collagen synthesis and, thus, reduced tensile strength at these time periods.

As was the case with the other phases of wound healing, some of the more recent research, although not specifically on the effects of estrogens on the remodeling phase of tissue repair, has investigated the influence of these hormones on some of the proteins, particularly collagen, that are involved in this phase of healing when injury does occur.

The remodeling of collagen is dependent upon the interplay of continued collagen synthesis and degradation[18], the degradation being controlled by a variety of collagenase enzymes which appear to be influenced by estrogen administration. Sato and co-workers[68] observed that treatment with 17β-estradiol decreased the level of procollagenase and prostromelysin produced by cultured rabbit uterine fibroblasts, but increased the production of TIMP by these cells. A study investigating the effects of estrogens on collagen metabolism in human cervical tissue in relation to cervical ripening for parturition[72] noted that collagenase activity was significantly elevated when estrone sulfate was added to the incubated cervical tissue. Kumar and Thampan[73] claimed that rat uterine collagenases which use collagen types I, III and V as substrates are regulated by estradiol, and Puistola and associates[74] demonstrated that estradiol also regulates the matrix metalloprotease-2 (MMP-2) gelatinase, which cleaves type IV collagen, in human granulosa–lutein cells.

Several investigations have also documented a role of estrogens in collagen synthesis in a variety of tissues, which again may be indirectly relevant to collagen synthesis in the remodeling phase of wound repair. Suzuki and Nakada[75] found that administration of 17β-estradiol increased collagen content in the prostate of rats, in accordance with the studies by Brincat and colleagues[14,17,76], which demonstrated that estrogen administration increased the collagen content of uninjured skin. Similarly, a recent study by Ashcroft and co-workers[77] showed that postmenopausal women who had never taken HRT had reduced matrix collagen deposition at 7 and 84 days post-wounding, whereas postmenopausal women who had taken HRT for at least 3 months had markedly increased levels of collagen deposition, similar to those observed in a premenopausal group. *In vitro* experiments carried out by these investigators indicated that this effect on wound healing was due to the estrogen component of HRT, possibly mediated by an increase in the activity of the cytokine transforming growth factor-β1[77].

However, in contrast to the above, estrogen administration resulted in a decrease in the collagen content of the temporomandibular joint disc of ovariectomized rats[78] and ovariectomy was not found to have an effect on the collagen content in the lower urinary tract smooth muscle of rabbits[79]. In accordance with these negative findings, Demirbilek and colleagues[80] demonstrated that combined administration of estradiol and progesterone to rats with esophageal burns resulted in significantly lower hydroxyproline levels and reduced collagen deposition compared to the control group. The authors believed that estradiol and progesterone inhibited new collagen synthesis following wounding to the esophageal tissue, but no data were available as to the effects of the latter following the administration of estrogen alone, or on its effects on collagenolysis.

CONCLUSION

In this chapter, the literature that is available regarding the involvement and influence of estrogens on the various phases of cutaneous repair has been presented and discussed. The investigations described demonstrate contradictory findings as to the effects of ovarian hormone deficiency, replacement or excess on the process of wound healing, making it difficult to draw valid conclusions from the studies. The discrepancies in the observed results may be explained by the usage of: (1) different species and gender of animal; (2) various types of hormone administered either alone or in combination with other sex hormones; (3) assorted routes of delivery of the hormone; (4) differing frequencies, doses and durations of treatment; (5) a diversity of methods for assessing healing; and (6) a variety of tissues and cell cultures in which the healing process was examined. Against this background, the varying and even contradictory results described in this chapter regarding the effects of estrogens on cutaneous repair are understandable and emphasize the need for further investigation in this field with a standardization of some of the above parameters.

There are estimated to be approximately 10 million postmenopausal women in the UK and 40 million in the USA, contributing 17% of the total population[81]. These statistics emphasize the importance of addressing the effects of ovarian hormone deficiency, and its replacement with HRT, on skin and its repair following injury, and the necessity to expand this area of research into the human population. Clinically, our aim should be to restore the integrity and function of wounded tissue as rapidly as possible after injury, and it is generally believed that a better understanding of this field could lead to improved care of cutaneous wounds, and the treatment of not only the wound but of the postmenopausal woman as a whole.

References

1. Lindsay R, Hart DM, MacLean A *et al.* Bone response to termination of estrogen treatment. *Lancet* 1978;1:1325–7
2. Brincat M, Kabalan S, Studd JWW, *et al.* A study of the decrease of skin collagen content, skin thickness and bone mass in the postmenopausal woman. *Obstet Gynecol* 1987;70:840–5
3. Stampfer MJ, Colditz GA, Willett WC, *et al.* Postmenopausal estrogen therapy and cardiovascular disease. Ten year follow-up from the Nurses' Health Study. *N Engl J Med* 1991;325:756–2
4. Brincat M, Studd JWW. Skin and the menopause. In Studd JWW, Whitehead MI, eds. *The Menopause*. Oxford: Blackwell, 1988:85–101
5. Allman RM, Damiano AM, Strauss MJ. Pressure ulcer status and post-discharge health care resource utilization among older adults with activity limitations. *Ad Wound Care* 1996;9:38–44

6. Calvin M. Thermal burns in the elderly: classification and pathophysiology. *J Geriatr Dermatol* 1995;3:149–57
7. Hasselquist MB, Goldberg N, Schroeter A, *et al.* Isolation and characterisation of the estrogen receptor in human skin. *J Clin Endocrinol Metab* 1980;50:76–82
8. Jee SH, Lee SY, Chiu HC, *et al.* Effects of oestrogen and oestrogen receptor in normal human melanocytes. *Biochem Biophys Res Comm* 1994;199:1407–12
9. Pedersen SB, Hansen PS, Lund S, *et al.* Identification of oestrogen receptor mRNA in human adipose tissue. *Eur J Clin Invest* 1996;26:262–9
10. Gulshan S, McCruden AB, Stimson WH, Oestrogen receptors in macrophages. *Scand J Immunol* 1990;31:691–7
11. Malet C, Gompel A, Yaneva H, *et al.* Oestradiol and progesterone receptors in cultured normal human breast epithelial cells and fibroblasts: immunocytochemical studies. *J Clin Endocrinol Metab* 1991;73:8–17
12. Venkov CD, Rankin AB, Vaughan DE. Identification of authentic oestrogen receptor in cultured endothelial cells. A potential mechanism for steroid hormone regulation of endothelial function. *Circulation* 1996;94:727–33
13. Punnonen R. Effect of castration and peroral estrogen therapy on the skin. *Acta Obstet Gynecol Scand* 1972;Suppl 21:7–44
14. Brincat M, Moniz CJ, Studd JWW, *et al.* Long term effects of the menopause and sex hormones on skin thickness. *Br J Obstet Gynaecol* 1985;92:256–9
15. Hooker CW, Pfeiffer CA. Effects of sex hormones upon body growth, skin, hair and sebaceous glands in the rat. *Endocrinology* 1943;32:69–70
16. Bolognia JL, Braverman IM, Rousseau ME, *et al.* Skin changes in menopause. *Maturitas* 1989;11:295–304
17. Brincat M, Moniz CF, Kabalan S, *et al.* Decline in skin collagen content and metacarpal index after the menopause and its prevention with sex hormone replacement. *Br J Obstet Gynaecol* 1987;94:126–9
18. Clark RAF. Wound repair; overview and general considerations. In Clark RAF, ed. *The Molecular and Cellular Biology of Wound Repair*, 2nd edn. London: Plenum Press, 1996:3–50
19. Loe H, Silness J. Periodontal disease in pregnancy. I. Prevalence and severity. *Acta Odont Scand* 1963;21:533–51
20. Cohen DW, Friedman J, Shapiro J, *et al.* A longitudinal investigation of the periodontal changes during pregnancy. *J Periodont Periodontics* 1969;40:563–70
21. Taubenhaus M, Amromin GD. Influence of steroid hormones on granulation tissue. *Endocrinology* 1949;44:359–67
22. Rigdon RH, Chrisman RB Jr. Effect of alpha oestradiol benzoate on local areas of inflammation in the skin of the rabbit. *Endocrinology* 1941;28:758–60
23. Shahrad P, Marks R. A pharmacological effect of oestrone on human epidermis. *Br J Dermatol* 1977;97:383–6
24. Brincat M, Versi E, Moniz CF, *et al.* Skin collagen changes in postmenopausal women receiving different regimens of estrogen therapy. *Obstet Gynecol* 1987;70:123–7
25. Brincat M, Versi E, O'Dowd T, *et al.* Skin collagen changes in postmenopausal women receiving oestradiol gel. *Maturitas* 1987;9:1–5
26. Lindhe J, Bjorn AL. Influence of hormonal contraceptives on the gingiva of women. *J Periodont Res* 1967;2:1–6
27. Lindhe J, Lundgren D, Stallard R, *et al.* Connective tissue alterations occurring during pregnancy as seen by vital dyes. *J Periodont* 1969;40:22–6
28. Hugoson A. Gingivitis in pregnant women. *Odont Rev* 1970;21:1–20
29. Hugoson A, Lindhe J. Gingival tissue regeneration in female dogs treated with sex hormones. *Odont Rev* 1971;22:425–40
30. Nyman S, Lindhe J, Zederfeldt B. Influence of estrogen and progesterone on tissue regeneration in oophorectomized rabbits. *Acta Chir Scand* 1971;137:131–9
31. Nyman S, Lindhe J, Zederfeldt B. The vascularity of wounded areas in estradiol and progesterone treated female rabbits. *Acta Chir Scand* 1971;137:631–7
32. Nyman S. Studies on the influence of estradiol and progesterone on granulation tissue. Granulation tissue formation and respiratory gas tensions in wound fluid in oestradiol and progesterone treated female rabbits. *J Periodont Res* 1971; 6(Suppl 7):12–13
33. Nyman S, Lindhe J, Zedefeldt B, *et al.* Vascular permeability in wounded areas of estradiol and progesterone treated female rabbits. *Acta Chir Scand* 1971;137:709–14
34. Nyman S, Zederfeldt B, Lewis DH. Blood flow in wounded areas of estradiol and progesterone treated female rabbits. *Acta Chir Scand* 1972;138:7–11
35. Lundgren D. Influence of estrogen and progesterone on exudation, inflammatory cell migration and granulation tissue formation in preformed cavities. *Scand J Plast Reconstr Surg* 1973;7:10–14
36. Pallin B, Ahonen J, Rank F, *et al.* Granulation tissue formation in ooophorectomized rats treated with female sex hormones: I. A histologic study. *Acta Chir Scand* 1975;141:702–9
37. Gouveia MA, Halbe HW, Schutze Filho N. The significance of female sex steroids on

the vascular permeability of the traumatised uterine serosa of rats. *Arch Gynecol Obstet* 1987; 241:121–6
38. Murthy CP, Prakash A, Pandit PN, *et al*. Effects of oestrogen on wound healing – an experimental study. *Indian J Surg* 1974;36:1–7
39. Tarantino MD, Kunicki TJ, Nugent DJ. The oestrogen receptor is present in human megakaryocytes. *Ann NY Acad Sci* 1994;714:293–6
40. Grodstein F, Stampfer MJ, Goldhaber SZ, *et al*. Prospective study of exogenous hormones and risk of pulmonary embolism in women. *Lancet* 1996;348:983–7
41. Daly E, Vessey MP, Hawkins MM, *et al*. Risk of venous thromboembolism in users of hormone replacement therapy. *Lancet* 1996;348:977–80
42. Rosenblum WI, El-Sabban F, Nelson GH. One day of oestradiol treatment enhances platelet aggregation at the site of microvascular injury without altering aggregation *ex vivo*. *Life Sci* 1988;42:123–8
43. Aune B, Oian P, Omsjo I, *et al*. Hormone replacement therapy reduces the reactivity of monocytes and platelets in whole blood – a beneficial effect on atherogenesis and thrombus formation? *Am J Obstet Gynecol* 1995;173:1816–20
44. Turk JL, Heather CJ, Diengdoh JV. A histochemical analysis of mononuclear cell infiltrates of the skin, with particular reference to delayed hypersensitivity in the guinea pig. *Int Arch Allergy Appl Immunol* 1976;29:278–89
45. Jansson G. Oestrogen-induced enhancement of myeloperoxidase activity in human polymorphonuclear leukocytes – a possible cause of oxidative stress in inflammatory cells. *Free Rad Res Comm* 1991;14:195–208
46. Magnusson U, Einarsson S. Effects of exogenous oestradiol on the number and functional capacity of circulating mononuclear and polymorphonuclear leukocytes in the sow. *Vet Immunol Immunopathol* 1990;25:235–47
47. Josefsson E, Tarkowski A, Carlsten H. Anti-inflammatory properties of oestrogen. I. *In vivo* suppression of leukocyte production in bone marrow and redistribution of peripheral blood neutrophils. *Cell Immunol* 1992;142:67–78
48. Ito I, Hayashi T, Yamada K, *et al*. Physiological concentration of oestradiol inhibits polymorphonuclear leukocyte chemotaxis via a receptor mediated system. *Life Sci* 1995;56:2247–53
49. Miyagi M, Aoyama H, Morishita M, *et al*. Effects of sex hormones on chemotaxis of human peripheral polymorphonuclear leukocytes and monocytes. *J Periodont* 1992;63:28–32
50. Calvin M, Dyson M, Rymer J, *et al*. The effects of ovarian hormone deficiency on the inflammatory phase of wound healing in a rat model. *Br J Obstet Gynacol* 1998; submitted.
51. Taylor FW, Dittmer TL, Porter DO. Wound healing and the steroids. *Surgery* 1952;31:683–90
52. Jorgensen O, Schmidt A. Influence of sex hormones on granulation tissue formation and on healing of linear wounds. *Acta Chir Scand* 1962;124:1–10
53. Portugal H, Lima A, Olivera GR, *et al*. The effect of sex steroids upon granulation tissue. *Int Arch Allergy* 1951;2:274–81
54. Robertson WB, Sanborn EC. Hormonal effects on collagen formation in granulomas. *Endocrinology* 1958;63:150–5
55. Lundgren D. Influence of estrogen and progesterone on vascularization of granulation tissue in preformed cavities. *Scand J Plast Reconstr Surg* 1973;7:85–90
56. Pallin B, Ahonen J, Zederfeldt B. Granulation tissue formation in oophorectomized rats treated with female sex hormones: II. Studies on the amount of collagen and on tensile strength. *Acta Chir Scand* 1975;141:710–14
57. Lindhe J, Birch J, Branemark P. Wound healing in estrogen treated female rabbits. *J Periodont Res* 1968;3:21–3
58. Hu SK, Mitcho YL, Rath NC. Effect of oestradiol on interleukin 1 synthesis by macrophages. *Int J Immunopharmacol* 1988;10:247–52
59. Sampson PM, Rochester CL, Freundlich B, *et al*. Cytokine regulation of human lung fibroblast hyaluronan (hyaluronic acid) production: evidence for cytokine-regulated hyaluronan (hyaluronic acid) degradation and human lung fibroblast-derived hyaluronidase. *J Clin Invest* 1992;90:1492–503
60. Cotran RS, Kumar V, Robbins SL, *et al*. Inflammation and repair. In Cotran RS, Kumar V, Robbins SL, *et al*., eds. *Robbins Pathologic Basis of Disease*, 5th edn. Philadelphia: WB Saunders, 1994:39–48
61. Shanker G, Sorci-Thomas M, Adams MR. Oestrogen modulates the inducible expression of platelet-derived growth factor mRNA by monocyte/macrophages. *Life Sci* 1995;56: 499–507
62. Katz MH, Kirsner RS, Eaglstein WH, *et al*. Human wound fluid from acute wounds stimulates fibroblast and endothelial cell growth. *J Am Acad Dermatol* 1991;25:1054–8
63. Battegay EF, Rupp J, Iruela-Arispe L, *et al*. PDGF-BB modulates endothelial proliferation and angiogenesis *in vitro* via PDGF β receptors. *J Cell Biol* 1994;125:917–28
64. Rappolee DA, Mark D, Banda MJ, *et al*. Wound macrophages express TGFα and other growth factors *in vivo*: analysis by mRNA phenotyping. *Science* 1988;241:708–12
65. Calvin M, Dyson M, Rymer J, *et al*. The effects of ovarian hormone deficiency on wound contrac-

tion in a rat model. *Br J Obstet Gynaecol* 1998;105:223–7
66. Levine AC, Ren M, Huber GK, *et al.* The effect of androgen, oestrogen and growth factors on the proliferation of cultured fibroblasts derived from human foetal and adult prostates. *Endocrinology* 1997;130:2413–19
67. Luo D, Lin Y, Liu X, *et al.* Effect of prostatic growth factor, basic fibroblast growth factor, epidermal growth factor and steroids on the proliferation of human foetal prostatic fibroblasts. *Prostate* 1996;28:352–8
68. Sato T, Ito A, Mori Y, *et al.* Hormonal regulation of collagenolysis in uterine cervical fibroblasts. Modulation of synthesis of procollagenase, prostromelysin and TIMPs by progesterone and oestradiol-17β. *Biochem J* 1991;275:645–50
69. Morales DE, McGowan KA, Grant DS, *et al.* Oestrogen promotes angiogenic activity in human umbilical vein endothelial cells *in vitro* and in a murine model. *Circulation* 1995;91:755–63
70. Schlaff WD, Gittlesohn AM, Cooley BC, *et al.* A rat uterine horn model of genital tract wound healing. *Fertil Steril* 1987;48:866–72
71. Calvin M. *The effects of ovariectomy on cutaneous wound healing in a rat model.* PhD thesis, University of London, 1997
72. Yoshida K, Tahara R, Nakayama T, *et al.* Effect of dehydroepiandrosterone sulphate, oestrogens and prostaglandins on collagen metabolism in human cervical tissue in relation to cervical ripening. *J Int Med Res* 1993;21:26–35
73. Kumar MP, Thampan RV. Dual hormonal involvement in the regulation of rat uterine collagenase activity. *Biochem Int* 1992;28:975–80
74. Puistola U, Westerlund A, Kauppila A, *et al.* Regulation of 72 kD type IV collagenase-matrix metalloproteinase-2 by oestradiol and gonadotrophin-releasing hormone agonist in human granulosa–lutein cells. *Fertil Steril* 1995;64:81–7
75. Suzuki H, Nakada T. Alteration of collagen biosynthesis and analysis of type I and type III collagens of prostate in young rats following sex hormone treatments. *Arch Androl* 1996;36:205–16
76. Brincat M, Moniz CF, Studd JWW, *et al.* Sex hormones and skin collagen content in postmenopausal women. *Br Med J* 1983;287:1337–8
77. Ashcroft GS, Dodsworth J, van Boxtel E, *et al.* Estrogen accelerates cutaneous wound healing associated with an increase in TGF-β1 levels. *Nat Med* 1997;3:1209–15
78. Abubaker AO, Hebda PC, Gunsolley JN. Effects of sex hormones on protein and collagen content of the temporomandibular joint disc of the rat. *J Oral Maxillofacial Surg* 1996;54:721–8
79. Persson K, Svane D, Glavind B, *et al.* Effects of ovariectomy on mechanical properties and collagen content in rabbit lower urinary tract smooth muscle. *Scand J Urol Nephrol* 1996;30:7–14
80. Demirbilek S, Bernay F, Rizalar R, *et al.* Effects of oestradiol and progesterone on the synthesis of collagen in corrosive oesophageal burns in rats. *J Pediatr Surg* 1994;29:1425–8
81. Wise PM, Krajnak KM, Kashon ML. Menopause: the aging of multiple pacemakers. *Science* 1996;273:67–70

5
The effect of estrogen deficiency on the bladder

A. Hextall and L. Cardozo

INTRODUCTION

The female genital and urinary tracts both arise from the primitive urogenital sinus and develop in close anatomical proximity from as early as the fourth week of embryological life. Human and animal studies have identified estrogen receptors in the tissues of the vagina, urethra, bladder and plevic floor. Sex hormones have a substantial influence on the female bladder throughout adult life with fluctuations in their levels leading to macroscopic, histological and functional changes. It is not surprising, therefore, that urinary symptoms may develop during the menstrual cycle, pregnancy and following the menopause. Estrogen deficiency, particularly when prolonged, is associated with a wide range of urogenital complaints including frequency, nocturia, incontinence, urinary tract infections and the 'urge syndrome'. These may co-exist with vaginal symptoms of dryness, itching, burning and dyspareunia.

EFFECT OF AGING ON THE BLADDER

Many women consider the development of urinary symptoms as they get older to be a normal phenomenon rather than the manifestation of a disease[1]. Indeed, in a study of Gjorup and colleagues[2], over 50% of women aged more than 75 years thought that their symptoms were normal for elderly people. Symptomatic and functional changes certainly do occur in the lower urinary tract as a result of the aging process, which are difficult to differentiate from those due to estrogen deficiency. Younger women tend to excrete the bulk of their fluid intake before they go to bed, whereas in the elderly, this pattern may be reversed. Postural effects lead to daytime pooling of extracellular fluid, especially in the ankles, and when this returns to the vasculature during the night there is a consequential increase in urine output. This, combined with an alteration in sleep patterns, may lead to nocturia.

Urodynamic studies have shown that the urethra and bladder become less efficient with age[3–5]. Elderly women have a reduced urine flow rate, increased urinary residual, higher first sensation of a desire to void and increased bladder capacity, although the latter may fall in the eighth and ninth decades[6]. In addition, detrusor pressures at urethral opening and closure during voiding fall in absolute terms as women become older[7]. Histologically, there is an age-related increase in fibrosis of the bladder neck[8] and collagen content in the human female bladder[9]. The number and diameter of muscle fibers in the pelvic floor also decrease with age[10], although neuronal damage secondary to childbirth may be a confounding factor[11,12].

The aging population are at risk of developing a number of illnesses which may present with lower urinary tract symptoms, including diabetes mellitus, congestive cardiac failure and renal disease. A patient with impaired mobility may develop incontinence of urine if suitable access to a toilet is not available, a situation which may be exacerbated if medications such as diuretics or hypnotics are being taken.

INFLUENCE OF SEX HORMONES ON THE LOWER URINARY TRACT

Estrogen receptors are consistently expressed in the squamous epithelium of the proximal and distal urethra and vagina, and trigone of the bladder in areas which have undergone squamous metaplasia (Figure 1)[13,14]. However, they are not present in the transitional epithelium of the bladder dome, reflecting the different embryological origin of this tissue (Figure 2). The pubococcygeous muscle of the pelvic floor is also a target site for estrogen[15,16]. Estrogens increase cell cycle activity in the female lower urinary tract[17], and this is demonstrated by an increase in the number of intermediate and superficial cells in the urethra and bladder[18] with similar changes also occurring in the vagina of postmenopausal women[19,20]. Alterations in urinary cytology during the menstrual cycle are comparable with those seen in vaginal cytology[21], changes which also occur in the urinary sediment following treatment with estrogens[22].

Progesterone receptors are expressed inconsistently in the lower urinary tract and may be dependent on the estrogen status of the woman[14]. Androgen receptors are found in both the female bladder and urethra, but their role is at present unclear[23].

Cyclical variations in urinary symptoms occurring during the menstrual cycle can be measured objectively using urethral pressure profilometry (UPP)[24]. The functional and anatomical lengths of the urethra increase midcycle and early in the luteal phase, reflecting serum estrogen concentrations. Changes also occur during pregnancy[25,26] which can partially be explained by an increase in urine output and pressure effects from the gravid uterus. However, the prevalence of detrusor instability antenatally is significantly greater than that found postpartum[27], suggesting a possible hormonal effect on the bladder thought to be mediated through progesterone[28].

EPIDEMIOLOGY

Urinary symptoms secondary to estrogen deficiency may only develop many years after the

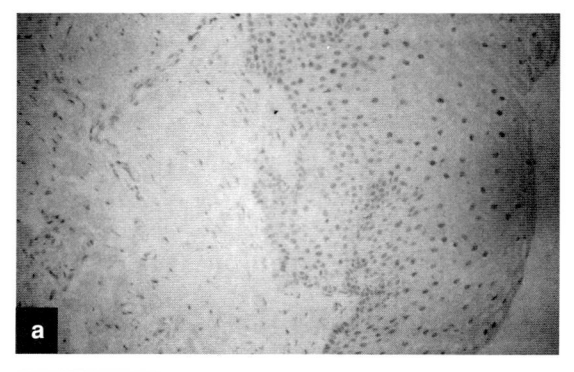

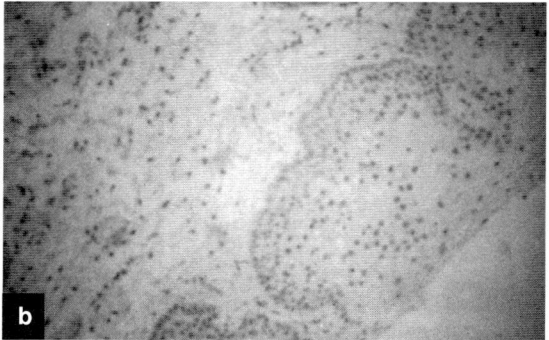

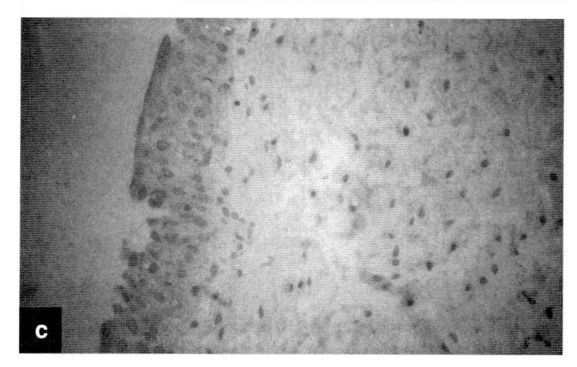

Figure 1 Estrogen receptors are expressed in squamous epithelium of the vagina (a) and urethra (b) but not transitional epithelium of the bladder dome (c). Reproduced from reference 14 with permission

menopause and, therefore, may be under-reported by both patient and doctor. Epidemiological studies have shown that the incidence of urogenital problems increases with age, with many women delaying seeking treatment for several years. In a study of 2045 women aged between 55 and 85 years, Barlow and colleagues[29] showed that urogenital symptoms had affected 48.5% of postmenopausal women at some time, but only 11% were currently affected by individual symptoms. At least two-thirds of women did not relate their vaginal or urinary complaint to the menopause. Iosif and Bekassy[30] studied 2200 women aged 61 years and also found that the incidence of lower genital tract disorders was high, with 49% of women having some symptoms. Urinary symptoms are certainly common after the climacteric, with one in five women attending a menopause clinic complaining of severe urgency, and nearly 50% of stress incontinence[31].

The prevalence of postmenopausal incontinence in the community is thought to be between 16 and 29% (Figure 3)[29,32,33]. While the aging process is clearly a significant etiological factor in the pathogenesis of urinary incontinence, there is conflicting evidence as to whether the menopause and estrogen deficiency are also important. Jolleys[34] surveyed 937 women registered with a rural general practice, and found that the prevalence of incontinence was most common in the 45–55-year age group, a period which includes the climacteric in most cases (Figure 4). Hilton[35] also found a similar pattern in hospital practice, with 40% of women referred to a urogynecology unit aged between 40 and 60 years, with a mean comparable with the average age of the menopause. In addition, 70% of the incontinent women studied by Iosif and Bekassy[30] related the onset of their urinary leakage to their final menstrual period. Urge incontinence, in particular, is found more commonly after the menopause, although the prevalence of stress incontinence starts to fall (Figure 5)[36]. Most studies, however, show that many women develop incontinence at least 10 years before the climacteric, with Jolleys[34] finding that significantly more premenopausal women were affected than postmenopausal women.

There are a number of different causes of urinary incontinence (Table 1), with elderly women particularly at risk of transient problems (Table 2).

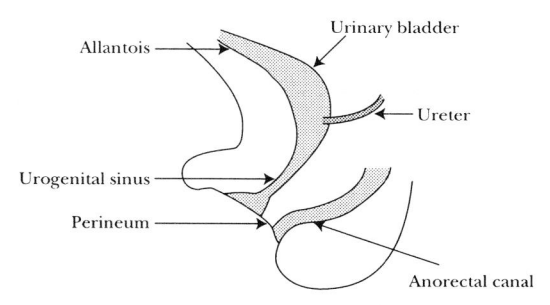

Figure 2 Embryology of lower urinary tract

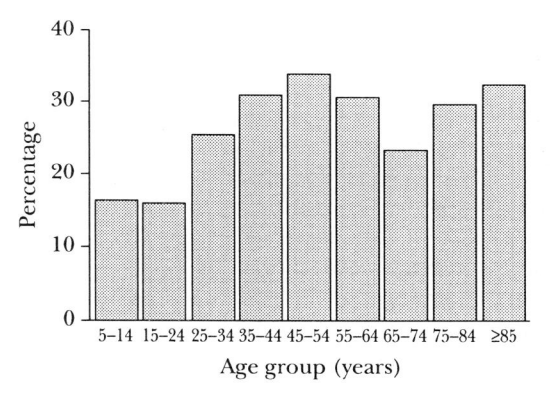

Figure 3 Prevalence of occasional or regular urinary incontinence in women. Adapted from reference 32

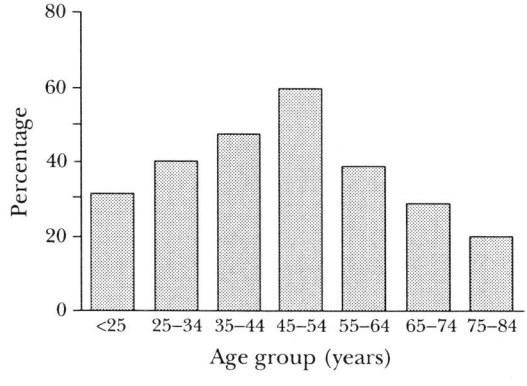

Figure 4 Prevalence of urinary incontinence with increasing age[34]

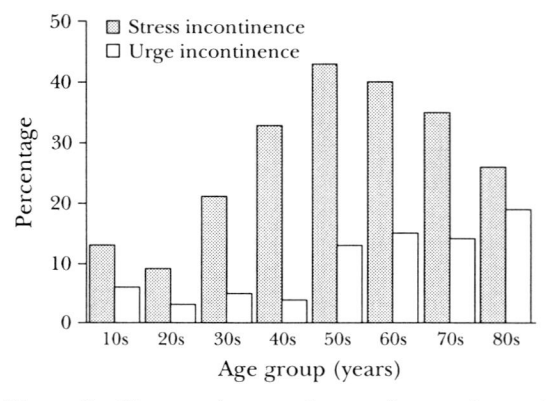

Figure 5 Changes in prevalence of stress incontinence and urge incontinence with increasing age[36]

Table 1 Common causes of female urinary incontinence

Genuine stress incontinence
Detrusor instability (detrusor hyper-reflexia)
Overflow incontinence
Fistulae (vesicovaginal, uterovaginal, urethrovaginal)
Urethral diverticulum
Functional (immobility)
Transient problems (Table 2)

Table 2 Transient causes of urinary incontinence in the elderly

Urinary tract infection
Fecal impaction
Estrogen deficiency
Restricted mobility
Drug therapy
Depression
Confusional state

Table 3 Mechanisms by which estrogens may treat female urinary incontinence

Increased urethral closure pressure
   increased urethral cell maturation
   increased urethral blood flow
   increased alpha-adrenergic receptor sensitivity in urethral smooth muscle
   stimulation of periurethral collagen production
Increased sensory threshold of bladder
Improved abdominal pressure transmission to proximal urethra
Reduced incidence of urinary tract infection
Improved mood and quality of life

ESTROGENS AND THE CONTINENCE MECHANISM

The estrogen-sensitive tissues of the bladder, urethra and pelvic floor all play an important role in the continence mechanism. For a woman to remain continent, the urethral pressure must exceed the intravesical pressure at all times except during micturition[37]. The urethra has four estrogen-sensitive functional layers which all play a part in the maintenance of a positive urethral pressure:

(1) Epithelium;
(2) Vasculature;
(3) Connective tissue;
(4) Muscle.

The cellular changes in the epithelial layer of the urethra which occur in response to estrogen have already been described above. There is evidence to suggest that the vasodilatory effect of estrogens which occurs in the systemic circulation[38] may also take place in the urogenital tract. Versi and Cardozo[39] have shown that the vascular pulsations seen on UPP, owing to blood flow in the urethral submucosa and urethral sphincter, increase in size in response to estrogen. Connective tissue metabolism is stimulated by estrogens, increasing the production of collagen in periurethral tissues and, therefore, possibly reversing the changes which occur as a result of aging[40]. Finally, the alpha receptors in the urethral sphincter are sensitized by estrogens[41], helping to maintain muscular tone. The estrogen status of the patient, therefore, can have a significant effect on urethral pressure[42], and this may be particularly important when there is already a degree of weakness.

ESTROGENS IN TREATMENT OF URINARY INCONTINENCE

There are a number of reasons why estrogens may be useful in the treatment of women with urinary incontinence (Table 3). As well as improving the 'maturation index' of urethral squamous epithelium[43], estrogens increase urethral closure pressure and improve abdominal pressure transmission to the proximal urethra[44–46]. The sensory threshold of the bladder may also be raised[47]. Salmon and colleagues[48] were the first to report the successful use of estrogens to treat urinary incontinence over 50 years ago. Intramuscular estrogen therapy was administered to 16 women with dysuria, frequency, urgency and incontinence for 4 weeks. Symptomatic improvement occurred in 12 women until treatment was discontinued, at which time the symptoms recurred. Further studies on larger numbers of patients[49,50] also showed impressive subjective improvement rates of between 39 and 70%.

There are a number of different causes of lower urinary tract disorders in postmenopausal women[51]. It is well recognized that there is a poor correlation between a woman's symptoms and the subsequent diagnosis following appropriate investigation[52]. Unfortunately, initial trials took place before the widespread introduction of urodynamic studies and, therefore, almost certainly included a heterogeneous group of individuals with a number of different pathologies. Lack of objective outcome measures also limits their interpretation.

ESTROGENS FOR STRESS INCONTINENCE

The role of estrogen in the treatment of stress incontinence has been controversial even though there are a number of reported studies. Some have given promising results, but this may be because they were observational, not randomized, blinded or controlled. The situation is further complicated by the fact that a number of different types of estrogen have been used with varying doses, routes of administration and durations of treatment. Two studies using oral estrogen have been reported recently. Fantl and co-workers[53] treated 83 hypoestrogenic women with urodynamic evidence of genuine stress incontinence and/or detrusor instability with conjugated equine estrogens 0.625 mg and medroxyprogesterone 10 mg cyclically for 3 months. Controls received placebo tablets. At the end of the study period, the clinical and quality-of-life variables had not changed significantly in either group. Jackson and associates[54] treated 57 postmenopausal women with genuine stress incontinence or mixed incontinence with estradiol valerate 2 mg or placebo daily for 6 months. There was no significant change in objective outcome measures although both the active and placebo group reported subjective benefit.

There have now been two meta-analyses performed which have helped to clarify the situation further. In the first, a report by the Hormones and Urogenital Therapy (HUT) Committee, the use of estrogens to treat all causes of incontinence in postmenopausal women was examined[55]. Of 166 articles identified which were published in English between 1969 and 1992, only six were controlled trials and 17 were uncontrolled series. The results showed that there was a significant subjective improvement for all patients and those with genuine stress incontinence. However, assessment of the objective parameters revealed that there was no change in the volume of urine lost. Maximum urethral closure pressure did increase significantly, but this result was influenced by only one study showing a large effect. In the second meta-analysis, Sultana and Walters[56] reviewed eight controlled and 14 uncontrolled prospective trials and included all types of estrogen treatment. They also found that estrogen therapy was not an efficacious treatment of stress incontinence but may be useful for the often associated symptoms of urgency and frequency.

Estrogen, when given alone, therefore, does not appear to be an effective treatment for stress incontinence. However, several studies have shown that it may have a role in combination with other therapies. Beisland and colleagues[57] treated 24 women with genuine stress incontinence using phenylpropanolamine (50 mg twice daily) and estriol (1 mg per day vaginally) separately and in combination. They found that the combination cured eight women and improved a further nine, and was more effective than either drug given alone. Hilton and colleagues[58] used estrogen (vaginal or oral) alone or in combination with phenylpropanolamine to treat 60 postmenopausal women with genuine stress incontinence in a double-blind, placebo-controlled study. Subjectively, the symptom of stress incontinence improved in all groups but, objectively, only in the women given combination therapy. This type of treatment may be particularly useful for women with mild stress incontinence or for those not suitable for surgery.

ESTROGENS FOR URGE INCONTINENCE

Estrogen has been used to treat postmenopausal urgency and urge incontinence for many years, but there have been very few controlled trials performed to confirm that it is of benefit. Walter and colleagues[59] found that a combination of estradiol 2 mg and estriol 1 mg daily cured the symptoms of urge incontinence in seven out of 11 women, whereas placebo cured only one of 10 patients. Samsioe and co-workers[60] also used oral estriol 3 mg daily, to treat 34 women aged 75 years in a double-blind placebo-controlled cross-over study. Overall, a substantial subjective improvement was found in the 12 women with urge incontinence and eight women with mixed incontinence. However, these reports need to be interpreted with caution because of the small patient numbers and lack of objective outcome measures, despite the known large placebo effect which occurs in treatment of this condition.

A double-blind multicenter study of 64 postmenopausal women with the 'urge syndrome' has failed to confirm these results[61]. All women underwent pretreatment urodynamic investigation to establish that they either had sensory urgency or detrusor instability. They were then randomized to treatment with oral estriol 3 mg daily or placebo for 3 months. Compliance was confirmed by a significant improvement in the maturation index of vaginal epithelial cells in the active but not the placebo group. Estriol produced subjective and objective improvements in urinary symptoms but it was not significantly better than placebo. In a further study, sustained-release 25 mg 17β-estradiol vaginal tablets (Vagifem, Novo Nordsk) or placebo were used to treat 110 postmenopausal women (Benness and associates, unpublished data). Urodynamic investigations confirmed that the women had either sensory urgency, detrusor instability or a normal study. At the end of the 6-month treatment period, the only significant differences between the active and placebo groups was an improvement in the symptom of urgency in the women who had a diagnosis of sensory urgency. It is possible that this low dose of local estrogen was reversing atrophic changes in the lower urinary/genital tract rather than treating the underlying pathology.

These studies may not have shown any benefit possibly because the wrong type of estrogen was used for too short a time period, or it may have been given by the wrong route. Estriol, although a naturally occurring estrogen, has little effect on the endometrium and does not prevent osteoporosis. It is also questionable, therefore, whether the low dose used in these studies is sufficient to treat urinary symptoms. Sustained-release 17β-estradiol vaginal tablets are well absorbed and have been shown to induce maturation of the vaginal epithelium within 14 days[62], but higher systemic levels may be needed for therapy to be effective.

ESTROGENS AND RECURRENT URINARY TRACT INFECTIONS

Alterations in the vaginal flora following the menopause place women at an increased risk of urinary tract infections, particularly if they are sexually active. There is a rise in vaginal pH and a fall in the number of lactobacilli, allowing colonization with gram-negative bacteria which act as uropathogens. Estrogen reverses these changes, an effect which enables it to be used for either treatment or prophylaxis.

Brandberg and colleagues[63] treated 41 elderly women with recurrent urinary tract infections using oral estriol and showed that their vaginal flora was restored to the premenopausal type and that they required fewer antibiotics. Kirkengen and associates[64] randomized 40 elderly women with recurrent urinary tract infections to receive either oral estriol 3 mg/day for 4 weeks followed by 1 mg/day for 8 weeks or matched placebo. After the first treatment period, there was no difference found between estriol and placebo. However, following the second treatment period, estriol was significantly better than placebo in reducing the incidence of urinary tract infections.

A randomized, double-blind, placebo-controlled study of 93 postmenopausal women has also shown that *intravaginal* estriol cream prevents recurrent urinary tract infections in those women presenting with this problem[65]. Midstream urine cultures were obtained at enrolment, monthly for 8 months and whenever urinary symptoms occurred. Changes in the vaginal pH and colonization with lactobacilli were present within the estriol group only, within 1 month of the start of treatment. The incidence of urinary tract infection in the group given estriol was significantly reduced, compared with that in the group given placebo (0.5 vs. 5.9 episodes per patient per year). Unfortunately, we have been unable to reproduce these results in a double-blind placebo-controlled study of *oral* estriol in the prevention of recurrent urinary tract infections in elderly women[66]. Although both estriol and placebo improved urinary symptoms during the trial, the incidence of urinary tract infection did not differ significantly between the two groups.

CONCLUSIONS

Estrogen has an important physiological effect on the female lower urinary tract, and its deficiency is an etiological factor in the pathogenesis of a number of conditions. The use of estrogens alone to treat urinary incontinence has given disappointing results, but when given in combination with alpha-adrenergic agonists they are more effective. Hormone replacement therapy does appear to improve irritative symptoms of frequency and urgency possibly by reversing urogenital atrophy. Treatment may need to be given for a long period of time before benefit is seen although, at present, the 'best' therapy is unknown. Estrogens may be effective when used for prophylaxis against recurrent urinary tract infections in postmenopausal women, but further studies are required to determine which route of administration is the most efficacious.

References

1. Svanberg A. The gerontological and geriatric study in Goteborg, Sweden. *Acta Med Scand* 1977;611:1–37
2. Gjorup T, Hendriksen C, Lund E, *et al.* Is growing old a disease? A study of the attitudes of elderly people to physical symptoms. *J Chron Dis* 1987;40:1095–8
3. Rud T, Anderson KE, Asmussen M, *et al.* Factors maintaining the urethral pressure in women. *Invest Urol* 1980;17:343–7
4. Rud T. Urethral pressure profile in continent women from childhood to old age. *Acta Obstet Gynecol Scand* 1980;59:331–5
5. Malone Lee J, Waheda I. The characterisation of detrusor contractile function in relation to old age. *Br J Urol* 1993;72:873–80
6. Collas DM, Malone Lee J. Age-associated changes in detrusor sensory function in women with lower urinary tract symptoms. *Int Urogynecol J* 1996;7:24–9
7. Wagg AS, Lieu PK, Ding YY, *et al.* A urodynamic analysis of age associated changes in urethral function in women with lower urinary tract symptoms. *J Urol* 1996;156:1984–8
8. Brocklehurst JC. Ageing of the human bladder. *Geriatrics* 1972;27:154
9. Susset JG, Servot-Viguier D, Lamy F, *et al.* Collagen in 155 human bladders. *Invest Urol* 1978;16:204–6
10. Kolbl H, Strassegger H, Riis PA, *et al.* Morphologic and functional aspects of pelvic floor muscles in patients with pelvic relaxation and genuine stress incontinence. *Obstet Gynecol* 1989;74:789–95
11. Smith ARB, Hosker GL, Warrell DW. The role of partial denervation of the pelvic floor in the etiology of genito-urinary prolapse and stress incontinence of urine. A neurophysiological study. *Br J Obstet Gynaecol* 1989;96:24–8
12. Allen RE, Warrell DW. The role of pregnancy and childbirth in partial denervation of the pelvic floor. *Neurourol Urodyn* 1992;6:183–4

13. Iosif CS, Batra S, Ek A, et al. Estrogen receptors in the human female lower urinary tract. *Am J Obstet Gynecol* 1981;141:817–20
14. Blakeman PJ, Hilton P, Bulmer JN. Mapping oestrogen and progesterone receptors throughout the female lower urinary tract. *Neurourol Urodyn* 1996;15:324–5
15. Ingelman-Sundberg A, Rosen J, Gustafsson SA, et al. Cytosol oestrogen receptors in urogenital tissues in stress incontinence women. *Acta Obstet Gynecol Scand* 1981;60:585–6
16. Smith P. Estrogens and the urogenital tract. *Acta Obstet Gynecol Scand* 1993;72 (Suppl):1–26
17. Blakeman PJ, Hilton P, Bulmer JN. Oestrogen status and cell cycle activity in the female lower urinary tract. *Neurourol Urodyn* 1996;15:325–6
18. Samsioe G, Jansson I, Meelstrom D, et al. Occurrence, nature and treatment of urinary incontinence in a 70 year old female population. *Maturitas* 1985;7:335–42
19. Smith PJB. The effect of oestrogens on bladder function in the female. In Campbell S, ed. *Management of the Menopause and Post Menopausal Years*. Lancaster: MTP Press, 1976:291–8
20. Semmens JP, Tsai CC, Semmens EC, et al. Effects of estrogen therapy on vaginal physiology during menopause. *Obstet Gynecol* 1985;66:15–18
21. McCallin PF, Taylor ES, Whitehead RW. A study of the changes in the urinary sediment during the menstrual cycle. *Am J Obstet Gynecol* 1950;60:64–74
22. Soloman C, Panagotopoulos P, Oppenheim A. The use of urinary sediment as an aid in endocrinological disorders in the female. *Am J Obstet Gynecol* 1958;76:56–60
23. Blakeman PJ, Hilton P, Bulmer JN. Androgen receptors in the female lower urinary tract. *Int Urogynecol J* 1997;8:S54
24. Van Geelen JM, Doesburg WH, Thomas CMG, et al. Urodynamic studies in the normal menstrual cycle: the relationship between hormonal changes during the menstrual cycle and the urethral pressure profile. *Am J Obstet Gynecol* 1981;141:384–92
25. Stanton SL, Kerr-Wilson R, Harris VG. The incidence of urological symptoms in normal pregnancy. *Br J Obstet Gynaecol* 1980;87:897–900
26. Cutner A, Carey A, Cardozo LD. Lower urinary tract symptoms in early pregnancy. *J Obstet Gynecol* 1992;12:75–8
27. Cutner A. *The Lower Urinary Tract in Pregnancy*. MD thesis, University of London, UK, 1993
28. Cutner A, Burton G, Cardozo LD, et al. Does progesterone cause an irritable bladder? *Int Urogynecol J* 1991;98:1181–3
29. Barlow DH, Cardozo LD, Francis RM, et al. Urogenital ageing and its effect on sexual health in older British women. *Br J Obstet Gynaecol* 1997;104:87–91
30. Iosif CS, Bekassy Z. Prevalence of genito-urinary symptoms in the late menopause. *Acta Obstet Gynecol Scand* 1984;63:257–60
31. Cardozo LD, Tapp A, Versi E. The lower urinary tract in peri- and postmenopausal women. In Samsioe G, Bonne Erickson P, eds. *The Urogenital Oestrogen Deficiency Syndrome*. Bagsverd, Denmark: Novo Industri AS, 1987:10–17
32. Thomas TM, Plymat KR, Blannin J, et al. Prevalence of urinary incontinence. *Br Med J* 1980;281:1243–5
33. Vetter NJ, Jones DA, Victor CR. Urinary incontinence in the elderly at home. *Lancet* 1981;2:1275–7
34. Jolleys JV. Reported prevalence of urinary incontinence in women in a general practice. *Br Med J* 1988;296:1300–2
35. Hilton P. *Urethral pressure measurement by microtransducer: observations on the methodology, the pathophysiology of stress incontinence and the effects of treatment in the female*. MD thesis, University of Newcastle-upon-Tyne, UK, 1981
36. Kondo A, Kato K, Saito M, et al. Prevalence of handwashing incontinence in females in comparison with stress and urge incontinence. *Neurourol Urodyn* 1990;9:330–1
37. Abrams P, Blaivas JG, Stanton SL, et al. The standardisation of terminology of lower urinary tract function. *Br J Obstet Gynaecol* 1990;97:1–16
38. Ganger KF, Vyas S, Whitehead M, et al. Pulsatility index in the internal carotid artery in relation to transdermal oestradiol and time since menopause. *Lancet* 1991;338:839–42
39. Versi E, Cardozo LD. Urethral instability: diagnosis based on variations in the maximum urethral pressure in normal climacteric women. *Neurourol Urodyn* 1986;5:535–41
40. Jackson S, Avery N, Shepard A, et al. The effect of oestradiol on vaginal collagen in postmenopausal women with stress urinary incontinence. *Neurourol Urodyn* 1996;15:327–8
41. Screiter F, Fuchs P, Stockamp K. Estrogenic sensitivity of alpha receptors in the urethra musculature. *Urol Int* 1976;31:13–19
42. Rud T. The effects of estrogens and gestagens on the urethral pressure profile in urinary continent and stress incontinent women. *Acta Obstet Gynecol Scand* 1980;59:265–70
43. Bergman A, Karram MM, Bhatia NN. Changes in urethral cytology following estrogen administration. *Gynecol Obstet Invest* 1990;29:211–13
44. Hilton P, Stanton SL. The use of intravaginal oestrogen cream in genuine stress incontinence. *Br J Obstet Gynaecol* 1983;90:940–4
45. Bhatia NN, Bergman A, Karram MM, et al. Effects of estrogen on urethral function in women with

urinary incontinence. *Am J Obstet Gynecol* 1989;160:176–81
46. Karram MM, Yeko TR, Sauer MV, *et al.* Urodynamic changes following hormone replacement therapy in women with premature ovarian failure. *Obstet Gynecol* 1989;74:208–11
47. Fantl JA, Wyman JF, Anderson RL, *et al.* Postmenopausal urinary incontinence: comparison between non-estrogen and estrogen supplemented women. *Obstet Gynecol* 1988;71:823–8
48. Salmon UL, Walter RI, Gast SH. The use of estrogen in the treatment of dysuria and incontinence in postmenopausal women. *Am J Obstet Gynecol* 1941;14:23–31
49. Musiani U. A partially successful attempt at medical treatment of urinary stress incontinence in women. *Urol Int* 1972;27:405–10
50. Schleyer-Saunders E. Hormone implants for urinary disorders in postmenopausal women. *J Am Geriatr Soc* 1976;24:337–9
51. Bent AE, Richardson DA, Ostergard DR. Diagnosis of lower urinary tract disorders in postmenopausal patients. *Am J Obstet Gynecol* 1983;145:218–22
52. Jarvis GJ, Hall S, Stamp S, *et al.* An assessment of urodynamic investigation in incontinent women. *Br J Obstet Gynaecol* 1980;87:184–90
53. Fantl JA, Bump RC, Robinson D, *et al.* Efficacy of estrogen supplementation in the treatment of urinary incontinence. *Obstet Gynecol* 1996;88:745–9
54. Jackson S, Shepherd A, Abrams P. The effect of oestradiol on objective urinary leakage in postmenopausal stress incontinence, a double blind placebo controlled trial. *Neurourol Urodyn* 1996;15:322–3
55. Fantl JA, Cardozo LD, McClish DK, *et al.* Estrogen therapy in the management of urinary incontinence in postmenopausal women: a meta-analysis. First report of the Hormones and Urogenital Therapy Committee. *Obstet Gynecol* 1994;83:12–18

56. Sultana CJ, Walters MD. Estrogen and urinary incontinence in women. *Maturitas* 1990;20:129–38
57. Beisland HO, Fossberg E, Moer A, *et al.* Urethral insufficiency in postmenopausal females: treatment with phenylpropanolamine and estriol separately and in combination. *Urol Int* 1984;39:211–16
58. Hilton P, Tweddel AL, Mayne C. Oral and intravaginal estrogens alone and in combination with alpha adrenergic stimulation in genuine stress incontinence. *Int Urogynecol J* 1990;12:80–6
59. Walter S, Wolf H, Barlebo H, *et al.* Urinary incontinence in postmenopausal women treated with estrogen. *Urol Int* 1978;33:135–43
60. Samsioe G, Jansson I, Mellstrom D, *et al.* Occurrence, nature and treatment of urinary incontinence in a seventy five year old female population. *Maturitas* 1985;7:335–42
61. Cardozo LD, Rekers H, Tapp A, *et al.* Oestriol in the treatment of postmenopausal urgency: a multicentre study. *Maturitas* 1993;18:47–53
62. Nilsson K, Heimer G. Low does oestradiol in the treatment of urogenital oestrogen deficiency – a pharmacokinetic and pharmacodynamic study. *Maturitas* 1992;15:121–7
63. Brandberg A, Mellstrom D, Samsioe G. Peroral estriol treatment of older women with urogenital infections. *Lakartidningen* 1985;82:3399–401
64. Kirkengen AL, Anderson P, Gjersoe E, *et al.* Oestriol in the prophylactic treatment of recurrent urinary tract infections in postmenopausal women. *Scand J Prim Health Care* 1992;10:139–42
65. Raz R, Stamm WE. A controlled trial of intravaginal estriol in postmenopausal women with recurrent urinary tract infections. *New Engl J Med* 1993;329:753–6
66. Cardozo LD, Benness CJ, Abbott D. Oestriol in the management of recurrent urinary tract infections in elderly women. *Br J Obstet Gynaecol* 1998; in press

6
Sexuality and the menopause

A. Graziottin

'No one dies from old skin, but maybe the soul does'.
A. M. Kligman, 1979[1]

INTRODUCTION

Human sexuality is a complex realm. It has strong biological roots, which determine and modulate the quality of body experience and its mental representation, through hormones and neurotransmitters[2–4]. Physical pleasure and pain are perceived within the body, through its sensory receptors, and depict the sensual scenario where affective and loving experiences, colored by mood swings, constitute a personal history over time[5,6]. Because every individual possesses a body, the body itself provides a common symbolic frame of reference in human thought[7]. This is particularly true in human sexuality, which may express the best of human emotions, desires, needs, loving perfumes and bonds, and the heights of psychic expression through words, memories, fantasies and phantasms, and even nostalgic and passionate poems, either written or designed in the skin or in the soul. Sensory experiences and biological facts blend with motivational-affective and -cognitive dynamics in the individual sexual experience[2–6]. This is all the more true around and after the menopause, when dramatic hormonal losses may threaten feminine identity, and female and couple sexuality, causing negative changes in libido, arousal and orgasm, worsening pelvic floor status and leading to dyspareunia, secondary vaginism, postcoital cystitis, vaginal hypoesthesia and finally, to sexual avoidance in many unfortunate women[2,4,5]. This dismissed, under-researched and undertreated aspect of female quality of life raises a provocative question: is female sexuality a medical issue or not? And is it more so in the menopause?

DIAGNOSTIC AND THERAPEUTIC BIASES

Unfortunately, sexology nowadays still shows the dichotomy that has affected neurology since the end of the 19th century, between 'psychology without body and medicine without soul'[8]. The majority of sexologists have psychological or humanistic training, and care more for psychodynamic implications of sexuality, too often dismissing the biological reality of the body. Doctors look at the body as an object, in a growing reification process, and too often forget the soul and the emotions, the psychic side that transforms a disease into an illness[9,10]. This is even more dramatic in the field of human female sexuality, because of persisting research and teaching biases that still pervade most of the academic world, with a few exceptions[4]. When a man complains of having a sexual problem, he undergoes a thorough clinical and instrumental evaluation, first of all from the medical point of view. The uro-andrologist is the doctor of choice. If a woman has a sexual problem, she is considered to have 'psychological' or relational problems. The gynecologist, who should be the doctor of choice to diagnose potential biological factors that may contribute to sexual problems, usually has no training at all in female clinical sexology.

THE 'BLIND' GYNECOLOGIST

Gynecologists, therefore, face a new challenge: to meet female expectations of a doctor willing to cure and care, even in the complex field of sexuality. No other physician has full clinical competence in respect of the genital area, the pelvic floor and the neuroendocrine changes involved in female sexuality as the gynecologist. No other doctor accompanies the female patient along such a lifelong path, full of so many emotionally and sexually significant events, as the gynecologist. Yet the majority of colleagues look at female physiology and pathology only from the strictly reproductive and/or 'physical' point of view, apparently totally unaware of the sexual function it implies, somehow affected by a selective, perception 'blindness'. They may be even more unaware of the many changes that illnesses or transitional periods, such as adolescence or menopause, may cause, starting from a biological aspect to involve a spectrum of psychodynamic and sexual consequences. They may also be unaware of the communicative difficulties of many elderly patients. These women feel ashamed and embarrassed to openly talk about sexual issues; they often do not even have the appropriate words and, therefore, need to be helped to ask and to be properly cured.

It is mandatory, therefore, for doctors who care, to open a new window in daily practice: to improve the ability to listen to sexual questions, to understand sexual implications of a clinical picture, to communicate openly on this issue, to be able to make a clinically competent diagnosis of the biological basis of a sexual problem and to suggest the best therapy. In the case of a menopausal patient, this window has three potential clinical scenarios: female sexual identity, female sexual function and couple relationship (Table 1). The biological aspects of these will now be discussed in turn, with a view to the psychosexual implications.

Table 1 Sexual changes during 'natural' menopausal transition

Female sexual identity
Involution of secondary sex characteristics, breast and genitals
Aging of sensory organs, more so for smell, taste and touch
Self-image crisis, secondary to the involution of:
  skin, hair and nails
  sweat and sebaceous glands, with loss of 'scent of woman'
  mucosae, with eye, mouth and vaginal dryness
Proprioceptive changes
Changes in mental perception of femininity

Female sexual function
Changes in libido, usually loss
Arousal difficulties
  mental
  non-genital peripheral
  genital
Orgasmic difficulties
After-sex (usually disappointing) memories

Couple relationship
Fading of biological sexual bonds (?)
Interfering male problems
  independent health and sexual problems
  real desirability of partner

FEMALE SEXUAL IDENTITY DURING MENOPAUSAL TRANSITION

'What is beautiful is good': the all-pervading force of this stereotype is real and increasing[11]. It is no longer limited to youth, and to the Greek ideal *kalòs kai agathòs*, but it is becoming mandatory for all ages. Women who face the menopausal transition in the western world, at the end of this millennium, have to (or feel they should) meet increasing expectations relating to the esthetic and cosmetic quality of their aging, an evergreen sexuality and a quality of relationship that should somehow maintain the rainbow of passion and enthusiasm of youth[12].

The media must take much of the responsibility for this shift in expectations from the realm of 'simple' health and well-being to the dreamy and delusional world of 'forever happiness'. Women adhere to this rainbow of hope for the future with different attitudes, related to personal family history, education, profession, income, family life and satisfaction, love and love affairs, quality of premenopausal sexual identity, sexual function and couple relationship, in addition to current health status and availability of properly suited hormonal replacement therapy (HRT)[2,5,13–16].

Women need to be helped in the complex task of facing a potential sexual identity crisis during the menopausal transition by a sensitive gynecologist who understands the importance of a persistently satisfying sexual identity and who does not dismiss as trivial female concerns about wrinkles, body weight gain or fear of aging. Tuning into these expectations may improve the quality of the doctor–patient relationship and increase compliance to HRT[16]. Well-suited HRT therapies, both systemic and/or local, represent the very first competent clinical answer to the desire to feel 'feminine forever'.

Biological and anagraphic age

Psychosexual attitudes to the menopausal transition are further complicated by a 'new' fact in the human life cycle: the increasing gap between anagraphic and biological age, a gap that can reach 15 years. Owing to an improvement in the general quality of life, attention to nutrients and quality of food intake, regular physical training, access to qualified medical care and diffusion of preventive health programs, men and women in good health look and feel usually younger than they are, and expect a quality of life adjusted to their inner emotional and energetic age, rather than to their anagraphic age. 'Health' is only a prerequisite for the new gold standard in aging, that is *joie de vivre*. Sexuality, the combination of good sexual identity, sexual function and love relationship, is the foremost area in which physical and emotional dimensions may blend to give a unique pleasure of living that women are increasingly reluctant to give up[12].

The intensity of the link between the body image of persistent feminine beauty and the inner self-perception in aging is amazing and still underevaluated. It has specifically been shown that physically attractive elderly women perceive themselves to be healthier, to have a greater feeling of well-being and a more positive outlook on life, and to be more cheerful, less depressed and definitely better adjusted[17]. This link suggests that there should probably be a change in the perspective and politics of women's education to the benefits of HRT. If a good inner self-perception is so potent from the psychoneuroendocrine point of view, then attention to this aspect of physical and mental health should no longer be overlooked[16].

Changes in the mirror

Femininity relates to the physical appearance of the body, with its primary and secondary sex characteristics, the emotional inner representation of it, mixed with stereotyped 'feminine' personality traits, and feedback messages from the environment. Menopause, with the underlying estrogen, progesterone and androgen deprivation, may threaten femininity perception on a multiple basis, where biological and emotional factors are strictly intertwined:

(1) The involution of secondary sex characteristics: breast and genital aging are perceived as a major threat of femininity, leading to reduced self-esteem, reduced self-confidence and reduced assertiveness. The vulnerability to this physical and symbolic wound is maximal in women who used to rely on physical beauty and seductiveness for their emotional equilibrium;

(2) Skin aging: the 'wear and tear' of the 'skin dress', maximum in thin women, may be perceived as a second major insult for feminine sexual identity, after the involution of secondary sex characteristics. Skin aging may appear through various objective alterations:

 (a) Elastosis: wrinkles, lax skin, lentigo, teleangectasiae, actinic keratosis;

 (b) Dry hypoelastic skin and pruritus;

 (c) Hair changes: graying of hair, hirsutism, alopecia, loss of pubic hair;

 (d) Nail changes: brittle nail and onychomycosis;

(e) Benign growths: skin tags, seborrheic keratosis, sebaceous hyperplasia, cherry angiomas;

(f) Miscellaneous conditions, such as acne rosacea and malignancies[11].

Many women confess to the listening gynecologist how they feel hurt by the dramatic aging of the skin, that seems to kill the soul of femininity, in the very first years after the menopause, unless they are treated with HRT. They perhaps feel deprived of sexual attraction because of the loss or whitening of the pubic hair, which they try to mask with tattoos or coloring; and perhaps they are thinking about additive mammoplasty to regain a magnificent breast, or about a facial lifting to minimize the wrinkles and aging. The flourishing industry of cosmetic and plastic surgery reveals how the 'identity' issue linked to physical appearance is strong and potent[1,17]. It could be said that these are not medical issues; but it is medical to contribute to the quality of life by medical prescriptions, i.e. suggesting HRT to sweeten the impact of aging and to give pertinent medical and non-medical advice to improve body self-perception and help the woman to accept unavoidable physical changes better. Moreover, some 'minor' signs, such as the loss of pubic hair, could be precious in recognizing a subgroup of women that could need a different kind of HRT. According to Sands and Studd[15], this loss could be a sign of 'female androgen deficiency syndrome' (FADS), a cluster of symptoms, including decrease of libido, diminished muscle mass and reduced vital energy, that could be significantly improved with androgen replacement therapy (ART).

Changes in sensory self-perception

Sensory organs are well-known windows for environmental sexual stimuli and the mental buildup of a person's self-perception and body image. Owing to their neuroectodermic origin, they are sensitive to sex steroids and may be considered as sexual targets and sexual determinants of libido[2]. Loss of estrogens may contribute to:

(1) Involution of skin sebaceous and sweat glands, with loss of the 'scent of woman' so typical of the fertile age and so important for the erotic cloud of pheromones that subtly surrounds the body, contributing to personal and the partner's libido, and 'smell identity' so important in the deep 'recognizing' of loved ones'[2];

(2) Mucosal involution, with its cohort of:

(a) Eye dryness, which may cause various ophthalmic complaints in 35% of postmenopausal women not on HRT[18];

(b) Mouth dryness, with tooth[19] and taste involution, that may reduce pleasure in kisses and oral intimacy, a totally understudied area to the present author's knowledge;

(c) Vaginal dryness with secondary arousal difficulties, dyspareunia, and even secondary vaginism and postcoital cystitis which may ultimately lead to a secondary loss of libido and/or frank sexual aversion[2,4,12,15,16];

(3) General involution of the sensory organs, partly dependent on estrogen deprivation[1,2,11,17–20], in addition to aging. This change is stronger for the involution of the olfactory epithelium, which is a perfect example of hormone-dependent neuroplasticity[20]. Its function is a key contributor to libido through the role of smell and perfumes in rhinencephalic and limbic circuits linked to sexual drive[2,20];

(4) Proprioceptive changes: self-perception is also dependent on the muscle tone and the proprioceptive information conveyed to the brain, contributing to the so-called 'sixth sense'[8]. Aging is characterized by a decrease in muscle mass, strength and flexibility. This process may be acutely worsened in women suffering from FADS[15]. Androgen replacement therapy, combined with physical training, may contribute to an

improvement in general well-being, better self-perception and self-esteem, body perception, assertiveness and, last but not least, libido[16].

Changes in mental self-perception

Femininity is not only dependent on body image, it is also built up through the emotional rethinking of the physical experience, through memories, nostalgia, dreams, love, fantasies, mood modulation of self-perception and feedback messages from others. Estrogens are specifically involved in the modulation of the affective view the woman has of herself and the surrounding world, as well as in affective disorders[2,3,12–16,21]. All these physical events depend on the optimal function of neurons. Psychoplasticity, a key sign of psychological well-being and health, requires neuroplasticity[22]. In women, estrogens prime the central nervous system, acting as neurotrophic and psychotrophic factors during female life[3,22]. Androgens thrill libido[2,15,21] and improve the quality of sexual motivation and mental arousal as well as the quality of clitoral and cavernosal response, which leads to an overall better sexual function. (The interplay between androgens and female sexuality is discussed in detail in Chapter 00.)

Physical femininity has a prerequisite of a well-balanced hormonal status. Nevertheless, feminine self-perception is strongly context-dependent. Vulnerability to sexual identity crisis during the menopausal transition may be further modulated by psychosocial factors[2,13–16,23–25].

CLINICAL IMPLICATIONS

Quality of skin and mucosal and sensory aging are informative windows on how the woman is facing the menopausal transition, from both the endocrine and the non-endocrine points of view. A badly aging body suggests to the gynecologist that he/she should:

(1) Look for other signs of hormone deprivation;

(2) Analyze the quality of food intake and possibly recommend nutritional improvement and integration with calcium, vitamins A, D, C and E and selenium, especially in the 'old-old' patient, in addition to prescribing a proper HRT (including ART in selected cases)[15];

(3) Recommend limited sun exposure to prevent photoaging[11], and increased physical fitness to improve the general trophism of the body, a stronger muscle tone and a higher mental tone, which all contribute to the physical perception of health, well-being and beauty[17];

(4) Actively ask about the quality of sexuality and the presence of arousal difficulties, vaginal dryness, coital pain or postcoital cystitis[2,26], secondary to vaginal and pelvic floor involution. In these cases, in addition to prescribing at least topical HRT and lubricants, he/she should look for the presence of a secondary vaginism and teach the woman how to actively relax the pubococcygeous muscle, to prevent sexual pain and a self-maintained worsening of the problem[26].

Attention to the quality of skin and body aging, and to the deterioration of the 'skin dress', is also an important factor in building a sensitive doctor–patient relationship and improving the quality of compliance to HRT[16]. 'If he/she cares about my skin, my body weight and the way I look and feel, he/she really understands what I am more afraid of in aging and really cares about me'[17].

Sometimes, the perceived, hurtful deterioration of personal beauty and attractiveness is reported to the listening doctor through the mirror of others' eyes: 'After the menopause I became invisible', or 'No man perceives me as a woman any more'. These concise expressions of a major sexual identity crisis, therefore, could appropriately be softened if an integrated management of the menopause is carried out[12].

The 'caring' gynecologist is expected to relate to the woman as a person who is facing an acute crisis in the long-lasting process of aging, and not simply to a 'prolapsed uterus', an 'osteoporotic skeleton' or an 'aging heart'.

In summary, attention to coherence of female sexual identity through the menopausal transition is a prerequisite for good sexual function in a growing number of women of the western world. The woman who is physically and emotionally satisfied with herself is more willing to accept courting and loving and more able to sweetly adjust to the changes that aging brings[2,12,17,25]. The relationship between sexual identity crisis during the menopause and sexual function disturbances deserves further investigation to better define their interplay, the prevalence of the two problems in the general female aging population and the identification of subgroups of women that may need different HRT and clinical approaches.

FEMALE SEXUAL FUNCTION

A growing consensus exists on the potential negative effect of the menopause on female sexual function[2,4,5,15,16,23–25,27–30]. Controversy exists regarding the prevalence of female sexual dysfunction during the menopausal transition and the specific role of hormonal loss, as many other psychosocial factors seem to have a causal and confounding role[23,24,27–29,31–33]. Methodological biases seem to be the major cause for the conflicting results[34].

In daily practice, the most frequent biologically rooted complaints that the gynecologist is required to diagnose and treat are:

(1) Loss of libido (Figure 1): Graziottin[2] discussed extensively elsewhere the biological roots of libido. Estrogens seem to have an *indirect* effect on libido, through their positive action on secondary sex characteristics, female sexual identity and self-perception, genital and pelvic floor trophism, physical quality of arousal and general well-being[3,4,5,12,16,17,21,22,27,35,36]. Androgens have a *direct* effect, as they specifically increase sexual motivation. In postmenopausal women, ART seems to be the best biological answer[3,12,15,16,28–30] when non-sexual hormones are within the normal range, when there are no other physical factors that may cause a secondary loss of sex drive and when this loss is general and not limited to the usual partner. In the latter case, lack of sex drive could be secondary to a 'perceptive wear and tear' of the couple-specific sexual attraction, which is not hormone-responsive.

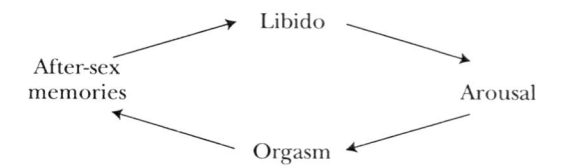

Figure 1 Cybernetic model of sexual function. This model, formulated by the present author, contributes to immediate comprehension of potential negative or positive feedback mechanisms operating in sexual function. Good libido easily leads to full mental, non-genital peripheral and peripheral arousal, facilitating orgasm. After-sex memories, full of vibrant emotions and physical satisfaction, light up libido again, with strong positive feedback. Conversely, weak libido leads to arousal difficulties, inadequate preparation of 'orgasmic platform' and overall delusional experience. After-sex negative thoughts and memories may further inhibit libido, with gradual block of the entire cascade of mental and neurochemical events. It is also clear that any negative event in any part of the circuit, i.e. dyspareunia secondary to arousal difficulties, may create negative feedback ending in definite loss of libido, which could be the very first complaint in clinical consultation. The clinician, therefore, should be alerted to potential problems in any critical component of sexual function, to make appropriate differential diagnosis and suggest best medical and psychosexual therapy

(2) Arousal difficulties: they may be central, non-genital peripheral and genital:

(a) Biological central difficulties may be secondary to estrogen and androgen loss, but they may be further worsened by depression, anxiety, chronic stress and insomnia[2], which may also be biologically rooted and worsened by estrogen deprivation. Reduced frequency of erotic dreams, of fantasies, of sexual day-dreams and of spontaneous mental arousal are the clinical consequences of central arousal difficulties.

(b) Problems in non-genital peripheral arousal may be better exemplified by 'touch-impaired' disorders. According to Sarrel and Whitehead[27], 35.71% of patients of their series described a change in touch perception suggestive of peripheral neuropathy that may lead to avoidance of skin contact during foreplay, so interfering with sexual arousal. Two usually underevaluated sites of touch-impaired disorders are nipple (personal unpublished data) and clitoris. Loss of clitoral feeling ('My clitoris is dead') was reported in 20.21% of the Sarrel and Whitehead series. In the present author's experience, systemic ART, in physiological doses, improves both nipple and clitoral responsiveness. At supraphysiological doses, it may cause nipple hypersensitivity and clitoral congestion to the extent of priapism, secondary to the androgenic effect on clitoral cavernosal bodies.

(c) As far as genital arousal is concerned, Levin[4] hypothesized that estrogens could be the 'permitting' factor for the action of vaso-intestinal peptide (VIP), the most important neurotransmitter that 'translates' sexual drive in vaginal lubrication. Without estrogen, vaginal dryness and dyspareunia are complained of by 35–50% of postmenopausal women[12,24,26,27]. In addition to estrogens, function itself, that is to have regular and continued sexual activity, has been found to protect against vaginal dryness[37]. Unfortunately, the body weight of women not on HRT having a regular sexual activity in postmenopause was not reported. To improve arousal, HRT is critical for thin postmenopausal women who cannot rely on extragonadal estrogen sources, as fatty women can, for pelvic floor trophism and vaginal vessel responsiveness. A second biological cause of arousal difficulties is vaginism, either primary or, more frequently, secondary to vaginal dryness and dyspareunia with secondary defensive spasm of the pubococcygeous muscle[26]. Vaginism may account for half the cases of postmenopausal dyspareunia[27]. Thorough examination of pelvic floor and perineal muscles should become part of routine gynecological examination, as well as care to teach the patient an adequate retraining to normalize the muscle elasticity and tonus and improve sexual responsiveness. The third most frequent cause of genital arousal difficulties is urinary incontinence. Women suffering from stress or urge incontinence secondary to detrusorial instability may suffer from occasional loss of urine during sex, and may become inhibited for fear that it might recur. Appropriate diagnosis and treatment of incontinence may contribute to a renewed self-confidence[27,38].

(3) Orgasmic difficulties: they may be the endpoint of a number of biological, as well as motivational-affective and -cognitive factors[2,5,27]. From the biological point of view, the diagnostic flow chart should look for loss of sexual hormones, with secondary libido and arousal problems, vaginal and vulvar trophism (including the clitoris) and pelvic floor status (see Table 2). Hypertonic conditions may cause dyspareunia, vaginism and postcoital cystitis[26], thus impairing the formation of the so-called 'orgasmic platform'[5] through the negative association of fear, anxiety and pain[26]. Hypotonic conditions, leading to vaginal hypoesthesia, also deserve a rehabilitative approach with Kegel exercises[5,39,40].

(4) Postcoital or postorgasmic memories: this exquisitely human phase may explain the positive or negative feedback mechanisms that modulate the circuit of sexual function. Negative feelings may restrict the sexual circuit, when pain or disappointment are the final feeling after sex. A simple question, 'How do you feel after sex?', may highlight where the problems are and indicate

Table 2 Semeiology of pelvic floor: tonus of pubococcygeous muscle and associated signs and symptoms

Hypertonus	Hypotonus
Postcoital cystitis	stress incontinence
Urethral syndrome	vaginal hypoesthesia
Vestibulitis	vaginal anesthesia
Dyspareunia	anorgasmia
Vaginismus	fecal incontinence
Stipsis	
Hemorrhoids	

whether they originate in the individual or in the couple relationship.

THE COUPLE RELATIONSHIP

Biological modifications, secondary to hormonal loss as well as to aging, may have a deep impact on the bases of physical attraction and affective bonding[2,3,5]. Male independent sexual problems may also affect the possibility of a satisfying perimenopausal sexuality. Last, but not least, the *real* desirability of an aging partner (taking into account such factors as being overweight, lack of attention to good hygiene, self-care and cure, the quality of courting and foreplay, general health and specific sexual problems, or lack of intimacy)[2] may further contribute to this fading of sexual life that worsens over the years. On the other hand, a new partner may contribute to an increase of libido, satisfaction and orgasm in the postmenopausal woman, which may be even better if the woman is given full biological equilibrium on account of HRT.

CONCLUSION

Sex hormones contribute to biological femininity, to the basic biology of sexual function and to biological signals, leading to the sexual attraction and affective bonding that run back and forth in the couple relationship.

Their action in these three key dimensions of human female sexuality are strongly context-dependent. This complex interaction may explain the objective methodological difficulties in asserting the relative importance of hormonal changes on psychosexual variations during and after the menopausal transition.

This difficulty is further worsened by the many biases that still persist in traditional academic social factors that interact in human sexuality and, specifically, in female sexual identity and function.

Patients who raise sexual issues are more often than not sent to the psychologist or sexologist. This is a most deplorable practice. The majority of problems related to female sexuality during the menopausal transition are biologically rooted and need a thorough clinical medical investigation and medical treatment, including a properly suited HRT, either systemic or local, before asking for psychosexual help.

Gynecologists should improve their skill in diagnosing and treating the biological aspects of the most common female sexual symptoms: loss of libido, arousal disorders, dyspareunia and anorgasmia. The best results will be obtained in sharing a 'twin competence' with a good psychosexologist, to whom patients with clear psychodynamic or relational problems should be referred for specific help, after having excluded or cured the potential biological roots of these problems.

References

1. Kligman AM. Perspectives and problems in cutaneous gerontology. *J Invest Dermatol* 1979;73: 39–46

2. Graziottin A. Libido. In Studd J, ed. *The Yearbook of the Royal College of Obstetricians and Gynaecologists.* London: RCOG Press, 1996:235–43

3. Pfaus JG, Everitt BJ. The psychopharmacology of sexual behavior. In Bloom FE, Kupfer DJ, eds. *Psychopharmacology, the Fourth Generation of Progress*. New York: Raven Press, 1995:743–58
4. Levin RJ. The mechanisms of human female sexual arousal. *Ann Rev Sex Res* 1992;3:1–48
5. Masters WH, Johnson VE, Kolodny RC. *Heterosexuality*. Glasgow: Harper Collins, 1994
6. Foucault M. *L'Usage des Plaisirs. L'Histoire de la Sexualité*, Vol. II. Paris: Gallimard, 1984
7. Douglas M. *Purity and Danger: an Analysis of Concepts of Pollution and Taboo*. Harmondsworth, UK: Penguin Books, 1970
8. Sachs O. *The Man Who Mistook his Wife for a Hat*. Milano: Adelphi, 1986 (in Italian)
9. Cassell EJ. *The Nature of Suffering and the Goals of Medicine*. New York: Oxford University Press, 1991
10. Lewis Wall L. After office hours: ritual meaning in surgery. *Obstet Gynecol* 1996;88:633–7
11. Coté J. Skin care and abnormal lesions. In Lorrain J, ed. *Comprehensive Management of Menopause, Part IV. Other Problems*. New York: Springer Verlag, 1994:351–7
12. Graziottin A. Menopausa e sessualità. In Marandola P, ed. *Andrologia e Sessuologia Clinica*. Pavia: La Goliardica, 1995:255–60
13. Raush JL. Psychobiological aspects of the menopause. In Lorrain J, ed. *Comprehensive Management of Menopause. Part IV. Other Problems*. New York: Springer Verlag, 1994:318–26
14. O'Leary Cobb J. Where the women are. In Lorrain J, ed. *Comprehensive Management of Menopause, Part IV. Other Problems*. New York: Springer Verlag, 1994:52–8
15. Sands R, Studd J. Exogenous androgens in postmenopausal women. *Am J Med* 1995; 98:76S–9S
16. Graziottin A. Risk reduction strategies. In Paoletti R, Crosignani PG, Kenemens P, Samsioe G, Soma M, Jackson AS, eds. *Women's Health and Menopause*. Amsterdam: Kluwer Academic, 1997:263–74
17. Kligman AM, Graham JA. The psychology of appearance in the elderly. In Kligman AM, ed. *Dermatology Clinics. The Aging Skin*, vol. 4. Philadelphia: W.B. Saunders, 1986:501–7
18. Metka M, Enzelsberger H, Knogler W, *et al.* Ophthalmic complaints as a climacteric symptom. *Maturitas* 1991;14:3–8
19. Grodstein F, Colditz GA, Stampfer MJ. Postmenopausal hormone use and tooth loss: a prospective study. *J Am Dent Assoc* 1996;127:370–7
20. Arimondi C, Vannelli GB, Balboni GC. Importance of olfaction in sexual life: morphofunctional and psychological studies in man. *Biomed Res (India)* 1993;4:43–52
21. Appleby L, Montgomery J, Studd J. Oestrogens and affective disorders. In Studd J, ed. *Progress in Obstetrics and Gynecology*, Vol. 9. Edinburgh: Churchill Livingstone, 1991:289–302
22. Birge SJ. The role of estrogen deficiency in the aging of the central nervous system. In Lobo RA, ed. *Treatment of Post-Menopausal Women: Basic and Clinical Aspects*. New York: Raven Press, 1994: 153–7
23. Dennerstein L, Smith AMA, Morse CA, *et al.* Sexuality and the menopause. *J Psychosom Obstet Gynecol* 1994;15:59–66
24. Channon LD, Ballinger SE. Some aspects of sexuality and vaginal symptoms during menopause and their relation to anxiety and depression. *Br J Med Psychol* 1986;59:173–80
25. Baldaro Verde J, Graziottin A. Ristrutturazione dell'identità femminile in menopausa negli anni novanta. In Bottiglioni F, de Aloysio D, eds. *Il Climaterio Femminile: Esperienze Italiane di un Decennio*. Bologna: Monduzzi Editore, 1988: 723–8
26. Graziottin A, Vaginismo. In Marandol P, ed. *Andrologia e Sessuologia Clinica*. Pavia: La Goliardica, 1995:247–54
27. Sarrel PM, Whitehead MI. Sex and menopause: defining the issues. *Maturitas* 1985;7:217–24
28. Davis SR, McCloud P, Strauss BJG, *et al.* Testosterone enhances estradiol's effects on postmenopausal bone density and sexuality. *Maturitas* 1995;21:227–36
29. Frock J, Money J. Sexuality and menopause. *Psychother Psychosom* 1992;57:29–33
30. Floter A, Nathorst-Boos J, Carlstrom K, *et al.* Androgen status and sexual life in perimenopausal women. *Menopause* 1997;4:95–100
31. Koster A, Garde K. Sexual desire and menopausal development. A prospective study of Danish women born in 1936. *Maturitas* 1993;16: 49–60
32. Laan E, van Lunsen RHK. Hormones and sexuality in postmenopausal women: a psychophysiological study. *J Psychosom Obstet Gynecol* 1998; in press
33. Kirchengast S, Hartmann B, Gruber D, *et al.* Decreased sexual interest and its relationship to body build in postmenopausal women. *Maturitas* 1996;23:63–71
34. Myers LS. Methodological review and meta-analysis of sexuality and menopause research. *Neurosci Biobehav Rev* 1995;19:331–41
35. Dennerstein L. Well-being, symptoms and menopausal transition. *Maturitas* 1996;23: 147–57
36. Bachmann GA. Influence of menopause on sexuality. *Int J Fertil Menopause Stud* 1995;40: 16–22
37. Pearce MJ, Hawton K. Psychological and sexual aspects of the menopause and HRT. *Baillières Clin Obstet Gynaecol* 1996; 10:385–99

38. Graziottin A. Aspetti psicologici e sessuali dell'incontinenza urinaria e delle alterazione della statica pelvica. In Minini GF, ed. *Icontinenza Urinaria Femminile e Prolasso Genitale: Dalla Diagnosi alla Terapia*. Brescia: Edizioni Clas International, 1991:27–31

39. Kegel AH. Sexual functions of the pubococcygeous muscles. *West J Surg Obstet Gynecol* 1952;60:521–4

40. Bourcier A. *Le Plancher Pelvien*. Paris: Vigot, 1989

7
Arthritis, estrogens and menopause

F. M. Cicuttini and T. D. Spector

INTRODUCTION

This review presents recent developments in the understanding of the roles of menopause, hormone replacement therapy (HRT) and hormonal factors on arthritis, focusing on the specific conditions osteoarthritis, rheumatoid arthritis, systemic lupus erythematosus and carpal tunnel syndrome. Joint symptoms are one of the principal components of the climacteric[1], with up to 50% of women experiencing climacteric symptoms complaining of joint symptoms[2]. These are often non-specific or common problems such as back pain or musculoskeletal pain syndromes such as fibromyalgia, which are associated with depression.

EPIDEMIOLOGICAL EVIDENCE FOR ASSOCIATION BETWEEN HORMONAL FACTORS AND OSTEOARTHRITIS

Osteoarthritis (OA) is a group of clinically heterogeneous disorders unified by the pathological features of hyaline cartilage loss and subchondral bone reaction. In women, OA more commonly affects multiple joints and is usually more severe than in men, affecting nearly one in three women to some extent[3]. The apparent prominence of women presenting with polyarticular symptoms in middle age has fueled speculation that there may be some relationship between the onset of OA and the menopause[4].

Kellgren and Moore described a form of 'menopausal arthritis' in a group of women with Heberden's nodes, characterized by a rapid onset of symptoms and multiple joint involvement (hands, spine and knees), and renamed the condition 'primary generalized osteoarthritis'[5]. In the population surveys of Lawrence, X-ray evidence of nodal generalized OA was three times higher in women than men in the age range 45–64 years[3]. Other hospital-based studies have shown a female/male ratio as high as 10:1, with a marked peak of age of onset at 50 years in women for nodal generalized OA[6]. Some[7], but not all[8] studies have shown that women who had a previous hysterectomy were found to have significantly higher rates of clinical signs of knee OA and first carpometacarpal OA than control women without hysterectomy[7], further supporting hormonal differences.

The trigger for the appearance of OA in middle age is unknown, but it is suggested that it may be the interaction of gynecological or hormonal factors. Whether these act in all cases of OA or are restricted to the so-called subtypes of OA ('menopausal OA' or 'generalized OA') is unclear.

Hormonal factors and osteoarthritis

The possible link between estrogens and OA has come from the suggestion that excess or unopposed estrogens might predispose cartilage and bone to OA. Estrogen receptors have been found on articular chondrocytes[6] and estrogen has been known to adversely affect several different animal models of OA[9]. Similarly, the antiestrogen drug, tamoxifen, has been reported to be beneficial in these same animal models[10]. Changes in estrogens perimenopausally may occur in a variety of ways. Whether it is the high unopposed estrogen levels *per se* or the increase in the estrogen/progesterone ratio which occurs leading up to the menopause that is responsible is not known. It certainly appears that estrogens may have a role in triggering the initial changes in proteoglycan in cartilage, either directly or via altering receptor sensitivity.

Endogenous sex steroid levels in women with generalized osteoarthritis

One might expect to find altered hormone levels in OA-affected women perimenopausally. A few small studies have examined urinary and serum sex-hormone levels in OA-affected women with inconsistent results[11,12]. Middle-aged women with generalized OA have been shown to have lower circulating sex hormone-binding globulin levels, implying that higher circulating free estrogens and androgens are present, suggesting a role in the etiopathogenesis of generalized OA[13]. In contrast, no association between endogenous hormone levels and severity of hand OA was observed when the age- and obesity-adjusted sex hormone concentrations were compared to the worst radiographic score of OA[12]. In a further study, there were no trends in the sex hormone concentrations, age at menarche or menopause, oral contraceptive use or hormone replacement use with increasing severity of hand OA in a case–control postal survey[14].

Other supportive evidence for a role for hormonal factors in osteoarthritis

Hormonal factors might explain why women, but not men, with OA have less osteoporosis and greater bone density than controls[15]. The protective effects of estrogens on osteoporosis are well known; similarly, osteoporosis and, therefore, oestrogen lack appear to be protective against OA[16].

In one study, significantly increased frequency of hysterectomy and menstrual problems was shown in women with OA compared to those with rheumatoid arthritis and population controls[17]. These results suggest that, although OA undoubtedly has a multifactorial etiology, an underlying hormonal imbalance of estrogen may be responsible for both the gynecological problems and the appearance several years later of OA in middle-aged women.

One common link between menstrual abnormalities and OA may be obesity. Overall, results to date suggest that the link between obesity and OA is more consistent in women and is strongest in OA of the knees and less conclusive in other joints[18]. Obesity in women is a known cause of hyperestrogenism and menorrhagia, and it is possible that obese women are more susceptible to both problems through this hormonal imbalance. It appears to be related to excess body weight rather than muscle bulk. Obesity in women is a known cause of hyperestrogenism via the peripheral formation of estrogen from androstenedione in the fat tissues. After the menopause, this route becomes the principal source of estrogens. Thus, the association between OA and obesity also suggests a role of endocrine influences in the development of OA.

Hormone replacement therapy and osteoarthritis

Several studies have observed a lower than expected risk of knee and hip OA in women on hormone replacement therapy (HRT)[14,19,20]. A meta-analysis of four prevalence studies which used a combined endpoint of knee and hip OA showed a pooled odds ratio of 0.76 (95% confidence interval, CI 0.63–0.91)[21]. In an 8-year follow-up study of current users of HRT in the Framingham study, the adjusted odds ratio for incident or progressive disease was 0.3 (95% CI 0.1–1.2, $p = 0.07$)[22]. The association between estrogen replacement therapy and incident symptomatic osteoarthritis was examined using a nested case–control design[23]. After controlling for obesity and healthcare utilization, past use of HRT was inversely associated with the risk of osteoarthritis (adjusted odds ratio 0.7; 95% CI 0.3–1.9).

A cross-sectional study of 4366 postmenopausal women examined whether postmenopausal estrogen replacement therapy is associated with a reduced risk of radiographic osteoarthritis of the hip[20]. Women who were currently using oral estrogen had a significantly reduced risk of any OA of the hip (adjusted odds ratio, OR 0.62; 95% CI 0.49–0.86) and moderate-to-severe manifestation of disease (OR 0.54; 95% CI 0.33–0.88). Current users who had taken estrogen for 10 years or longer had a greater reduction in the risk of OA of the hip (OR 0.57; 95% CI 0.40–0.82) compared with that of users for less than 10 years (OR 0.75; 95% CI 0.47–1.24). This supports a role for estrogen replacement therapy in postmenopausal women to protect against OA of the hip. Results from a cross-sectional study of 1003 women also showed an inverse association between HRT use and radiological OA of the knee[24]. The effect in the hand joints was weaker.

Despite attempting to adjust for confounders, women who use and remain on HRT are not the same as women who do not. For example, HRT is often used to protect against osteoporosis. There is some evidence for an inverse relationship between osteoporosis and osteoarthritis. Despite some studies attempting to adjust for such differences, residual confounding may remain. Randomized controlled trials are lacking in this area and will provide the strongest evidence, but the thought that HRT can modify such a common disease is exciting.

RHEUMATOID ARTHRITIS

Rheumatoid arthritis (RA) is a multifactorial disease with a prevalence of about 1% in which both environmental and genetic factors play a role. A role for sex hormones is suggested by a number of features of this disease[25]. Rheumatoid arthritis is characterized by striking age–sex disparities. In a population of 564 patients with RA, the onset of symptoms was studied in relation to age, sex and last menstrual period for women[26]. The median age of first symptoms was 45 years in women and 50 in men. The individual interval between menopause and first symptoms had a Gaussian distribution with mean at time 0, indicating that the average woman developed the first symptoms at the time of her menopause. The female/male (F/M) ratio of all patients was 2.3:1; with increasing age, the F/M ratio decreased from 3.7:1 before 30 years of age to 1 after the sixth decade of life, with a peak at the age of 40–44 years. These observations have suggested a possible effect of age-related changes in sex hormone levels on the pathogenesis of RA

Age at menopause and rheumatoid arthritis

A number of large studies have shown no association between ages at menarche and menopause in the development of RA[27,28]. Risk factors for RA were examined in a cohort of 121 700 female nurses aged 30–55, followed in the Nurses' Health Study. During 883 187 person-years of follow-up, 217 new cases of RA were identified. There were no significant associations between parity, age at birth of the first child, menopause or obesity, and the incidence of RA[28].

Sex hormones and rheumatoid arthritis

The association between sex hormones and rheumatoid arthritis has been examined in a number of studies. In one study, the concentrations of sex hormones were studied in 45 women with RA, 26 of whom were premenopausal and 19 of whom were postmenopausal. The two groups were compared with 40 control women (20 premenopausal and 20 postmenopausal). The average plasma concentrations of estradiol, progesterone and androgens were comparable in the premenopausal women with RA and the control group of premenopausal women. On the other hand, the plasma concentration of androgens was higher in the postmenopausal women with RA compared to the postmenopausal controls[29]. These data have suggested a role for androgens in this disease.

Dehydroepiandrosterone (DHEA), an adrenal product, is the major androgen in women. Its production is strikingly dependent upon age. Peak production is in the second and third decades, but levels decline precipitously thereafter. Levels of DHEA are low in both men and women with RA[30,31]. Recent data have suggested that levels of this hormone may be depressed before the onset of disease. The role of DHEA in immune diseases, however, remains controversial. It is unclear whether the low levels of DHEAs in RA are a consequence of chronic illness or immune dysfunction, or a defect of adrenal androgen synthesis[30]. In one recent study of 68 patients with RA, the level of DHEAs inversely correlated with disease duration, a radiographic grading score, the Health Assessment Questionnaire score, duration of morning stiffness, and a clinical score of disease activity and severity (the Spread/Severity index). The lack of correlation between disease activity and DHEA levels gives support to the hypothesis that this may relate to the chronic disease state.

Effect of hormone replacement therapy on rheumatoid arthritis

Evidence from case–control studies

Non-contraceptive hormone use has not been shown to affect a woman's risk of developing RA in case–control studies[32,33]. A recent population-based case–control study found that the age-adjusted relative risk among women who had ever used non-contraceptive estrogens was 1.04 (95% CI 0.70–1.55), and among women who had ever used progestins it was 0.66 (95% CI 0.40–1.08)[32]. There was little evidence of a dose–duration relationship.

Evidence from cohort studies

No increased incidence of RA was observed when two cohorts of women aged 35–64 (1075 estrogen replacement therapy users and 3251 women from general practice registers) were compared[34]. Similar results were obtained in the Nurses' Health Study when a cohort of 121 700 female nurses aged 30–55 was followed[28].

Evidence from randomized controlled trials

Whether estrogen replacement therapy (HRT) affects disease activity in postmenopausal women with RA was examined in a placebo-controlled double-blind study of 62 patients with RA, 22 on placebo and 40 on estrogen replacement therapy (transdermal estradiol patches twice weekly for 48 weeks plus norithisterone tablets when clinically indicated)[35]. In the HRT group, there was significant improvement in well-being as assessed by the Nottingham Health Care Profile and in the articular index. However, there were no significant changes in laboratory markers erythrocyte sedimentation rate (ESR) or C-reactive protein (CRP) in either group. In this study, transdermal HRT was well tolerated, increased well-being, reduced articular index and increased lumbar spine bone density over a 1 year period in postmenopausal women with RA. Although no laboratory evidence was found of a disease-modifying effect, there were symptomatic benefits and improvements in bone density, suggesting that HRT may be a valuable adjunct to conventional antirheumatic therapy in RA.

SYSTEMIC LUPUS ERYTHEMATOSUS

Systemic lupus erythematosus (SLE) is a multifactorial disease with both genetic and environmental etiologies. It is a disease of marked female prevalence, and abnormal estrogen metabolism has been described in women with SLE. Clinical and animal studies suggest a role for female hormones in increasing the risk for SLE[36].

Estrogen has been suspected of causing changes in the lupus disease process by an as yet undetermined mechanism. A number of potential mechanisms may be involved. For example, significant elevations in interleukin-1 (IL-1) and tumor necrosis factor-α secretion in mice with experimental SLE and reductions in IL-2, IL-4 and interferon-γ levels, compared with the levels detected in health controls, were recently observed[37]. Treatment with either the antiestradiol antibody or with tamoxifen restored the levels of all these cytokines to the normal levels observed in the control mice, suggesting a role for estrogen in cytokine modulation.

Changes in sex hormone metabolism seem to play a role in the expression of SLE[38]. Epidemiological studies have demonstrated an increased risk of developing SLE in women using estrogens for more than 10 years[37]. Onset or aggravation of symptoms has been described in case reports and small retrospective series of SLE patients. Although oral contraceptives containing estrogen can induce flares in a small proportion of SLE patients, estrogen replacement therapy is generally well tolerated, although there are a few individual case reports of severe adverse reactions.

Hormone replacement therapy in systemic lupus erythematosus

Despite its obvious benefits, many physicians are reluctant to prescribe HRT to patients with SLE. A retrospective study in 60 postmenopausal women with SLE including 30 HRT users and 30 never-users was performed[39]. The patients were studied for 12 months after the initiation of HRT. The two groups were well matched for disease characteristics. The HRT users experienced significant improvements in general well-being, libido and depression. There was no significant difference in any other parameter measured. There was no increase in the number of thromboembolic events in the user group, despite seven patients having a positive thrombophilia screen. This study found that, in a stable postmenopausal SLE, HRT was safe and well tolerated.

Counseling of women on the use of postmenopausal hormones should include a discussion of these risks and benefits in addition to the risks of cardiovascular disease, uterine and breast cancer, and osteoporosis. Patients with stable SLE may use estrogen provided there is close follow-up, particularly during the first 6 months of treatment. Treatment with estrogen is contraindicated in SLE patients with a history of thromboembolism, and those testing positively for phospholipid antibodies, and in the presence of severe organ involvement.

CARPAL TUNNEL SYNDROME

The carpal tunnel syndrome is five times more common in women than in men[40]. It often occurs in women associated with pregnancy and the menopause, but its pathophysiology is not well understood. Carpal tunnel syndrome may also be precipitated by iatrogenic menopause[41,42]. Conservative treatment is recommended, although some individuals eventually progress to surgical decompression of the nerve. Hormone replacement therapy has been shown to be associated with improvement of symptoms in some postmenopausal women[2,43]. However, all the studies are observational and no randomized trials have yet been performed.

CONCLUSION

The menopause coincides with the appearance of many of the common arthritic conditions and with the lessening of severity of others such as SLE. Because of the insidious development of the arthritides, it is difficult to study the role of the timing of the menopause in these diseases. In addition, the low-grade aches and pains experienced at the menopause make distinguishing specific and non-specific symptoms difficult. Nevertheless, the hormonal changes that ensue are likely to modify many of these diseases, and hormonal manipulation can have beneficial or detrimental effects on a number of common joint diseases of which surgeons and physicians need to be aware.

References

1. Neugarten BL, Kraines RJ. 'Menopausal symptoms' in women of various ages. *Psychosom Med* 1965;27:266–73
2. Hall GM, Spector TD, Studd JW. Carpal tunnel syndrome and hormone replacement therapy. *Br Med J* 1992;8:304–82
3. Lawrence JS. *Rheumatism in Populations*. London: Heinemann, 1977

4. Silman AJ, Newman J. Obstetric and gynaecological factors in susceptibility to peripheral joint osteoarthritis. *Ann Rheum Dis* 1996;55:671–3
5. Kellgren JH, Moore R. Generalised osteoarthritis and Heberdens nodes. *Br Med J* 1952;1:181–7
6. Tsai CL, Liu TK. Osteoarthritis in women: its relationship to estrogen and current trends. *Life Sci* 1992;50:1737–44
7. Spector TD, Hart DJ, Brown P, *et al.* Frequency of osteoarthritis in hysterectomized women. *J Rheumatol* 1991;18:1877–83
8. Samanta A, Jones A, Regan M, *et al.* Is osteoarthritis in women affected by hormonal changes or smoking? *Br J Rheumatol* 1993;32:366–70
9. Rosner IA, Goldberg VM, Getzy L, *et al.* Effects of estrogen on cartilage and experimentally induced osteoarthritis. *Arthritis Rheum* 1979;22:52–8
10. Rosener IA, Goldberg VM, Moskowitz RW. Estrogens and osteoarthritis. *Clin Orthop* 1986;213:77–83
11. Wathen NC, Perry LA, Rubenstein E, *et al.* A relationship between sex hormone binding globulin and dehydroepiandrosterone sulphate in normally menstruating females. *J Gynaecol Endocrinol* 1987;1:47–55
12. Cauley JA, Kwoh CK, Egeland G, *et al.* Serum sex hormones and severity of osteoarthritis of the hand. *J Rheumatol* 1993;20:1170–5
13. Spector TD, Perry LA, Jubb RW. Endogenous sex steroid levels in women with generalised osteoarthritis. *Clin Rheumatol* 1991;10:316–19
14. Samanta A, Jones A, Regan M, *et al.* Is osteoarthritis in women affected by hormonal changes or smoking? *Br J Rheumatol* 1993;32:366–70
15. Lindsay R. Estrogen deficiency. In Riggs BL, Melton LJ, eds. *Osteoporosis: Etiology, Diagnosis and Management*, 2nd edn. Philadelphia: Lippincott-Raven, 1995:133–60
16. Hart D, Mootooswamy I, Doyle D, *et al.* The relationship between osteoarthritis and osteoporosis in the general population: the Chingford Study. *Ann Rheum Dis* 1994;53:158–62
17. Spector TD, Brown GC, Silman AJ. Increased rates of previous hysterectomy and gynaecological operations in women with osteoarthritis. *Br Med J* 188;297:899–901
18. Cicuttini FM, Baker JR, Spector TD. The association of obesity with osteoarthritis of the hand and knee in women: a twin study. *J Rheumatol* 1996;23:1221–6
19. Hannan MT, Felson DT, Anderson JJ, *et al.* Estrogen use and radiographic osteoarthritis of the knee in women. The Framingham Osteoarthritis Study. *Arthritis Rheum* 1990;33:525–32
20. Nevitt MC, Cummings SR, Lane NE, *et al.* Association of estrogen replacement therapy with the risk of osteoarthritis of the hip in elderly white women. Study of Osteoporotic Fractures Research Group. *Arch Int Med* 1996;156:2073–80
21. Nevitt MC, Felson DT. Sex hormones and the risk of osteoarthritis in women: epidemiological evidence. *Ann Rheum Dis* 1996;55:673–6
22. Zhang YQ, McAlindon T, Hannan MT, *et al.* A longitudinal study of the relationship of estrogen replacement therapy (ERT) to the risk of radiographic knee osteoarthritis (OA). In *Abstracts of the ASRC National Scientific Meeting*, 1995
23. Oliveria SA, Felson DT, Klein RA, *et al.* Estrogen replacement therapy and the development of osteoarthritis. *Epidemiology* 1996;7:415–19
24. Spector TD, Nandra D, Hart DJ, *et al.* Is hormone replacement therapy protective for hand and knee osteoarthritis – The Chingford Study. *Ann Rheum Dis* 1997;56:432–4
25. Wilder RL. Adrenal and gonadal steroid hormone deficiency in the pathogenesis of rheumatoid arthritis. *J Rheumatol* 1996;44(Suppl):10–12
26. Goemaere S, Ackerman C, Goethals K, *et al.* Onset of symptoms of rheumatoid arthritis in relation to age, sex and menopausal transition. *J Rheumatol* 1990;17:1620–2
27. Brun JG, Nilssen S, Kvale G. Breast feeding, other reproductive factors and rheumatoid arthritis. A prospective study. *Br J Rheumatol* 1995;34:542–6
28. Hernandez Avila M, Liang MH, Willett WC, *et al.* Reproductive factors, smoking, and the risk for rheumatoid arthritis. *Epidemiology* 1990;1:285–91
29. Arnalich F, Benito-Urbina S, Gonzalez Gancedo P, *et al.* Increase in plasma androgens in menopausal women with rheumatoid polyarthritis. *Rev Rhum Mal Osteoartic* 1990;57:509–12
30. Hall GM, Perry LA, Spector TD. Depressed levels of dehydroepiandrosterone sulphate in postmenopausal women with rheumatoid arthritis but no relation with axial bone density. *Ann Rheum Dis* 1993;52:211–14
31. Deighton CM, Watson MJ, Walker DJ. Sex hormones in postmenopausal HLA-identical rheumatoid arthritis discordant sibling pairs. *J Rheumatol* 1992;19:1663–7
32. Koepsell TD, Dugowson CE, Nelson JL, *et al.* Non-contraceptive hormones and the risk of rheumatoid arthritis in menopausal women. *Int J Epidemiol* 1994;23:1248–55
33. Carette S, Marcoux S, Gingras S. Postmenopausal hormones and the incidence of rheumatoid arthritis. *J Rheumatol* 1989;16:911–13
34. Spector TD, Brennan P, Harris P, *et al.* Does estrogen replacement therapy protect against rheumatoid arthritis? *J Rheumatol* 1991;18:1473–6
35. MacDonald AG, Murphy EA, Capell HA, *et al.* Effects of hormone replacement therapy in

rheumatoid arthritis: a double blind placebo-controlled study. *Ann Rheum Dis* 1994;53:54–7
36. Liang MH, Karlson EW. Female hormone therapy and the risk of developing or exacerbating systemic lupus erythematosus or rheumatoid arthritis. *Proc Assoc Am Physicians* 1996;108:25–8
37. Dayan M, Zinger H, Kalush F, *et al.* The beneficial effects of treatment with tamoxifen and anti-oestradiol antibody on experimental systemic lupus erythematosus are associated with cytokine modulations. *Immunology* 1997;90:101–8
38. Ostensen M. Use of estrogen in women with systemic lupus erythematosus – should, should not? *Nidsskr Nor Laegeforen* 1996;116:3237–9
39. Arden NK, Lloyd ME, Spector TD, *et al.* Safety of hormone replacement therapy (HRT) in systemic lupus erythematosus (SLE). *Lupus* 1994;3:11–13
40. Milford L. Carpal tunnel and ulnar tunnel syndromes and stenosing tenosynovitis. In Crenshaw AH, ed. *Campbell's Operative Orthopoedics*, 7th edn. St Louis, MO: CV Mosby, 1987: 459–68
41. Bjorkqvist SE, Lang AH, Punnonen R, *et al.* Carpal tunnel syndrome in ovariectomized women. *Acta Obstet Gynecol Scand* 1977;56:127–30
42. Pascual E, Giner V, Arostegui A, *et al.* Higher incidence of carpal tunnel syndrome in oophorectomized women. *Br J Rheumatol* 1991;30:60–2
43. Confino-Cohen R, Lishner M, Savin H, *et al.* Response of carpal tunnel syndrome to hormone replacement therapy. *Br Med J* 1991;303:1514

8
Contraception for women over forty

A. E. Gebbie

INTRODUCTION

Health-care professionals often have difficulty in giving women over 40 years good advice on issues relating to fertility regulation. All methods of contraception become increasingly effective when used by older women but no single method exists that meets all preferences. Older women themselves may have longstanding fears about using certain methods at their age, and many may be tempted to abandon contraception altogether because of declining fertility with age. Reliable contraception is particularly important for women of this age as, when an unplanned pregnancy occurs, there may be devastating psychosocial consequences for the individual woman and her family.

The average age of the menopause is 50 years and, in the UK at the present time, there is growing enthusiasm for use of hormone replacement therapy (HRT) in symptomatic perimenopausal women. Differences between hormonal contraception and HRT are frequently misunderstood and, since HRT is not reliably contraceptive, a contraceptive method must be recommended in addition for women taking HRT who have not yet reached the natural menopause. Advising women taking HRT when to stop contraception poses particular difficulty.

FERTILITY IN OLDER WOMEN

Although the menopause marks the end of reproduction, natural decline in fertility begins much earlier. In the 1920s, natural fertility rates were observed in studies of the Hutterite sects in North America who did not practice contraception and enjoyed a high standard of living. Increasing intervals between conceptions were observed in older Hutterite women and, by the age of 40 years, half had delivered their last child, although only 1% would be expected to be postmenopausal[1]. However, these data probably do not fully represent the biological potential of women's reproductive systems, as confounding factors such as coital frequency, subfertility and early pregnancy losses were not taken into consideration[2].

Data from studies on gynecologically normal women with azoospermic husbands, who were undergoing artificial insemination by donor, provide a good indicator of fecundability related to age. The decline in conception rates was slight but significant after 30 years of age, and more marked after 35 years[3]. The monthly conception rate for women under 24 years was 30% compared with 14% for women aged 40–45 years[4].

Oocyte quality is likely to be the main factor in the age-related decline in fertility. After the age of 37 years, oocytes disappear faster from the ovaries and are more susceptible to aneuploidy and mitochondrial mutations[5]. Transvaginal imaging of the ovaries in one study showed an age-related decline in follicle numbers, with a decrease of about 60% between 22 and 42 years[6].

The oldest woman to give birth following spontaneous conception was 57 years and 129 days (*Guinness Book of Records*). Advances in assisted conception techniques using donor oocytes have made pregnancies possible in postmenopausal women[7] and, in the USA in 1997, a woman gave birth to a live child at the age of 63 years. Several studies have demonstrated similar conception and pregnancy loss rates in 'younger' and 'older' groups of women undergoing egg donation from the same source[8]. This supports the theory that aging of oocytes is the limiting factor in conception for these older women rather than diminished ability of the older uterus to sustain a pregnancy.

HORMONAL FACTORS

Longitudinal studies of endocrine changes in women, irrespective of age, indicate a strong correlation between regular cycles and the occurrence of ovulation[9]. Subtle changes do occur, however, in components of the reproductive axis in the regular cycles of women in the perimenopausal transition. Many women note shortening of their cycle length (less than 24 days) as the first perimenopausal change. These regular but shortened cycles are ovulatory but associated with a relatively higher follicle-stimulating hormone (FSH) concentration in the follicular phase of the cycle[10]. Elevated day 2 or 3 FSH concentrations are indicative of diminished ovarian reserve and are highly predictive of poor outcome in women undergoing *in vitro* fertilization[11]. In addition, concentrations of the glycoprotein hormone inhibin, produced by ovarian granulosa cells, decrease significantly in the follicular phase in women over 40 years of age, providing a very early index of declining ovarian function[12].

As a woman progresses through the perimenopause, menstrual cycles become increasingly erratic and unpredictable, associated with fluctuating sex steroid and gonadotropin hormone levels. Spells of amenorrhea may be followed by regular menstruation, implying ovulation and a theoretical risk of conception. Long, anovulatory cycles are frequently associated with menorrhagia. The economic cost of menstrual dysfunction in women in the perimenopause is significant in terms of absenteeism from employment and the number of consultations in primary care. The permanent cessation of menstruation marks the menopause and is a diagnosis made in retrospect, 1 year following the last menstrual period.

PREGNANCY IN OLDER WOMEN

Many women in western countries now choose to delay childbearing in the pursuit of career and educational goals, made possible with use of effective contraception. Women over 35 years have traditionally been believed to have more serious adverse pregnancy outcomes than younger women. Recent studies, however, have found little evidence for this once the data are corrected for pre-existing disease such as hypertension, when associated with a high standard of obstetric practice[2]. Spellacy and colleagues reported no perinatal maternal mortality in women over 40 years receiving optimum obstetric care[13]. Specific antepartum and intrapartum complications do, however, appear to be more prevalent in older women, and Bobrowski and Bottoms found that women over 35 years had a significantly higher risk of pre-eclampsia, gestational diabetes, induction of labour and Cesarean section[14]. Older women appeared slightly more likely to have a low birth-weight infant, although risk of poor neonatal outcome was not appreciably increased[15].

The incidence of clinically recognizable spontaneous abortion in women over 40 years is of the order of 30%. This may well represent a gross underestimate of the overall rate, as many early miscarriages may be occult. The age-related increase in spontaneous abortion corresponds to fetuses that are both chromosomally normal and abnormal. The gradual increase in risk of trisomic miscarriage begins about the age of 29 years[2], and the incidence of Down's syndrome reaches 1/40 by the age of 45 years compared with 1/600 for all pregnancies.

Of particular note is that women over the age of 40 years are more likely to seek termination of pregnancy under the terms of the UK 1967 Abortion Act than any other age group (Figure 1)[16]. Although terminations in women aged over 40 years only represent 3.2% of the total terminations performed in 1995, they account for over 40% of all pregnancies in this age group.

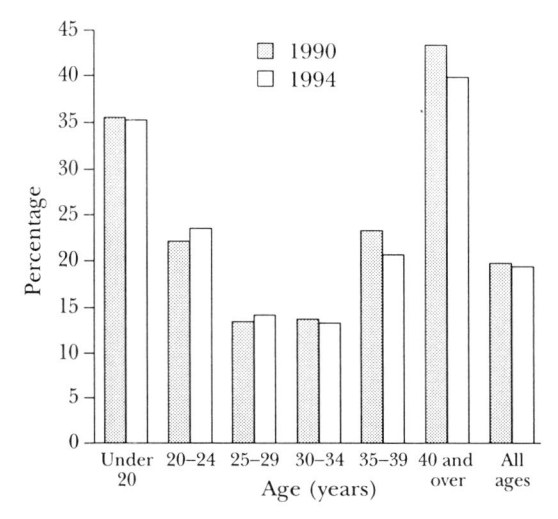

Figure 1 Percentage of all conceptions leading to legal terminations, England and Wales residents, 1990 and 1994. Reproduced from reference 16, with permission

SEXUAL FUNCTION

Frequency of coitus is strongly and inversely associated with age (Figure 2)[17]. Wellings and colleagues, in their large survey of sexual lifestyles in the British population, found frequency of coitus to peak in the mid-20s age group and, thereafter, show a gradual decline, more marked for women than for men[18]. Length of relationship was also found to be closely associated with frequency of sex at all ages, the number of episodes of coitus being much lower in longer relationships. The excitement of a relatively new partnership presumably influences the frequency of sexual activity in the early years of a relationship.

The prevalence of sexual dysfunction is high in women in their 40s and is probably more related to psychological, interpersonal and sociocultural influences rather than biological factors. Sexual activity may also be influenced by factors such as frequent or heavy menstruation. An older male partner's sexual dysfunction can also cause sexual difficulties for women[19], and both men and women may find a gradual reduction in the speed and intensity of their sexual responses with the aging process itself[20]. In

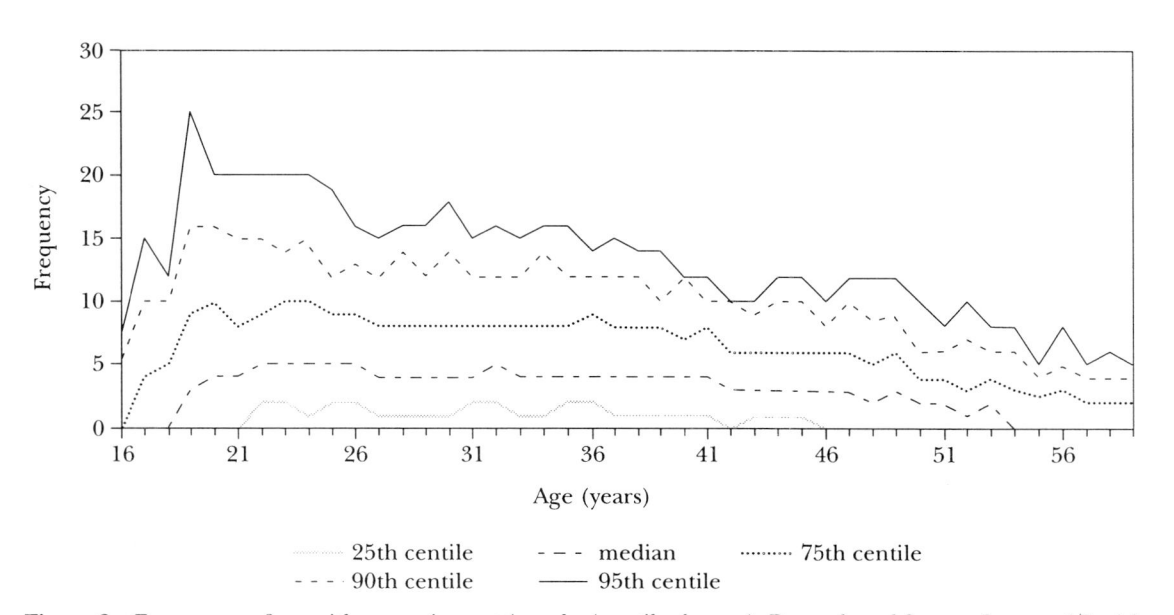

Figure 2 Frequency of sex with a man in past 4 weeks (centiles by age). Reproduced from reference 17, with permission

contrast, some older women find an improvement in sexual function related to a new partner, greater leisure time or more privacy. Frequency of intercourse appears to be positively associated with the effectiveness of the contraceptive method used[21], although Graham and co-workers found an adverse effect of the combined oral contraceptive pill on sexual interest in women in Scotland but no adverse sexual effect with the progestogen-only pill[22]. Several studies have demonstrated that couples relying on a permanent sterilization procedure, particularly vasectomy, find their sex life is enhanced by the removal of the fear of pregnancy[23].

METHODS OF CONTRACEPTION

Wellings and colleagues found striking changes in patterns of contraceptive usage with age (Table 1). Relatively low rates of use of combined oral contraception (COC) and intrauterine contraception were demonstrated in women over 34 years, in contrast to a rise in the popularity of female and male sterilization procedures. Worldwide, COC remains primarily a method of contraception used by young women. Use of condoms declined overall with age although in older couples who had not been sterilized, they were relatively more popular. Increased use of condoms in the general population reflects health promotion campaigns to reduce sexually transmissible infections including human immunodeficiency virus (HIV) and acquired immunodeficiency syndrome (AIDS), although this is often perceived to be of less concern to older women. Oddens and colleagues found that 73% of women believed that COC was associated with weight gain and had doubts about its safety[24]. Many women also had ambivalent attitudes to intrauterine devices (IUDs), and 72% thought that they caused pelvic infection. The popularity of barriers other than male condoms has declined since the 1960s with the advent of effective methods of hormonal, non-coitus related contraceptives. The high uptake of sterilization procedures in the UK reflects many deep-seated fears and prejudices against currently available reversible contra- ceptive methods.

Barrier methods

Condoms are one of the oldest forms of contraception, and individuals, irrespective of age,

Table 1 Method of contraception used in past year by age (%). Reproduced from reference 17, with permission

	16–24	25–34	35–44	45–59	All ages
Pill	64.1	43.6	11.3	2.5	28.8
IUD	3.1	8.9	9.3	3.8	6.6
Condom	41.9	31.0	20.7	12.8	25.9
Diaphragm	1.0	3.9	2.3	1.3	2.3
Pessaries	0.5	1.0	1.1	0.3	0.8
Sponge	0.1	0.2	0.1	0.0	0.1
Douche	0.2	0.1	0.1	0.2	0.1
Safe period	2.3	2.5	2.1	0.7	1.9
Withdrawal	6.6	4.3	3.6	3.0	4.2
Female sterilization	0.4	6.2	17.8	17.9	11.0
Vasectomy	1.1	7.4	24.3	15.0	12.6
Abstinence	1.7	1.6	0.6	0.1	1.0
Other method	0.9	0.9	0.5	0.5	0.7
None	9.5	12.7	16.2	45.3	21.1
Base* (n)	1692	2667	2344	2208	8911

*Excludes respondents with no heterosexual partners in past year: percentages sum to more than 100% because more than one contraceptive method could have been reported; IUD, intrauterine device

should be advised to consider their use in new relationships for personal protection against sexually transmissible infection. Condom use is limited, however, by factors such as decreased sensitivity and sexual enjoyment. Older couples are generally better at using condoms more conscientiously but rarely find them sufficiently user-friendly to start using them for the first time in later life. Sensitivity to latex condoms can occasionally occur in either partner and hypoallergenic condoms are available. Various oil-based vaginal products, including some estrogen and antifungal creams, can drastically affect the tensile strength of latex condoms and lead to condoms bursting.

The diaphragm or Dutch cap is the most commonly used female barrier in the UK, and there have been no significant improvements or variations in diaphragms for many decades. Although overall failure rates of the diaphragm are relatively high[25], older women use diaphragms more reliably and have significantly lower failure rates. Use of diaphragms without spermicide is associated with unacceptably high failure rates[26], so adjunctive spermicidal agents are always recommended and may provide additional lubrication if vaginal dryness is a problem. The presence of uterovaginal prolapse, particularly a cystocele, may make secure retention of a diaphragm difficult, but a cervical or vault cap may overcome this problem. Diaphragms offer significant protection against pelvic inflammatory disease and cervical neoplasia, although symptomatic urinary tract infection is more common in diaphragm users.

Studies of the efficacy of the female condom indicate that it has failure rates similar to those of other barrier methods[27]. Many women find its appearance unesthetic, and it is never likely to find widespread popularity. Manufactured of polyethylene and not latex rubber, it is less likely to burst during intercourse and is unaffected by oil-based vaginal products[28]. The vaginal contraceptive sponge has a higher failure rate than a diaphragm and can only really be recommended at times of extremely low fertility, such as in conjunction with hormone replacement therapy and during long spells of amenorrhea in the perimenopause. Beckman and Harvey found that many women discontinued using the sponge because of vaginal irritation[29], and it has recently been withdrawn from the US market because of allegations that unsafe manufacture has led to an increased risk of infection.

Intrauterine devices

Worldwide, the IUD is the second most popular method of reversible contraception after COC. Its uptake in developed countries is very variable, ranging from less than 1% of married women of reproductive age in the USA to over 30% in some Scandinavian countries. The modern IUD is a highly effective and convenient method of contraception for older women and rivals the efficacy of female sterilization[30]. In terms of comparative costs, the copper-bearing IUD appears to be one of the most cost-effective methods of contraception over 5 years of use[31]. The large inert devices, the Lippes loop and the Saf-T coil, are no longer commercially available, although some older women may still have them *in situ*. Trials of many of the currently available high-load copper IUDs have shown an effective intrauterine life span of up to 10 years[32]. If an IUD is inserted after a woman's 40th birthday, this device may effectively remain *in situ* until the woman reaches the menopause[33]. Devices should always be removed from postmenopausal women because of the very occasional occurrence of systemic sepsis originating from an infected IUD. A frameless IUD, the Gyne-Fix, consisting of six copper sleeves on a prolene thread, is now available, and research to date indicates a low expulsion rate combined with reduced dysmenorrhea[34].

Recent research clearly demonstrates that IUDs cause neither ectopic pregnancy nor pelvic infection. Overall, IUDs protect against all types of pregnancy, but in the event of an IUD failure, there is an increased risk of ectopic pregnancy[35]. When an IUD is used by a woman in a stable, mutually monogamous relationship, there is no increased risk of pelvic infection[32]. The IUD, therefore, is a recommendable choice for older women who are more likely to be in a stable relationship and at lower risk of exposure to sexually transmissible infection. Many women using copper-bearing IUDs experience a modest increase in menstrual blood loss of around 50 ml[36] and increased dysmenorrhea. For most women, this is an acceptable trade-off for the other advantages of an IUD. However, it may be unacceptable to an older woman who has pre-existing dysfunctional menstrual bleeding, menorrhagia or pelvic pain. Removals for bleeding do become more frequent in the peri-menopause, and this is generally attributed to hormonal changes and their sequelae and not causally linked to the IUD[37].

Levonorgestrel-releasing system

The levonorgestrel-releasing intrauterine system (LNG-IUS) combines the advantages of both hormonal and intrauterine contraception and may be a particularly appropriate method for some older women. Modeled on the Nova-T plastic frame, it has a central reservoir which contains 52 mg of levonorgestrel, released at a steady rate of 20 µg per 24 h. This daily dosage of progestogen is the lowest dose of any progestogen-containing contraceptive (Table 2). It is as effective as female sterilization, the risk of ectopic pregnancy is particularly low and it has a protective effect against pelvic infection in common with other hormonal methods[38].

In contrast with conventional IUDs, the LNG-IUS confers positive health benefits and is associated with a dramatic reduction in menstrual blood loss of as much as 90%[39]. It is the most effective medical treatment of menorrhagia, and for many women may be a real alternative to hysterectomy[40]. Irregular bleeding and spotting are very common in the first 3–6 months of use, but improve significantly thereafter. Hormonal side-effects include acne and headache and those in common with other progestogen-only methods (Table 3). Good counseling about this prior to insertion is essential. The LNG-IUS is broader within its insertion tube than the Nova-T (4.8 mm cf. 3.7 mm) but, in parous women, insertion should not pose any practical difficulty. Other potential applications for the LNG-IUS include treatment of endometrial hyperplasia, as the progestogen component of HRT[41] and part of a therapeutic strategy for premenstrual syndrome.

Sterilization

Over one-half of couples in the UK aged over 40 years rely on a permanent, sterilization procedure for contraception. Vasectomy is slightly more popular in younger age groups and, thereafter, female sterilization becomes more common[18] as couples are presumably influenced in their choice of method by the natural decline in female fertility. Individuals seeking sterilization must be carefully counseled on the possible, very small, failure rate and the permanency of the procedure. Sterilization of older women is less likely to lead to regret and request for reversal.

Female sterilization involves the mechanical blockage of the Fallopian tubes, and is generally performed laparoscopically under general anesthesia. Women discontinuing COC at the time of sterilization may find a noticeable increase in subsequent menstrual blood loss, although there is no evidence that sterilization *per se* increases risk of menstrual dysfunction and hysterectomy[42]. Sterilization can be performed in women of any age up to the menopause, but

Table 2 Daily doses of levonorgestrel in contraception

Levonorgestrel-releasing IUS	20 µg
Progestogen-only pill	30 µg
Norplant	70 µg the first year
	30 µg thereafter
Combined pill (both with ethinylestradiol)	
Microgynon 30	150 µg
Eugynon 30	250 µg

IUS, intrauterine system

Table 3 Menstrual and gynecological problems associated with use of any progestogen-only methods of contraception

Amenorrhea
Polymenorrhea
Irregular menstrual cycles
Functional ovarian cysts
Mood swings
Acne

those approaching the menopause should probably be advised to use an alternative method until they achieve natural sterility. The US Collaborative Review of Sterilization Group in a recent, very large prospective study found cumulative failure rates of female sterilization substantially higher than most previously reported[43]. Over a 10-year period following sterilization, the probability of failure overall was 18.5 per 1000 procedures, of which laparoscopic spring-clip procedures had the highest probability of failure (36.5 pregnancies per 1000 procedures). The older a woman was at the time of procedure, the less likely the risk of sterilization failure.

Vasectomy is a simple technique often performed under local anesthesia, involving bilateral division of the vas deferens. It is undoubtedly technically easier and associated with fewer complications than female sterilization. The health effects of vasectomy have been extensively studied, and the procedure is considered to have an excellent record for safety and effectiveness. However, recent epidemiological studies have linked vasectomy to a small increased risk of testicular and prostate cancer. Much of the controversy is due to inconsistent results in these studies and the lack of plausible biological mechanisms[44]. Research will need to continue to elucidate this possible relationship between vasectomy and cancer, but the findings to date do not justify any change in family-planning practice[45].

Natural methods of fertility regulation

Natural family planning depends on a woman's ability to identify the fertile phase of each menstrual cycle and refrain from vaginal intercourse during this phase. Fertility awareness techniques include the rhythm method, measuring basal body temperature, monitoring cervical mucus changes (Billing's method) and multiple index systems. Effectiveness depends largely on motivation and older couples are more likely to comply with periodic abstinence from intercourse. Natural family planning may sometimes be the only method of contraception acceptable for religious or ethical reasons. Difficulty with interpretation of the signs of ovulation occurs when the menstrual cycle becomes shortened or anovulatory during the menopausal transition.

The new Persona monitor for fertility awareness is a hand-held device which measures urinary concentrations of estrone and luteinizing hormone. A computer within the monitor analyzes the hormonal patterns of a woman's cycle and calculates fertile phases when abstinence is required. Its high cost at the present time means it is unlikely to make a great impact on contraceptive choice[46].

Combined oral contraception

Combined oral contraception is the most popular method of reversible contraception worldwide, and is of very high efficacy in women of all ages. The primary mode of action of COC is suppression of ovulation, with changes in cervical mucus and endometrium as a secondary effect. A significant reduction in dosage of both estrogen and progestogen components has occurred since its introduction to the UK in 1961. The modern, low-dose preparations containing 20–35 μg estrogen undoubtedly have an improved safety profile as a result. Nowadays, COC offers excellent contraceptive protection and other non-contraceptive benefits which may make it a particularly appropriate choice for healthy older women.

COC and risk of arterial disease

In the late 1960s, a definite causal relationship between COC use and an increased risk of myocardial infarction (MI) and thrombotic stroke was identified, and found to be potentiated by other risk factors, particularly cigarette smoking. This relationship was attributed to the effect of estrogen increasing risk of thrombosis and, to a lesser extent, the effect of synthetic progestogens on arterial wall disease. The effect of estrogens on coagulation factors is clearly dose-dependent, and a relative risk of MI of only 1.1 with current use of low-dose (30 μg) COC compared to a risk of 4.1 with current use of preparations containing 50 μg estrogen has been found[47]. Smoking undoubtedly increases risk, and a recent WHO Collaborative Study found that acute myocardial infarction was extremely rare in non-smoking young women who use COC[48]. Women who smoke must always be advised to discontinue COC at the age of 35 years, as the WHO study clearly showed a substantial degree of excess risk of MI among older women who smoke. Recent data on stroke in users of low-dose COC found no statistically significant increase in risk, although the overall rate of COC use among older women in the study was low[49].

Combined oral contraceptives containing the third-generation progestogens (desogestrel, norgestimate and gestodene) were thought to produce fewer adverse effects on lipid and carbohydrate metabolism and, therefore, to be particularly suitable for older women. Third-generation COC has, as yet, to be shown to have any clinical benefit over older pills in terms of reduction of arterial disease.

COC and risk of venous thromboembolism

Combined oral contraception increases risk of venous thromboembolism by an estrogen-induced, dose-dependent alteration of clotting factors tending to promote coagulation. Three separate studies have indicated that COC containing third-generation progestogens is associated with a doubling of risk of venous thromboembolism (VTE) compared with COC containing the older progestogens[50]. Risk overall of VTE was small: at worst, 30 per 100 000 women taking third-generation preparations compared with 15 per 100 000 in women taking older equivalent preparations. This compared with a risk in healthy women not taking hormones of 5 per 100 000 and a risk in pregnancy of 60 per 100 000[51]. Based on these data, which were unpublished at the time, the UK Committee of Safety of Medicines in 1995 recommended that all women wanting to use COC should be prescribed preparations containing second-generation progestogens unless they were previously intolerant of these. Confirmation of these epidemiological studies has now come with recent laboratory data which demonstrate evidence of resistance to the blood's natural anticoagulation system (acquired activated protein-C resistance) in COC users, which is more marked in women using third-generation COC compared with users of second generation COC[52]. Advising older women which COC preparation to take and weighing up potential cardiovascular benefit and thromboembolic risk, therefore, has become more complex. Based on our present knowledge, the older, second-generation preparations would probably be best for healthy, low-risk older women.

COC and risk of breast cancer

The possible association between breast cancer and hormonal contraception is an important public health question as well as one of great importance to individual women selecting their method of contraception. Numerous studies have shown no overall association between breast cancer and use of COC[53]. A weak association had been found between development of breast cancer under the age of 36 years and previous COC use. The Collaborative Group on Hormonal Factors in Breast Cancer, which reported in 1996, pooled the results of 54 case–control studies and concluded that women who were using or had recently stopped using COC had a slightly increased risk of breast cancer (odds ratio 1.24 for current users and 1.16 for women who stopped using the pill 1 or 4 years before)[54]. No increase in risk of breast cancer was seen after 10 years of stopping the pill, and the breast cancers in COC users were clinically less advanced than among non-users. For older women currently taking COC, this small increase in risk is of more concern, as the background incidence of breast cancer is higher, particularly in developed countries[55]. For many older women, however, the other advantages of COC may outweigh this small increased risk of breast cancer.

Non-contraceptive health benefits of COC to older women

Combined oral contraception users have a reduced incidence of many gynecological problems which are particularly pertinent for older women (Table 4), and they are less likely to

Table 4 Menstrual and gynecological advantages associated with use of combined oral contraception

Regular, predictable menstrual periods
Reduction in menstrual blood loss
Reduction in dysmenorrhea
Improvement in premenstrual syndrome
Reduced incidence of benign ovarian cysts
Reduced incidence of fibroids
Suppression of endometriosis
Protective effect against endometrial cancer
Protective effect against ovarian cancer

require major and minor gynecological surgery, notably hysterectomy. It is well established that COC offers protection against types of gynecological cancer, a fact that is frequently overlooked in discussions with women considering COC. A strong protective effect against epithelial ovarian cancer has been demonstrated, reducing risk by around 40% and persisting for at least 15 years after discontinuing COC[56]. A protective effect against endometrial cancer which is maintained for a similar length of time after discontinuing COC has also been shown. Use of COC will prevent loss of bone mineral density in the perimenopause, and there is some evidence that premenopausal women using low-dose COC will stabilize or even increase their bone mass compared with that of non-users[57].

Progestogen-only contraception

A variety of delivery systems now exist for giving very low- to high-dose progestogen-only contraception and offering women a wide choice of hormonal contraceptives. Progestogen-only pills (POPs or mini-pills), injectables, subdermal implants and progestogen-releasing IUDs are all now available commercially. Progestogens exert a contraceptive effect by several local mechanisms which include altering cervical mucus to hinder sperm penetration, inducing changes in the endometrium which affect the survival of a blastocyst or prevent implantation, and altering tubal mobility. In addition, there is varying suppression of ovulation with different progestogen dosages, which tends to disrupt the menstrual cycle in an unpredictable way. Erratic bleeding and other hormonal side-effects influence the acceptability of all progestogen-only methods and may affect compliance (Table 2). Abnormal bleeding in older women using progestogen-only contraception may occasionally be associated with underlying pathology which should not be overlooked.

Progestogen-only methods of contraception are particularly useful for older women who smoke or have cardiovascular risk factors which contraindicate COC. They are not contraindicated in women with hypertension, gallstones, migraine or diabetes. Progestogen-only methods appear to have little or no effect on coagulation factors and can be used by women with a history of thromboembolic disease[58]. Effects on lipid parameters appear limited even with higher-dose progestogen methods[59].

Progestogen-only pills

Progestogen-only pills (POPs) are generally an under-used and under-studied method of contraception, and contain a lower total amount of progestogen than COC.

There is very little difference in efficacy, cycle control and side-effects between the different brands. Efficacy of the POP increases substantially with age, and the failure rate in a women in her 40s compares favorably with the failure rate of the combined pill in young women[60]. It is a recommendable choice for older women with contraindications to COC but who like an oral method. Between 15 and 40% of cycles in POP users are anovulatory[61], and this is reflected in the unpredictable and erratic bleeding pattern in some women. The incidence of amenorrhea in POP users increases with age, but is not associated with significant hypo-estrogenism until the onset of the menopause, in contrast to Depo-Provera. There is no evidence to suggest that use of the POP increases risk of breast cancer, but women with breast cancer should probably avoid all hormonal contraceptives as it is simply not known what effect they have on the course of the disease.

Injectables

Depot medroxyprogesterone acetate (Depo-Provera, DMPA) and norethisterone enanthate

(NET-EN) are long-acting progestational contraceptives, the latter having a shorter duration of action. Since its introduction in the 1960s, Depo-Provera has been the subject of various campaigns relating to feminist and consumer concerns over its potential for misuse, which have had a major effect on its worldwide availability and usage. Concerns have also been expressed about the relationship between Depo-Provera and breast cancer, but there is now general consensus that there is no significant overall increase in the risk in Depo-Provera users but a possible very small risk in long-term users[62]. Depo-Provera, in common with all progestogen-only methods, is protective against endometrial cancer and probably ovarian cancer.

Amenorrhea is common with prolonged use of Depo-Provera and, in some older women, can lead to confusion about onset of the menopause. Some concerns exist that long-term Depo-Provera use is associated with hypoestrogenism and loss of bone mineral density in premenopausal women[63]. This issue is as yet unresolved, but it is probably good practice to advise women to discontinue Depo-Provera at the age of 45 years to allow time for recovery of bone density prior to the menopause. In women with amenorrhea of longer than 5 years' duration, particularly those with other risk factors for osteoporosis, a serum estradiol should be checked and bone densitometry performed. If both of these give low results, an alternative method of contraception should be advised or 'add back' estrogen replacement offered in conjunction with Depo-Provera. Transdermal 50 μg estrogen patches applied twice per week give a bone-conserving dose.

Norplant

Norplant consists of six flexible capsules containing the synthetic progestogen, levonorgestrel, which are inserted subdermally in the upper arm under local anesthesia and last for 5 years. Norplant can be an extremely effective and acceptable contraceptive for older women[64], although data sheets in the UK arbitrarily recommend use in women aged 18–40 years. In common with all progestogen-only contraceptives, Norplant has an unpredictable effect on menstrual pattern, and 5–10% of users report symptoms of headache, mood changes, weight gain and altered hair and skin consistency, which significantly affect long-term compliance[65].

STOPPING CONTRACEPTION

Women are generally advised to continue contraception for 1 year following their last spontaneous menstrual period if over the age of 50 years. Women under the age of 50 years should continue with contraception for 2 years following their last period, to exclude the likelihood of a further ovulation. Hormone levels are generally unhelpful in the perimenopause because of marked fluctuations, and women must not be advised to discontinue contraception purely on the basis of an isolated elevated FSH concentration or short period of amenorrhea.

Hormonal contraception

In older women taking COC, the symptoms and signs of the menopause are masked. The hypothalamo–pituitary axis is suppressed by COC, with inhibition of FSH secretion. To date, no method has been developed to ascertain ovarian status in women using COC. Clinicians generally recommend discontinuation of COC at the age of 50 years, with institution of a barrier method or a POP to allow evaluation of the menstrual cycle, and FSH measurement after approximately 6 weeks. Some studies have indicated that an elevated FSH level, after 1 week of COC, may be a reliable indicator of postmenopausal status[66,67].

Annual FSH estimation is recommended in amenorrheic POP users after the age of 45 years, to detect the onset of the menopause and to give accurate advice on when POP can be discontinued. The POP does not suppress FSH secretion. In the presence of elevated FSH concentration, the woman should be advised to continue with the POP for 1 further year. The presence of regular cycles in an older POP user indicates cyclical ovarian activity and the need for ongoing contraception.

There is considerable interest in the development of COC preparations containing 17β-estradiol (E_2), which induce fewer adverse effects on the cardiovascular system than those containing ethinylestradiol. Hormone replacement therapy preparations can be safely prescribed to older women who smoke, are hypertensive or have ischemic heart disease where COC is contraindicated. In contrast with earlier epidemiological data, recent case–control studies now indicate a small causal relationship between current use of HRT and idiopathic venous thromboembolism[68]. Development of COC containing natural estrogens has so far been unsuccessful because of a high incidence of irregular bleeding and difficulty maintaining high levels of E_2 over 24 h. A small study found that 3 mg E_2 in combination with desogestrel achieved anovulation in all subjects, although there was breakthrough bleeding in between 26 and 42% of the cycles studied[69].

Hormone replacement therapy

Many women now start HRT for relief of menopausal symptoms prior to the menopause. Once established on HRT, it becomes impossible to assess accurately when the natural menopause has occurred. Conventional HRT cannot be relied on for contraception, and perimenopausal women may ovulate on HRT, particularly in the first few months of therapy[70]. High-dose HRT regimens, particularly using the transdermal and subcutaneous routes of estrogen administration, have been demonstrated to suppress ovulation[71]. Sexually active women who are not relying on a sterilization procedure and commence HRT prior to the menopause should be advised still to use contraception. Barrier methods, an IUD and the POP can be continued in conjunction with HRT. Although there are no scientific data to confirm efficacy of the POP in this context, it is now quite widely recommended.

Advising women on HRT when to stop contraception is complex. This should be determined for individual women depending on their menstrual patterns at the time of starting HRT, their ages and how long they have been taking HRT. Contraception can be arbitrarily continued to the age of 55 years, which is the assumed upper age limit for complete loss of fertility. Alternatively, women can have a short break from HRT of around 6 weeks to assess their menstrual pattern and have their FSH concentration measured. An FSH concentration within the menopausal range accompanied by amenorrhea would indicate very low fertility, and contraception should be used for 1 further year[72].

ACKNOWLEDGEMENT

The author would especially like to thank Dr Nancy Loudon for checking the manuscript.

References

1. Eaton JW, Mayer AJ. The social biology of very high fertility among the Hutterites. The demography of a unique population. *Hum Biol* 1953;25: 206–64
2. Maroulis GB. Effect of aging on fertility and pregnancy. *Semin Reprod Endocrinol* 1991;3: 165–75
3. CECOS, Schwarz D, Mayaux MJ. Female fecundity as a function of age. Results of artificial insemination in 2193 nulliparous women with azoospermic husbands. *N Engl J Med* 1982;306: 404–6
4. Stovall DW, Toma SK, Hammond MG. The effect of age on female fecundity. *Obstet Gynecol* 1991; 77:33–6

5. Gosden R, Rutherford A. Delayed childbearing. *Br Med J* 1995;311:1585
6. Reuss ML, Kline J, Santos R, *et al.* Age and the ovarian follicle pool assessed with transvaginal ultrasonography. *Am J Obstet Gynecol* 1996;174: 624–7
7. Borini A, Bafaro G, Violini F, *et al.* Pregnancies in postmenopausal women over 50 years old in an oocyte donation program. *Fertil Steril* 1995;63: 258–60
8. Navot D, Drews MR, Bergh PA, *et al.* Age-related decline in female fertility is not due to diminished capacity of the uterus to sustain embryo implantation. *Fertil Steril* 1994;61:97–101
9. Metcalf MG. The approach of the menopause: a New Zealand study. *NZ Med J* 1988;101:103–6
10. Burger HG, Dudley EC, Hopper JL, *et al.* The endocrinology of the menopausal transition; a cross-sectional study of a population based sample. *J Clin Endocrinol Metab* 1995;80:3537–45
11. Balasch J, Creus M, Fabregues F, *et al.* Inhibin, follicle-stimulating hormone, and age as predictors of ovarian response in *in-vitro* fertilization cycles stimulated with gonadotropin-releasing hormone agonist–gonadotropin treatment. *Am J Obstet Gynecol* 1996;5:1226–30
12. Seifer DB, Lambert-Messerlian G, Hogan JW, *et al.* Day 3 serum inhibin-β is predictive of assisted reproductive technologies outcome. *Fertil Steril* 1997;67:110–16
13. Spellacy WN, Miller SL, Winegar A. Pregnancy after 40 years of age. *Gynaecology* 1986;83:452–4
14. Bobrowski RA, Bottoms SF. Underappreciated risks of the elderly multipara. *Am J Obstet Gynecol* 1995;172:1764–7
15. Berkowitz GS, Skovron ML, Lapinski RH, *et al.* Delayed childbearing and the outcome of pregnancy. *N Engl J Med* 1990;322:659–64
16. Office for National Statistics. *Population Trends* 1997;87:17
17. Wadsworth J, *et al.* Sexual health for women: some findings of a large national survey discussed. *Sex Marital Ther* 1995;10:169–88
18. Wellings K, Field J, Johnson A, *et al. Sexual Behaviour in Britain. The National Survey of Sexual Attitudes and Lifestyles.* London: Penguin Books, 1994
19. Bachmann GA. Sexual function in the perimenopause. *Obstet Gynecol Clin North Am* 1993; 20:379–89
20. Bancroft J. Sexuality and family planning. In Loudon N, Glasier A, Gebbie A, eds. *Handbook of Family Planning and Reproductive Health Care*, 3rd edn. London: Churchill Livingstone, 1995: 339–62
21. Trussell J, Westoff CF. Contraceptive practice and trends in coital frequency. *Fam Plann Persp* 1980;12:246–9
22. Graham CA, Ramos R, Bancroft J, *et al.* The effects of steroidal contraceptives on the well-being and sexuality of women: a double-blind, placebo-controlled, two-centre study of combined and progestogen-only methods. *Contraception* 1995;52:363–9
23. Hart AJL, Dean RF. A retrospective study of one hundred vasectomies carried out at the FPA. *Br J Sex Med* 1980;7(67):10–14
24. Oddens BJ, Visser AP, Vemer HM, *et al.* Contraceptive use and attitudes in Great Britain. *Contraception* 1993;49:73–86
25. Bounds W. Contraceptive efficacy of the diaphragm and cervical caps use in conjunction with a spermicide – a fresh look at the evidence. *Br J Fam Plann* 1994;20:84–7
26. Smith C, Farr G, Feldblum PJ, *et al.* Effectiveness of the non-spermicidal fit-free diaphragm. *Contraception* 1995;51:289–91
27. Trussel J, Sturgen K, Stickler J, *et al.* Comparative contraceptive efficacy of the female condom and other barrier methods. *Fam Plann Perspect* 1994; 24:66–72
28. Webb A. The female condom – a reappraisal three years on. *Br J Fam Plann* 1996;21:127
29. Beckmann LJ, Harvey SM. Factors affecting the consistent use of barrier methods of contraception. *Obstet Gynecol* 1996;88(Suppl):65S–71S
30. Schmidt F, Sivin I, Waldman S. The copper T 380 IUD. In Bardin CW, Mishell DR, eds. *Proceedings from the Fourth International Conference on IUDs.* Boston: Butterworth-Heinemann, 1994:298
31. Trussell J, Leveque JA, Loenig JD, *et al.* The economic value of contraception: a comparison of 15 methods. *Am J Public Health* 1995;85:494
32. Chi I. What we have learned from recent IUD studies: a researcher's perspective. *Contraception* 1993;48:81–108
33. Tacchi D. Long term use of copper intrauterine devices. *Lancet* 1991;336:182
34. Wildemeersch D, Van der Pas H, Thiery M, *et al.* The Copper-Fix: a new concept in IUD technology. *Adv Contracept* 1988;4:197–205
35. Sivin I. Dose- and age-dependent ectopic pregnancy risks with intrauterine contraception. *Obstet Gynecol* 1991;78:291–8
36. Tatum HJ, Connell EB. Intrauterine contraceptive devices. In Filshie M, Guillebaud J, eds. *Contraception – Science and Practice.* London: Butterworth, 1989
37. Kuzuh-Novak M, Andolsek L. IUD use after 40 years of age. *Adv Contracept* 1988;4:85–9
38. Toivonen J, Luukainen T, Allonen H. Protective effect of intrauterine release of levonorgestrel on pelvic infection: three years comparative experience of levonorgestrel- and copper-releasing intrauterine devices. *Obstet Gynecol* 1991;77: 261–4

39. Andersson K, Rybo G. Levonorgestrel-releasing intra-uterine device in the treatment of menorrhagia. *Br J Obstet Gynaecol* 1990;97:690–4
40. Barrington JW, Bowen-Simpkins P. The levonorgestrel intrauterine system in the management of menorrhagia. *Br J Obstet Gynaecol* 1997;104:614–16
41. Suhonen SP, Holmstrom T, Allonen HO, *et al.* Intrauterine and subdermal progestin administration in postmenopausal hormone replacement therapy. *Fertil Steril* 1995;63:336–42
42. Chi IC. Is tubal sterilization associated with an increased risk of subsequent hysterectomy but decreased risk of ovarian cancer? A review of recent literature. *Adv Contracept* 1996;12: 77–99
43. Peterson HB, Xia Z, Hughes JM, *et al.* The risk of pregnancy after tubal sterilization: findings from the US Collaborative Review of Sterilization. *Obstet Gynecol Surv* 1996;51(Suppl):S8–S19
44. Schwingl PJ, Guess HA. Vasectomy and cancer: an update. *Gynaecol Forum, Med Forum Int* 1996; 1:25–8
45. *International Planned Parenthood Statement on Vasectomy and Prostate Cancer.* IPPF Medical Bulletin 27, 1993:2
46. Glasier A. *Persona.* IPPF Medical Bulletin 31, 1997:3–4
47. Thorogood M, Mann JI, Murphy M, *et al.* Is oral contraceptive use still associated with an increased risk of fatal myocardial infarction? Report of a case control study. *Br J Obstet Gynaecol* 1991;98:1245–53
48. WHO Collaborative Study of Cardiovascular Disease and Steroid Hormone Contraception. Acute myocardial infarction and combined oral contraceptives: results of an international multicentre case–control study. *Lancet* 1997;349:1202–9
49. Pettiti DB, Sidney S, Bernstein A, *et al.* Stroke in users of low-dose oral contraceptives. *New Engl J Med* 1996;335:8–15
50. Weissn N. Third generation oral contraceptives: how risky? (commentary). *Lancet* 1995;346:1570
51. Guillebaud J. Advising women on which pill to take (leader). *Br Med J* 1995;311:1111–12
52. Rosing J, Tans G, Nickolaes AF, *et al.* Oral contraceptives and venous thrombosis: different sensitivities to activated protein C in women using second- and third-generation oral contraceptives. *Br J Haematol* 1997;97:233–8
53. World Health Organization. *Oral Contraceptives and neoplasia.* Report of a WHO scientific group. WHO Technical Report Series. Geneva: WHO, 1992:817
54. Collaborative Group on Hormonal Factors in Breast Cancer. Breast cancer and hormonal contraceptives: collaborative reanalysis of individual data on 53 297 women with breast cancer and 100 239 women without breast cancer from 54 epidemiological studies. *Lancet* 1996;346:1713–27
55. Meirik O. *The Pill and Breast Cancer: New Information.* IPPF Medical Bulletin 30, 1996:1–2
56. Cancer and Steroid Hormone Study. The reduction in the risk of ovarian cancer associated with oral contraceptive use. *N Engl J Med* 1987;316:650–655
57. DeCherny A. Bone-sparing properties of oral contraceptives. *Am J Obstet Gynecol* 1996;174:15–20
58. *IPPF Statement on Contraception for Women with Medical Disorders.* IPPF Medical Bulletin 29, 1995:1–4
59. Fraser I. Progestogen-only contraception. In Loudon N, Glasier A, Gebbie A, eds. *Handbook of Family Planning and Reproductive Health Care.* London: Churchill Livingstone, 1995:91–118
60. Vessey MP, Lawless M, Yeats, D. Progestogen-only oral contraception. Findings in a large prospective study with special reference to effectiveness. *Br J Fam Plann* 1985;10:117–21
61. Chi IC. The safety and efficacy issues of progestin-only oral contraceptives – an epidemiological perspective. *Contraception* 1993;47:1–21
62. Meirik O. Updating DMPA safety. Preface to an issue on DMPA and cancer. *Contraception* 1994;49:185–8
63. Cundy T, Evans M, Roberts H, *et al.* Bone density in women receiving depot medroxyprogesterone acetate for contraception. *Br Med J* 1991;30:13–16
64. Sivin I. Contraception with Norplant implants. *Hum Reprod* 1994;9:1818–26
65. Bromham D. Contraceptive implants. *Br Med J* 1996;312:1555–6
66. Castracane VD, Gimpel T, Goldzieher JW. When is it safe to switch from oral contraceptives to hormonal replacement therapy? *Contraception* 1995;52:371–6
67. Creinin MD. Laboratory criteria for menopause in women using oral contraceptive. *Fertil Steril* 1996;66:101–4
68. Daly E, Vesskey JP, Hawkins MM, *et al.* Risk of venous thromboembolism in users of hormone replacement therapy. *Lancet* 1996;348:977–80
69. Csemiczky G, Dieben T, Coeling Bennink HJ, *et al.* The pharmacodynamic effects of an oral contraceptive containing 3 mg micronized 17β-oestradiol and 0.150 mg desogestrel for 21 days, followed by 0.030 mg desogestrel only for 7 days. *Contraception* 1995; 54:333–8
70. Gebbie AE, Glasier A, Sweeting V. Incidence of ovulation in perimenopausal women before and during hormone replacement therapy. *Contraception* 1995;52:221–2

71. Smith RNJ, Studd JWW, Zamblera D, et al. A randomised comparison over 8 months of 100 µg and 200 µg twice weekly doses of transdermal oestradiol in the treatment of severe premenstrual syndrome. *Br J Obstet Gynaecol* 1995;102:475–84

72. Whitehead M, Godfree V. *Hormone Replacement Therapy – Your Questions Answered*. Edinburgh: Churchill Livingstone, 1992

9
Epidemiology of phytoestrogens and cancer

M. S. Morton and K. Griffiths

INTRODUCTION

Breast cancer and carcinoma of the prostate belong to a group of hormone-dependent cancers that would also include tumors of the ovary and endometrium. These cancers comprise a major proportion of the so-called 'western diseases'. The incidence of and mortality from these cancers are high in the western world relative to the rates associated with Asian populations such as the Chinese, Japanese, Thai and Filipino, and somewhat higher than those for people in countries surrounding the Mediterranean. Cardiovascular disease and osteoporosis follow a similar pattern and would also be considered 'western diseases'.

EPIDEMIOLOGY OF HORMONE-DEPENDENT TUMORS

Breast cancer

Carcinoma of the breast is the principal cause of the death from cancer in women in the developed countries of the west, particularly in the United States and Northern Europe. A recent report[1] confirms that the highest incidence rates are exclusively within the United States with an annual rate of 104.2 cases per 100 000 population observed for white women in the Bay Area of San Francisco. Outside the United States, the highest rates occur in Porto Allegre in Brazil (78.5/100 000) and in Geneva (73.5/100 000). Very much lower rates are reported in Asia with an annual rate of 17.6/100 000 in Yamagata, Japan and 9.5/100 000 in Qidong, China. In England and Wales, breast cancer constitutes 28% of all female cancers with 25 000 women annually presenting and 15 000 dying from the condition each year[2].

Endometrial cancer

In the United States, cancer of the corpus uteri is the third most common cancer in women, with about 40 000 new cases diagnosed annually[2]. The incidence rates differ world-wide by about 25 times between 29.9 and 1.2 per 100 000[3]. White women of the United States occupy a top position for women with an incidence rate of over 20, Hawaiian women in Hawaii also belonging to this top group. Most Canadian and European populations, as well as the black and Asian populations of the United States, are represented in a broad middle group displaying incidence rates from 10 to 20. The Asian populations of Japan, China and India show low incidence rates between 1 and 4, but British, East European, Canadian and South American populations all have incidence rates below 10. The mortality rate from endometrial cancer is much lower than that of incidence. In the Cancer Surveillance, Epidemiology and End Results (SEER) areas of the United States for the years 1973–77, the age-adjusted mortality rate was 4.4/100 000 and the annual age-adjusted incidence rate was 29.7[2].

Comparing the rank order of incidence rates of breast and endometrial cancers, the following similarities are apparent: 19 of 30 populations with top rates of breast cancer incidence also occupy a top position for incidence of endometrial cancer. Fifteen of 20 populations with low breast cancer incidence are also represented at the bottom of the list for endometrial cancer[2]. The figures for incidence and mortality rates should ideally only include women with intact uteri, but this has not always been the case. By 1975, almost one-third of American women over 50 years of age had had a hysterectomy[4]. The incidence rate, adjusted for prior hysterectomy, would be 15 points higher than that of the unadjusted rate in Connecticut[5].

Ovarian cancer

The highest incidence of ovarian cancer is found in Switzerland (St Gall, 17.0/100 000). Iceland (16.6/100 000), Sweden (14.6/100 000), Denmark (14.9/100 000) and Norway (14.6/100 000) also occupy top positions. In the United States, the incidence of ovarian cancer, like that of breast cancer, is higher in white women than in blacks with the highest incidence (13.1/100 000) observed for white women in San Francisco and Hawaii[6]. Most European, Australian and North American populations have incidences in the range 10–12. For Italian, Spanish and Portuguese women, the incidence is somewhat lower than this. The Asian populations of India, China and Japan have the lowest incidences, between 4 and 6/100 000; for women in Qidong in The People's Republic of China, the incidence of ovarian cancer is only 1.5/100 000.

Prostate cancer

Prostatic cancer is already a serious healthcare problem and is one of the most commonly diagnosed cancers in the west[7-9]. World-wide, the incidence in rising annually by approximately 2–3%[2,10]. The lifetime risk of developing prostate cancer is nearly 10% in North American men[1]. A recent report[11] indicates that, in the United States, carcinoma of the prostate is now the second most common cancer after skin cancer in the male population, and the second most common cause of death from cancer after that of the lung. In 1996, 317 000 new cases of prostate cancer were diagnosed in the United States and 42 000 men died from the disease during that year[12].

The highest mortality rates from prostatic cancer are found in the black male population of the United States, twice that of Whites[2,3,13]. The age-adjusted mortality rates per 100 000 vary in different areas of the country, from 18.9 for white males in Arkansas to 55.5 for black men in North Carolina and the District of Columbia. The rate is 30 times less in Osaka, Japan and 120 times less in Shanghai, China than that for black males in North America[6,8,14]. The low prevalence of carcinoma of the prostate in Japanese men is noteworthy as their mean life-expectancy and socioeconomic standards are as high as their counterparts in the west. Epidemiological studies of migrating populations, particularly those populations migrating from China and Japan to Hawaii or to mainland United States, show that the risk of developing prostate or breast cancer increases from a low rate to one closer to that of the indigenous population within a few generations[15-17]. Data from the migrant studies are amassed sufficiently quickly to suggest that the differences can be attributable to dietary and environmental factors and not to the genetic characteristics of the different peoples.

DIET AND CANCER

The significant differences in the incidences of specific types of cancer in particular countries or regions of the world have directed attention to the possible influence of dietary components on the biological processes concerned with carcinogenesis. As a result of many epidemiological studies, it has often been implied that certain of these dietary factors may be 'causative' with regard to certain cancers, whereas others are seen to some extent as 'protective' agents. Some estimates suggest that approximately 35% of cancer deaths may be attributable to dietary habits; Doll and Peto[18] provide some support for this estimate but suggest that a range of 10–70% would be more appropriate.

In general terms, the 'western diet' is characterized by a high fat consumption, whereas the 'fiber' intake is low. In contrast, the proportion of the total calorific intake related to fat in the more vegetarian-style 'eastern diet' is comparatively low, and the fiber content is much higher. Predictably, therefore, western diseases such as cancers of the breast and prostate, and also colorectal cancer and cardiovascular disease, have been associated with fat as a causative factor. Recently, it has been recognized that constituents of the eastern diet may be protective against certain diseases and it is the lack of such constituents, rather than a high fat intake, that is the important factor. The concept is, therefore, that components in the Asian diet and possibly also in the Mediterranean and vegetarian diets are protective against the development of these diseases that are so prevalent in western developed countries. The traditional Asian diet, and to a lesser extent the Mediterranean and vegetarian diets also, are not only low in fat/high in fiber, they are also a rich source of weak, dietary plant estrogens. These plant or phytoestrogens are excreted in large amounts in the urine of Chinese, Japanese[19] and vegetarian[20] men and women, and have many interesting properties which single them out as possible cancer-protective agents in these populations. Two groups of compounds, namely the isoflavonoids and mammalian lignans, have attracted particular attention. Some of these diphenolic phytoestrogens possess weak estrogenic and antiestrogenic activity and, therefore, the potential for exerting an influence on hormone-dependent cancers such as those of the breast and prostate[21].

ESTROGENIC SUBSTANCES IN PLANTS

Isoflavonoids

The presence in plants of non-steroidal substances with estrogenic activity has been recognized for some time, and many hundreds of plants manifest some degree of estrogenic activity[22,23]. Soybean and red clover are members of the leguminosae family and are a major source of isoflavonoids[23–25]. Soya is consumed daily in large amounts in a number of forms in China and Japan and in Asia generally. Soybeans contain the glucoside conjugates of the isoflavonoids genistein, daidzein and glycitein, which can be metabolized by gut bacteria to their respective aglycones. Genistein can be further metabolized to the non-estrogenic p-ethylphenol and daidzein is converted to the estrogenic isoflavan, equol. Recently, other metabolites, such as dihydrodaidzein and dihydrogenistein, have been identified[26]. The aglycones and their metabolites are then absorbed and appear in blood and urine, primarily as glucuronide conjugates, but also as sulfates[21]. Daidzein and genistein were isolated from soya beans more than 60 years ago[27] and 100 g of fat-free soybeans may yield up to 300 mg of genistein[28]. Generally, the presence of isoflavonoids in plants is limited to legumes, although they have recently been identified in beer and bourbon[29,30] and may be more widely distributed than was previously thought.

Lignans

Lignans are another group of polyphenolic plant compounds[23]. The plant precursors matairesinol and secoisolariciresinol are metabolized after ingestion by intestinal microflora to give rise to the weekly estrogenic enterolactone and enterodiol, respectively. The lignans are absorbed from the gut to appear in blood and other body fluids[21]. Plant lignans are widely distributed in nature and precursors are found in many cereals, grains, fruits and vegetables, but the richest source is linseed (flaxseed) and other oilseeds such as sesame[31].

Flavonoids

The flavonoids are closely related in structure to the isoflavonoids, the former having a 2-phenylchroman nucleus and the latter a 3-phenylchroman nucleus[32]. Recently, several commonly occurring plant flavonoids have been shown to possess weak estrogenic activity[32]. Unlike isoflavonoids, flavonoids are ubiquitous in nature, and are found in high concentration in many fruits, vegetables and crop species. In particular, apigenin and kaempferol, both of which are estrogenic, are regarded as two of the major flavonoids because of their common occurrence among plants, and their significant concentrations when they are present. Apigenin, for example, is found in the leaves, seeds and fruits of flowering plants, with up to 7% of dry weight in leafy vegetables. Tea leaves are an excellent source of apigenin[32].

Isoflavonoids and lignans are normal constituents of body fluids and have been identified in most animal and human body fluids by gas chromatography–mass spectrometry (GC–MS)[21]. They are present in urine[20,33], plasma[34], saliva[35] and semen[36]. Analysis of expressed prostatic fluid found that enterolactone and equol were constituents[35,37], suggesting that dietary estrogens can accumulate in the prostate.

The levels of isoflavonoids are high in the urine and plasma of the Japanese and Chinese[19,38], whose traditional foodstuffs contain large amounts of soya in the forms of bean curd (tofu), soybean milk, miso and tempeh. The concentration of lignans is high in the urine of vegetarians[20] whose diet contains whole grain cereals, vegetables and fruits. In western subjects fed 40 g soya daily, the urinary excretion of equol was found to increase 1000-fold above control levels[25,39]. The concentrations of flavonoids in plasma and urine of different populations have yet to be determined and is an obvious program for future research. However, as tea, fruit and vegetables are the principal sources of flavonoids, it is probable that Asians, with their high consumption of tea, and vegetarians have significant circulating levels of these compounds.

BIOLOGICAL PROPERTIES OF ISOFLAVONOIDS AND LIGNANS

Estrogenic activity

The mammalian lignans enterolactone and enterodiol, the isoflavonoids daidzein, genistein, glycitein, coumestrol and equol and the flavonoids apigenin, kaempferol and phloretin all possess weak estrogenic activity[32,40–42]. Some antiestrogenic properties have also been described[43,44].

Genistein stimulates uterine growth in ovariectomized mice[45], sheep[46] and rats[47]. In mice, genistein is approximately 100 000 times less effective than diethylstilbestrol (DES) in stimulating uterine growth[48]. Based on competitive binding to human tumor cell receptors, however, genistein is only 50 times less potent than estradiol[48]. Affinity for estradiol receptors, *in vitro*, clearly indicates a much higher potency for genistein than *in vivo* uterine weight gain assays. Transport and metabolic effects may be responsible for these differences. A recent report demonstrates that genistein binds with a higher affinity than tamoxifen to the newly discovered estrogen receptor β[49,50]. The significance of this isoform of the estrogen receptor to future research on hormone-dependent cancers remains to be elucidated.

In contrast to these estrogenic effects, Folman and Pope[44] reported that both genistein and coumestrol, *in vivo*, can act as antiestrogens by inhibiting the DES-promoted uterine weight gain in immature albino mice. In a more recent report, the citrus flavonoid naringenin has demonstrated similar properties[51]. In rats cotreated with estradiol plus naringenin, significant decreases in estradiol-induced uterine wet weight, DNA synthesis, progesterone receptor binding and peroxidase activity were observed. High concentrations of genistein (> 10 μmol/l) are able to inhibit the growth of MCF-7 cells. In addition, prolonged exposure of these cells to genistein resulted in a decrease in estrogen receptor mRNA as well as a decreased response to stimulation by estradiol[52]. The natural isoflavone kievitone is a more potent inhibitor of proliferation than genistein of the estrogen receptor-positive (MCF-7 and T47D) and estrogen receptor-negative (SKBR3) cell lines[53]. Kievitone is present in red kidney beans.

Cancers of the breast and prostate are initially hormone-dependent in that, if the source of hormone is removed, by castration for example, the tumor will regress. A large proportion of the hormones estradiol and testosterone circulating in plasma are bound to transport proteins such as sex hormone-binding globulin (SHBG) and only about 2% is unbound, and this is considered to be the biologically active fraction which passively diffuses into the target cells[54]. As weak estrogens, phytoestrogens stimulate the synthesis of SHBG in the liver[55]. Therefore, any increase in the concentration of SHBG, by phytoestrogens for example, causes a reduction in the free fraction of the growth-promoting steroid hormone. Higher plasma levels of SHBG and decreased concentrations of free testosterone have recently been reported for vegetarian men when compared to an omnivorous group[56], and also for Chinese and Japanese men[57].

Inhibition of steroid-metabolizing enzymes

Inhibition of aromatase

The aromatase enzyme is responsible for the irreversible conversion of C19 androgens into C18 estrogens. In a recent study, the lignan enterolactone was shown to be a moderate inhibitor of aromatase activity in placental microsomes[58]. Enterolactone was found to bind at or near to the active site of the aromatase, thereby competing with the androgen substrate of the enzyme. Unpublished studies from the Tenovus Institute also show that the isoflavonoids biochanin A, coumestrol, genistein and equol are moderate inhibitors of aromatase in genital skin fibroblasts. The flavonoid apigenin is a potent inhibitor of ovarian aromatase activity in the rainbow trout[59].

The aromatase activity of adipose and muscle tissue is the major source of estrogen in the postmenopausal woman, and elevated aromatase activity has been observed in adipose tissue adjacent to breast cancer[60]. With estrogen synthesis in adipose tissue considered to be implicated in breast cancer progression in the postmenopausal patient, aromatase inhibitors such as aminoglutethamide have been used as a form of second-line breast cancer therapy[61,62]. Plant estrogens, as aromatase inhibitors, may act as a natural form of therapy in Asian postmenopausal women. In western women, breast cancer incidence continues to rise after the menopause, whereas in Asian women, a slight decrease is observed.

Inhibition of 17β-hydroxysteroid dehydrogenase

The enzyme system 17β-hydroxysteroid dehydrogenase catalyzes the interconversion of 17-keto and 17-hydroxy steroids and several isozymes have been identified[63,64]. Thus, the metabolism of testosterone to androstenedione and that of estrone to estradiol is under the control of 17β-hydroxysteroid dehydrogenases. Coumestrol and genistein inhibit the 17β-hydroxysteroid dehydrogenase type I enzyme and, hence, the conversion of estrone to estradiol[65]. In the report of Evans and colleagues[66], several isoflavonoids and lignans were shown to inhibit the conversion of testosterone to androstenedione, with the lignan enterolactone the most potent inhibitor. From this study also, the IC$_{50}$ of an eight-compound cocktail of isoflavonoids and lignans was only 0.7 µmol/l of each compound. Daidzein, genistein, formononetin and biochanin A are strong inhibitors of β-hydroxysteroid dehydrogenases of *Pseudomonas testosteronii*[67]. Diadzein was shown to inhibit the oxidation not only of testosterone, but also that of pregnenolone, pregnanolone, estradiol, epiandrosterone and dehydroepiandrosterone. In addition, many plant estrogens are also inhibitors of the 5α-reductase enzymes[66].

As early breast and prostate cancers are dependent on hormones for growth, the ability of natural dietary compounds to alter either the biological availability or metabolism of these hormones may, over a lifetime's exposure to phytoestrogens, have a significant effect on the development of breast and other cancers in Asian populations.

Phytoestrogens and the menstrual cycle

In carefully controlled intervention trials in premenopausal women of soya-modified hormonal status[68], specifically luteinizing hormone (LH) and follicle-stimulating hormone (FSH) levels were suppressed mid-cycle and peak luteal-phase progesterone concentrations were delayed over a single menstrual cycle. In addition, the length of the follicular phase of the menstrual cycle was increased resulting in a delay in menstruation. None of these changes was observed when soya was replaced with Arcon F, an isoflavone-free soya product[69], providing evidence that phytoestrogens are the biologically active compounds of soya products. In postmenopausal women, 60 g/day soya over a 4-week period suppressed LH levels, while 40 g/day linseed daily over a 6-week period caused a significant suppression of both LH and FSH[70]. Phytoestrogen-rich diets, therefore, exert a weak estrogenic effect on the hypothalamic–pituitary–gonadal axis, resulting in an increase in the follicular phase of the menstrual cycle, and may be potentially beneficial with respect to risk factors for breast cancer. Estrogen exposure and the cumulative number of cycles a woman experiences over her premenopausal years are two important risk factors for breast cancer[71]. Mean cycle length in western countries, where breast cancer risk is high, is 28–29 days, while the average cycle length in Japan, where the breast cancer risk is much lower, is 32 days[72].

In addition to the properties listed above which influence hormone metabolism, dietary isoflavonoids and lignans have many other non-hormonal characteristics which may affect the carcinogenesis process.

Inhibition of tyrosine-specific protein kinases

Tyrosine kinases are necessary for the function of several growth factor receptors, including those for epidermal growth factor (EGF), platelet-derived growth factor, insulin and insulin-like growth factors[73]. In addition, several retroviral oncogenes such as *src*, *abl*, *fps*, *yes*, *fes* and *ros* code for tyrosine-specific protein kinases[74]. Tyrosine phosphorylation plays an important role in cell proliferation and cell transformation and tyrosine kinase-specific inhibitors may well be used as anticancer agents[75,76]. The isoflavonoid genistein has been shown to be a specific inhibitor of tyrosine kinase activity[77]. In addition, the flavonoids apigenin and kaempferol reverse the transformed phenotypes of v-H-ras NIH3T3 cells, an effect mediated via inhibition of tyrosine kinase[78].

Furthermore, genistein induces apoptosis in human breast tumor cells[79], inhibits invasion of murine mammary carcinoma cells[80] and enhances adhesion of endothelial cells[81]. Genistein is a potent inducer of tumor cell differentiation in many types of leukemia and melanoma cells and inhibits effectively their proliferation[82]. Recently, Uckun and colleagues[83] took advantage of this property in treating mice with B-cell precursor (BCP) leukemia by targeting genistein to the B-cell specific receptor CD19 with a monoclonal antibody. At less than 10% of the maximum tolerated dose, more than 99.999% of human BCP leukemia cells were killed which led to 100% long-term event-free survival from an otherwise fatal leukemia.

Inhibition of DNA topoisomerases

The DNA topoisomerases are enzymes which alter the conformation of DNA and are crucial to cell division[84]. By a process involving strand cleavage, strand passage and religation, these enzymes are able to untangle supercoiled DNA. Genistein is a potent inhibitor of these enzymes and is considered to act by stabilization of a putative 'cleavable complex' between DNA and the topoisomerase enzyme[85]. The flavonoids quercetin, fisetin and morin also inhibit DNA topoisomerases I and II, while kaempferol inhibits only DNA topoisomerase II[86]. Inhibition of the topoisomerases is now the target for the design of new anticancer drugs. In addition, genistein is cytostatic, arresting cell cycle progression in G2-M[87,88], and induces apoptosis in immature human thymocytes by inhibiting DNA topoisomerase II[85]. The flavonoid apigenin induces morphological differentiation and G2-M arrest in rat neuronal cells[89].

Inhibition of angiogenesis

Angiogenesis, or neovascularization, involves the generation of new capillaries, a process invoking the proliferation and migration of endothelial cells. Normally, the process is restricted to wound healing, but it is also enhanced in association with cancer growth. Folkman and co-workers[90–92] report that new capillary blood vessels are necessary for a cancer to expand beyond 2 mm in size. Angiogenesis, therefore, exercises an important role in cancer progression and is essentially seen as the growth towards a focus of cancer, of capillary sprouts and columns of endothelial cells from pre-existing capillaries. The process is probably promoted by the production of growth factors by the cancer cells, and fibroblast growth factor (FGF), or members of the FGF family, are recognized as potent angiogenic agents. Genistein inhibits angiogenesis and endothelial cell proliferation[93]. In wound healing, the process is regulated by a balance between angiogenic factors and restraining factors such as transforming growth factor-β (TGF-β). Restraining the process of angiogenesis could inhibit cancer progression, and cortisone and heparin treatment has been reported to suppress the metastatic capacity of experimental tumors by this means[91]; significantly, genistein may have a similar influence. These effects may relate to the inhibition of the tyrosine kinase-associated FGF receptor[77].

Antioxidant activity

Flavonoids, isoflavonoids and lignans are all polyphenolic compounds and can function as effective antioxidants and radical scavengers. Genistein is a good inhibitor of ultraviolet (UV) light-induced oxidative DNA damage and is also a potent scavenger of hydrogen peroxide and superoxide anion[94]. Compounds such as quercetin and cyanidin have antioxidant potentials four times that of trolox, the vitamin E analog. Removing the ortho-dihydroxy substitution, as in kaempferol, for example, or reducing the 2,3 double bond in the C-ring, as in catechin or epicatechin, decreases the antioxidant activity by more than 50%, although these structures are still more effective than α-tocopherol or ascorbate[95]. In addition, flavonoids such as catechin inhibit the oxidation of low-density lipoprotein, an effect consistent with the ability of some flavonoids of similar structure to inhibit lipoxygenases[96].

Inhibition of tumorigenesis

Soybean isoflavones and lignans inhibit experimental carcinogenesis in a wide variety of systems. Of 26 animal studies in which diets containing soy or soybean isoflavones were employed, 17 (65%) reported protective effects[97,98]. No studies reported that soy intake increased tumor development. Most of the studies reporting no inhibition of tumorigenesis employed soya protein isolate (SPI), the preparation of which includes treatment with alkali and is responsible for a 4–6-fold reduction in isoflavone concentration[28]. Of particular interest are the studies of Lamartiniere and colleagues[99,100]. In these, rats were given genistein on days 2, 4 and 6 or 16, 18 and 20 postpartum and, on day 50, they were exposed to the carcinogen, dimethylbenz(a)anthracene. The rats receiving genistein had a longer latency to first mammary tumor and lower incidence and multiplicity of tumors than control animals. A positive correlation was observed between chemoprevention and reduced cellular proliferation, and differentiation of terminal ductal structures. Many *in vitro* tumor model systems are also growth- inhibited by isoflavonoids and lignans, including those for both breast and prostate cancers[101,102]. Genistein and biochanin A, a precursor of genistein, at high concentrations inhibit the growth of estrogen receptor-positive (MCF-7) and estrogen receptor-negative breast cancer cells (MDA-468)[101]. In addition, isoflavonoids and flavonoids inhibit the bioactivation of potent chemical carcinogens. Biochanin A inhibits the metabolic activation of benzo(a)pyrene[103] and the flavonoid catechins from green and black tea inhibit the activation of the potent tobacco carcinogen 4-(methylnitrosoamino)-1-(3-pyridyl)-1-butanone (NNK) and subsequent lung tumorigenesis in A/J mice[104].

SUMMARY

Asian and, to a lesser extent, vegetarian and Mediterranean populations have lower incidences of hormone-dependent cancers than western people who are omnivores. The lower-risk populations consume large amounts of weak estrogens in their diet. Soya is a rich source of isoflavonoid phytoestrogens and it has recently been estimated that the traditionally eating Chinese consumes, on average, 35 times more soya than their western counterparts. Barnes and associates[105] estimate that oriental populations consume 20–80 mg of genistein per day, whereas the dietary intake of genistein in the United States is only 1–3 mg/day. The former figures for daily oriental exposure to genistein are probably an overestimate as Fukutake and co-workers[106] calculate, on the basis of data on the average annual consumption of soybeans and related products, the daily intake of genistein and genistin by Japanese to be 1.5–4.1 and 6.3–8.3 mg per person, respectively. Vegetarians consume large amounts of fruits, vegetables and cereals, foods which contain the weakly estrogenic lignans. These plant estrogens can effect hormone metabolism and availability, and have several other properties which can influence the carcinogenic process. They have been measured in biological fluids by GC–MS, and Asians and vegetarians have high plasma and urinary concentrations of these compounds. A lifetime exposure to isoflavonoids and lignans may, in part, be responsible for the lower levels of hormone-dependent cancers and other degenerative diseases in Asian, vegetarian and Mediterranean populations.

ACKNOWLEDGEMENTS

The authors are grateful to the Tenovus Organisation and also to the University Hospital of Wales Healthcare Trust for generous financial support. They also acknowledge the assistance of Mrs Pat Davies.

References

1. Boyle P, Maisonneuve P. Diet. In Waxman J, ed. *Hormonal Carcinogenesis*. Cambridge: Cambridge University Press, 1998: in press
2. Dhom G. Epidemiology of hormone-dependent tumors. In Voigt KD, Knabbe C, eds. *Endocrine Dependent Tumors*. New York: Raven Press, 1991: 1–42
3. Muir C, Waterhouse J, Mack T, *et al*. *Cancer Incidence in Five Continents*, Vol. V. Lyon: IARC Scientific Publications, No. 88, 1987
4. Lyon JL, Gardner JN. The rising frequency of hysterectomy: its effects on uterine cancer rates. *Am J Epidemiol* 1977;105:439
5. Marrett L, Elwood JM, Meigs JW. Recent trends in the incidence of cancer of the uterine corpus in Connecticut. *Gynecol Oncol* 1978;6:183–95
6. Parkin DM, Muir CS, Whelan SL, *et al*. *Cancer Incidence in Five Continents*, Vol. VI. Lyon: IARC Scientific Publications, No. 120, 1992
7. Silverberg E, Boring CC, Squires TS. Cancer statistics. *Cancer J Clinicians* 1990;40:9–26
8. Zaridze DG, Boyle P, Smans M. International trends in prostate cancer. *Int J Cancer* 1984;33:223–30
9. Sondik E. Incidence, survival and mortality trends in prostate cancer in the United States. In Coffey DS, Resnick MI, Dorr FI, *et al*. eds. *A Multidisciplinary Analysis of Controversies in the Management of Prostate Cancer*. New York: Plenum Press, 1981:9–16
10. Boyle P. Evolution of an epidemic of unknown origin. In Denis L, ed. *European School of Oncology Monograph*. Heidelberg: Springer-Verlag, 1994: 5–11
11. World Health Organization. Trends in Prostate Cancer 1980–1988. *WHO Weekly Epidemiol Rec* 1992;67:281–8
12. Boyle P, Napalkov P, Barry MJ, *et al*. Epidemiology and natural history of prostate cancer. In Murphy G, Griffiths K, Denis L, *et al*. eds. *First International Consultation on Prostate Cancer, Monaco, 1996*. Paris: Scientific Communication International, 1997:1–31
13. Zaridze DG, Boyle P. Cancer of the prostate: epidemiology and aetiology. *Br J Urol* 1987;59: 493–503
14. Skeet RG. Epidemiology of urological tumours. In Williams DI, Chisholm GD, eds. *Scientific*

Foundations of Urology, Vol. II. London: William Heineman Medical Books, 1976:199–211
15. Haenzel W Kurihara M. Studies of Japanese migrants. I. Mortality from cancer and other diseases among Japanese in the United States. *J Natl Cancer Inst* 1968;40:43–68
16. Buell P. Changing incidence of breast cancer in Japanese–American women. *J Natl Cancer Inst* 1973;51:1479–83
17. Shimizu H, Ropp RK, Bernstein L, et al. Cancers of the breast and prostate among Japanese and white immigrants in Los Angeles County. *Br J Cancer*, 1991;63:963–6
18. Doll R, Peto R. The causes of cancer: quantitative estimates of avoidable risks of cancer in the United States today. *J Natl Cancer Inst* 1981;66:1191–308
19. Adlercreutz H, Honjo H, Higashi A, et al. Urinary excretion of lignans and isoflavonoid phytoestrogens in Japanese men and women consuming traditional Japanese diet. *Am J Clin Nutr* 1991;54:1093–100
20. Adlercreutz H, Fotsis T, Bannwart C, et al. Determination of urinary lignans and phytoestrogen metabolites, potential antiestrogens and anticarcinogens, in urine of women on various habitual diets. *J Steroid Biochem* 1986;5:791–7
21. Setchell KDR, Adlercreutz H. Mammalian lignans and phytoestrogens. Recent studies on their formation, metabolism and biological role in health and disease. In Rowland IR, ed. *Role of Gut Flora in Toxicity and Cancer*. London: Academic Press, 1988:315–45
22. Bradbury RB, White DC. Oestrogens and related substances in plants. *Vit Horm* 1954;12:207–33
23. Price KR, Fenwick GR. Naturally occurring oestrogens in food – a review. *Food Add Contam* 1985;2:73–106
24. Verdeal K, Brown RR, Richardson T, et al. Affinity of phytoestrogens for estradiol-binding proteins and effect of coumestrol on growth of 7,12-dimethylbenz(a)anthracene-induced rat mammary tumors. *J Natl Cancer Inst* 1980;64:285–90
25. Axelson M, Sjovall J, Gustafsson BE, et al. A dietary source of the non-steroidal oestrogen equol in man and animals. *J Endocrinol* 1984;102:49–56
26. Joannou GE, Kelly GE, Reeder AM et al. A urinary profile of phyto-oestrogens. The identification and mode of metabolism of new isoflavonoids. *J Steroid Biochem Mol Biol* 1995;54:167–84
27. Walz E. Isoflavon-und Sapogenin-Glucoside in Sojahispida. *Justus Liebigs Ann Chem* 1931;489:118–55
28. Coward L, Barnes NC, Setchell KDR, et al. Genistein, daidzein and their β-glycoside conjugates: antitumor isoflavones in soybean foods from American and Asian diets. *J Agric Food Chem* 1993;41:1961–7
29. Rosenblum ER, Campbell IM, Van Thiel DH, et al. Isolation and identification of phytoestrogens from beer. *Alcoholism: Clin Exp Res* 1992;16:843–5
30. Van Thiel DH, Galvao-Teles A, Monteiro E, et al. The phytoestrogens present in de-ethanolized bourbon are biologically active: a preliminary study in a postmenopausal woman. *Alcoholism: Clin Exp Res* 1991;15:822–3
31. Thompson LU, Robb P, Serraino M, et al. Mammalian lignan production from various foods. *Nutr Cancer* 1991;16:43–52
32. Miksicek RJ. Commonly occurring plant flavonoids have estrogenic activity. *Mol Pharmacol* 1993;44:37–43
33. Kelly GE, Nelson C, Waring MA, et al. Metabolites of dietary (soya) isoflavones in human urine. *Clin Chim Acta* 1993;223:9–22
34. Morton MS, Wilcox G, Wahlqvist ML, et al. Determination of lignans and isoflavonoids in human female plasma following dietary supplementation. *J Endocrinol* 1994;142:251–9
35. Finlay EMH, Wilson DW, Adlercreutz H, et al. The identification and measurement of 'phytooestrogens' in human saliva, plasma, breast aspirate or cyst fluid, and prostatic fluid using gas chromatography–mass spectrometry. *J Endocrinol* 1991;129(Suppl):49
36. Dehennin L, Reiffsteck A, Joudet M, et al. Identification and quantitative estimation of a lignan in human and bovine semen. *J Reprod Fertil* 1982;66:305–9
37. Morton MS, Chan PSF, Cheng C, et al. Lignans and isoflavonoids in plasma and prostatic fluid in men: samples from Portugal, Hong Kong and the United Kingdom. *Prostate* 1997;32:122–9
38. Adlercreutz H, Markkanen H, Watanabe S. Plasma concentrations of phyto-oestrogens in Japanese men. *Lancet* 1993;342:1209–10
39. Setchell KDR, Borriello SP, Hulme P, et al. Nonsteroidal oestrogens in dietary origin: possible roles in hormone-dependent disease. *Am J Clin Nutr* 1984;40:569–78
40. Pope GS, Wright HG. Oestrogenic isoflavones in red clover and subterranean clover. *Chem Ind* 1954;1019–20
41. Bickoff EM. Estrogen-like substances in plants. In Hissaw FL, ed. *Physiology of Reproduction, Proceedings of the 22nd Annual Biology Colloquium*. Corvallis: Oregon State University Press, 1961;93–118

42. Song TT, Hendrich S, Murphy PA. Estrogenic activity of glycitein, a soy isoflavone. *FASEB J* 1997;A601:3472
43. Waters AP, Knowler JT. Effect of a lignan (HPMF) on RNA synthesis in the rat uterus. *J Reprod Fertil* 1982;66:379–81
44. Folman Y, Pope GS. The interaction in the immature mouse of potent oestrogens with coumestrol, genistein and other utero–vaginotrophic compounds of low potency. *J Endocrinol* 1966;34:215–25
45. Bickoff EM, Booth AN, Lyman RI, *et al.* Coumestrol, a new estrogen isolated from forage crops. *Science* 1957;126:969–70
46. Braden AWH, Hart NK, Lamberton JA. The estrogenic activity and metabolism of certain isoflavones in sheep. *Aust J Agric Res* 1967;18:335–48
47. Noteboom WD, Gorsky J. Estrogenic effects of genistein and coumestrol diacetate. *Endocrinology* 1963;73:736–9
48. Bickoff EM, Livingstone Al, Hendrickson AP, *et al.* Relative potencies of several oestrogen-like compounds found in forages. *Agric Food Chem* 1962;10:410–12
49. Gustafsson J-A. Estrogen receptor-β – getting in on the action. *Nature Med* 1997;3:493–4
50. Kuiper GGJM, Carlsson B, Grandien K, *et al.* Comparison of the ligand binding specificity and transcript distribution of estrogen receptors α and β. *Endocrinology* 1997;138:863–70
51. Ruh MF, Zacharewski T, Connor K, *et al.* Naringenin, a weakly estrogenic bioflavonoid that exhibits antiestrogenic activity. *Biochem Pharmacol* 1995;50:1485–93
52. Wang TT, Sathyamoorthy N, Phang JM. Molecular effects of genistein on estrogen receptor mediated pathways. *Carcinogenesis* 1996;17:271–5
53. Hoffman R. Potent inhibition of breast cancer cell lines by the isoflavonoid kievitone: comparison with genistein. *Biochem Biophys Res Comm* 1995;211:600–6
54. Vermeulen A, Rubens R, Verdonck L. Testosterone secretion and metabolism in male senescence. *J Clin Endocrinol Metab* 1972;34:730–5
55. Adlercreutz H, Hockerstedt K, Bannwart C, *et al.* Effect of dietary components, including lignans and phytoestrogens on enterohepatic circulation and liver metabolism of estrogens and on sex hormone binding globulin (SHBG). *J Steroid Biochem* 1987;27:1135–44
56. Belanger A, Locong A, Noel C, *et al.* Influence of diet on plasma steroids and sex hormone-binding globulin levels in adult men. *J Steroid Biochem* 1989;32:829–33
57. Vermeulen A. Metabolic effects of obesity in men. *Verhan-Koninklijke Acad Gen Belgie* 1993;55:393–7
58. Adlercreutz H, Bannwart C, Wahala K, *et al.* Inhibition of human aromatase by mammalian lignans and isoflavonoid phytoestrogens. *J Steroid Biochem Mol Biol* 1993;44:147–53
59. Pelissero C, Lenczowski MJ, Chinzi D, *et al.* Effects of flavonoids on aromatase activity, an *in vitro* study. *J Steroid Biochem Mol Biol* 1996;57:215–23
60. O'Neill JS, Miller WR. Aromatase activity in breast adipose tissue from women with benign and malignant breast diseases. *Br J Cancer* 1987;56:601–4
61. Lonning PE, Kvinnsland S. Mechanism of action of aminoglutethimide as endocrine therapy for breast cancer. *Drugs* 1988;35:685–70
62. Miller WR. Aromatase inhibitors. *Endocr Relat Cancer* 1996;3:65–79
63. Tait GH, Newton CJ, Reed MJ, *et al.* Multiple forms of β17-hydroxysteroid oxidoreductase in human breast tissue. *J Mol Endocrinol* 1989;2:71–80
64. Reed MJ. Oestradiol 17β-hydroxysteroid dehydrogenase: its family and function. *J Endocrinol* 1991;129:163–5
65. Makela S, Pentanen M, Lehtimaki J, *et al.* Estrogen-specific 17beta-hydroxysteroid oxidoreductase type I (E.C.1.1.1.62) as a possible target for the action of phytoestrogens. *Proc Soc Exp Biol Med* 1995;208:51–9
66. Evans BAJ, Griffiths K, Morton M. Inhibition of 5α-reductase and 17β-hydroxysteroid dehydrogenase in genital skin fibroblasts by dietary lignans and isoflavonoids. *J Endocrinol* 1995;147:295–302
67. Keung WM. Dietary phytoestrogens are potent inhibitors of beta-hydroxysteroid dehydrogenase of *P. testosteronii*. *Biochem Biophys Res Comm* 1995;215:1137–44
68. Cassidy A, Bingham S, Setchell K. Biological effects of isoflavones present in soy in premenopausal women: implications in the prevention of breast cancer. *Am J Clin Nutr* 1994;60:333–40
69. Cassidy A, Bingham S, Setchell K. Biological effects of isoflavones in young women – importance of the chemical composition of soya products. *Br J Nutr* 1995;74:597–601
70. Cassidy A, Faughnan M, Hughes R, *et al.* Endocrine modifying effects of phytoestrogens in postmenopausal women and middle aged men. *Am J Clin Nutr* 1998; in press
71. Spicer DV, Krecker EA, Pike MC. The endocrine prevention of breast cancer. *Cancer Invest* 1995;13:495–504

72. Henderson BE, Ross RK, Judd HL, *et al.* Do regular ovulatory cycles increase breast cancer risk? *Cancer* 1985;56:1206–8
73. Hunter T, Cooper JA. Protein tyrosine kinases. *Ann Rev Biochem* 1985;54:897–930
74. Bishop JM. Cellular oncogenes and retroviruses. *Ann Rev Biochem* 1985;52:301–54
75. Schlessinger J, Schreiber AB, Levi A, *et al.* Regulation of cell proliferation by epidermal growth factor. *Crit Rev Biochem* 1983;14:93–111
76. Kenyon GL, Garcia GA. Design of kinase inhibitors. *Med Res Rev* 1987;7:389–416
77. Akiyama T, Ishida J, Nakagawa S, *et al.* Genistein, a specific inhibitor of tyrosine-specific protein kinases. *J Biol Chem* 1987;262:5592–5
78. Kuo ML, Lin JK, Huang TS, *et al.* Reversion of the transformed phenotypes of v-H-ras NIH3T3 cells by flavonoids through attenuating the content of phosphotyrosine. *Cancer Lett* 1994;87:91–7
79. Kiguchi K, Glesne D, Chubb CH, *et al.* Differential induction of apoptosis in human breast cells by okadaic acid and related inhibitors of protein phosphatases 1 and 2A. *Cell Growth Diff* 1994;5:995–1004
80. Scholar EM, Toews ML. Inhibition of invasion of murine mammary carcinoma cells by the tyrosine kinase inhibitor, genistein. *Cancer Lett* 1994;87:159–62
81. Tiisala S, Majuri ML, Carpen O, *et al.* Genistein enhances the ICAM-mediated adhesion by inducing the expression of ICAM-1 and its counter receptors. *Biochem Biophys Res Comm* 1994;203:443–9
82. Constantinou A, Huberman E. Genistein as an inducer of tumour cell differentiation: possible mechanism of action. *Proc Soc Exp Med Biol* 1995;208:109–15
83. Uckun FM, Evans WE, Forsyth CJ, *et al.* Biotherapy of B-cell precursor leukemia by targetting genistein to CD19-associated tyrosine kinases. *Science* 1995;267:886–91
84. Cummings J, Smyth JF. DNA topoisomerase I and II as targets for rational design of new anticancer drugs. *Ann Oncol* 1993;4:533–43
85. McCabe MJ Jr, Orrenius S. Genistein induces apoptosis in immature human thymocytes by inhibiting topoisomerase-II. *Biochem Biophys Res Comm* 1993;194:944–50
86. Constantinou A, Mehta R, Runyan C, *et al.* Flavonoids as DNA topoisomerase antagonists and poisons: structure–activity relationships. *J Nat Prod* 1995;58:217–25
87. Spinozzi F, Pagliacci MC, Migliorati G, *et al.* The natural tyrosine kinase inhibitor genistein produces cell cycle arrest and apoptosis in Jurkat T-leukemia cells. *Leuk Res* 1994;18:431–9
88. Matsukawa Y, Marui N, Sakai T, *et al.* Genistein arrests cell cycle progression at G2-M. *Cancer Res* 1993;53:1328–31
89. Sato F, Matsukawa Y, Matsumoto K, *et al.* Apigenin induces morphological differentiation and G-2M arrest in rat neuronal cells. *Biochem Biophys Res Comm* 1994;204:578–84
90. Folkman J, Watson K, Ingber D, *et al.* Induction of angiogenesis during the transition from hyperplasia to neoplasia. *Nature (London)* 1989;339:58–61
91. Folkman J. Toward an understanding of angiogenesis: search and discovery. *Perspect Biol Med* 1985;29:10–36
92. Weidner M, Semple JP, Welch WR, *et al.* Tumour angiogenesis and metaplasia – correlation in invasive breast cancer. *N Engl J Med* 1991;324:1–8
93. Fotsis T, Pepper M, Adlercreutz H, *et al.* Genistein, a dietary-derived inhibitor of *in vitro* angiogenesis. *Proc Natl Acad Sci USA* 1993;90:2690–4
94. Wei H, Cai Q, Rahn RO. Inhibition of UV light- and Fenton reaction-induced DNA damage by the soybean isoflavone genistein. *Carcinogenesis* 1996;17:73–7
95. Rice-Evans CA, Miller NJ, Bolwell PG, *et al.* The relative antioxidant activities of plant-deirved polyphenolic flavonoids. *Free Rad Res* 1995;22:375–83
96. Mangiapane H, Thomson J, Salter A, *et al.* The inhibition of the oxidation of low density lipoprotein by (+)-catechin, a naturally occurring flavonoid. *Biochem Pharmacol* 1992;43:445–50
97. Messina MJ, Persky V, Setchell KDR, *et al.* Soy intake and cancer risk: a review of the *in vitro* and *in vivo* data. *Nutr Cancer* 1994;21:113–30
98. Hawrylewicz EJ, Zapata JJ, Blair WH. Soy and experimental cancer: animal studies (review). *J Nutr* 1995;125(Suppl 3):698S–708S
99. Lamartiniere CA, Moore JB, Holland M, *et al.* Neonatal genistein chemoprevents mammary cancer. *Proc Soc Exp Biol Med* 1995;208:120–3
100. Lamartiniere CA, Moore JB, Brown NM, *et al.* Genistein suppresses mammary cancer in rats. *Carcinogenesis* 1995;16:2833–40
101. Peterson G, Barnes S. Genistein inhibition of the growth of human breast cancer cells: independence from estrogen receptors and the multi-drug resistant gene. *Biochem Biophys Res Comm* 1991;179:661–7
102. Peterson G, Barnes, S. Genistein and Biochanin A inhibit the growth of human prostate cancer cells but not epidermal growth factor receptor tyrosine autophosphorylation. *Prostate* 1993;22:335–45
103. Chae YH, Ho DK, Cassady JM, *et al.* Effects of synthetic and naturally occurring flavonoids on

metabolic activation of benzo(a)pyrene in hamster cell cultures. *Chem–Biol Int* 1992;82:181–93

104. Shi ST, Wang ZY, Smith TJ, *et al.* Effects of green tea and black tea on 4-(methylnitrosoamino)-1-(3-pyridyl)-1-butanone bioactivation, DNA methylation and lung tumorigenesis in A/J mice. *Cancer Res* 1994;54:4641–7

105. Barnes S, Peterson TG, Coward L. Rationale for the use of genistein-containing soy matrices in chemoprevention trials for breast and prostate cancer. *J Cell Biochem* 1995;Suppl 22:181–7

106. Fukutake M, Takahashi M, Ishida K, *et al.* Quantification of genistein and genistin in soybeans and soybean products. *Food Chem Tox* 1996;34:457–61

10
Ovum donation for premature menopause

H. I. Abdalla and A. K. S. Kan

INTRODUCTION

Women with premature menopause are ideally suited for ovum donation because, without functioning ovaries, better control can be achieved of their hormonal milieu without interference from cyclical ovarian hormones. However, the performance of ovum donation raises logistic, scientific and ethical problems. This chapter will try to address these issues and give an overview of this very interesting subject.

PREMATURE MENOPAUSE

Premature menopause should ideally be defined as ovarian failure occurring two standard deviations in years before the mean menopausal age of the study population. As the epidemiological studies necessary to make such a definition meaningful are rarely, if ever, available, it is not surprising that a number of arbitrary age-related definitions of premature ovarian failure have arisen. These range from onset before 35 years[1,2] to onset before 45 years[3]. The most commonly accepted definition is ovarian failure before the age of 40 years[4-7] which is the definition we have adopted. Premature menopause affects between 1 and 3% of women up to the age of 40. It is associated with 10–20% of primary amenorrhea and up to 18% of secondary amenorrhea. The condition, thus, is not rare, affecting over 110 000 women in the UK alone[8].

In most cases, a definite etiology cannot be established. Among the identifiable causes, genetic disorders predominate in cases that present early, while autoimmune disorders are more common in those with later onset[4,9,10] (Table 1).

HISTORICAL ASPECT

The concept of using donated gametes to achieve pregnancy, however, is not new. In 1884, Pancoast reported the first pregnancy using

Table 1 Causes of premature menopause

Genetic
Chromosomal
　Turner's syndrome
　pure gonadal dysgenesis
　familial
Metabolic
　17α-hydroxylase deficiency
　galactosemia
　myotonic dystrophy
Immunological
　Di George syndrome
　ataxia telangiectasia
　mucocutaneous fungal infections

Autoimmune diseases

Infections

Environmental

Iatrogenic
Surgical
Chemotherapy
Irradiation

Idiopathic

donated sperm[11]. The relative inaccessibility of female gametes and the difficulties of achieving synchrony between the ovulatory process in the donor and endometrial development in the recipient resulted in a delay of 99 years before the first pregnancy using a donated embryo was reported[12]. The following year, Lutjen and colleagues reported the first ongoing pregnancy using *in vitro* fertilization of a donated oocyte in a patient with primary ovarian failure[13]. In 1987, Yovich and co-workers reported pregnancies following tubal transfer of donated zygotes[14]. In 1988, Asch emulated his original work by recording the first pregnancy following the transfer of donated oocytes[15]. The successful application of cryopreservation followed later in the same year, when Abdalla and Leonard reported the first successful birth following zygote intrafallopian transfer of a cryopreserved zygote derived from a donated oocyte[16]. Donated ova, thus, may now be transferred as gametes to the Fallopian tubes or, following fertilization, as pronuclear-stage zygotes or embryos (either fresh or frozen) to the Fallopian tubes or the endometrial cavity.

PROCEDURE

In a natural cycle, the synchronization between embryonic and endometrial development is dependent on the cyclical production of ovarian hormones by the woman. In an ovum donation cycle, the events of ovarian stimulation of the donor and the endometrial preparation of the recipient are two separate events. Correct endometrial development appears to be the critical parameter when assessing the efficacy of different regimens of hormone replacement therapy. The effective oral dose of estradiol appears to be between 2 and 8 mg/day, while the effective progesterone dose lies between 25 and 100 mg/day intramuscularly or 300 mg/day per vaginum. The successful implementation of the fixed steroid dosages as opposed to incremental dosages has made protocols simpler[17], but the perfect protocol is yet to be designed and, as there are certain to be individual variations in response to therapy, the importance of a pretreatment 'dummy' cycle to evaluate histological[18] and endocrinological responses cannot be overstated.

EFFICACY

Most oocyte donation programs have experienced a higher pregnancy rate than usually seen in regular *in vitro* fertilization[19], which suggests that either the quality of the oocytes or of the endometrium is superior. To clarify this issue, de Ziegler and Frydman analyzed the results of transfers of 136 cryopreserved embryos originating either from donated oocytes (18 transfers) or from regular *in vitro* fertilization (IVF) (118 transfers). The transfer of embryos originating from donated oocytes took place following the administration of exogenous estradiol and micronized progesterone. Transfers of embryos originating from IVF took place either in a natural cycle (53 transfers) or after suppression of ovarian function by the luteinizing hormone-releasing hormone (LHRH) analog and the administration of hormonal replacement regimens similar to those for oocyte donation. The pregnancy rate after transfer of embryos originating from IVF was 9% per transfer, which was significantly less than the pregnancy rate of 33% per transfer seen after the transfer of embryos originating from donated oocytes. This suggested that the difference in embryo implantation is not related to ovarian hyperstimulation but that either the embryos originating from donated oocytes are of higher quality or the endometrium is less receptive in IVF patients[20].

The relative importance of the endometrium was studied by Davies and colleagues[21] who prospectively followed 15 patients with primary ovarian failure and who had 21 embryo transfers following *in vitro* fertilization of donated oocytes. All patients had endometrial biopsies taken in a preceding cycle of hormonal replacement therapy. Sixty-one per cent showed delayed maturation compared with the expected appearances for the day of the cycle as assessed by optical microscopy. Patients who conceived had a significantly better endometrial response than those who did not, and 71% (five of seven patients) conceived when the endometrium was 'in phase' (less than 2 days delay).

The authors concluded that endometrial receptivity is a key factor in conception. Endometrial receptivity, however, is not necessarily related to the age of the recipient. Paulson and associates[22] found that, in 418 fresh ovum donation cycles, there was no statistically significant difference in the pregnancy rate attributable to the recipients' age, thus implying that endometrial receptivity is unaltered by age. This is in support of Sauer and colleagues' finding that endometrial biopsy specimens from women both below and above the age of 40 receiving hormone replacement therapy are histologically indistinguishable from normal endometria[23].

On the other hand, Schwartz and co-workers[24] concluded that embryo quality is the most reliable predictor of pregnancy outcome as it was significantly better in pregnant cycles in all four categories of patients, including 12 fresh ovum donation cycles, 10 frozen–thawed ovum donation cycles, 214 standard IVF cycles and 30 frozen–thawed autologous embryo cycles, when compared to non-pregnant cycles, whereas the endometrial echo was only significantly thicker in pregnant versus non-pregnant patients in the standard IVF cycles.

The other factor that might affect the outcome of oocyte donation is the method of embryo transfer. In 1989, Borrero and colleagues reported the first pregnancy obtained using gamete intrafallopian transfer (GIFT) with donated oocytes[25]. Since then, intrafallopian transfer of gametes or, more commonly, zygotes has been used by other groups. Intrafallopian transfer has been shown to be more successful whether the pronuclear embryos (zygotes) were used fresh or after being frozen[26]: in this study, however, the groups were not comparable, as those who received intrauterine transfer had blocked Fallopian tubes with associated adhesions and possibly reduced uterine blood flow. The stage at which the embryo is transferred to the tube is apparently important, as a pregnancy rate of 81.8% has been reported by Rotsztejn and associates[27] when cleaved embryos were transferred to the Fallopian tubes in patients who suffered from premature ovarian failure. These results are far superior to those from any other method of treatment with assisted conception. This success rate represents a 33.3% chance of one implanted embryo developing into a gestational sac, as the authors reported 14 gestational sacs in these nine patients out of 42 embryos transferred. They have postulated that these improved results could be related to: (1) early exposure of the embryo to the Fallopian tube; (2) synchronous arrival in the uterine cavity for implantation; (3) transfer to the tube avoiding the potential mechanical problems associated with uterine transfer.

Fertility in women is known to decline with age[28], strikingly so after 35 years[14]; fecundity being all but lost by the age of 45 years[15]. This reproductive failure might result from either an inadequate endometrium or poor oocyte quality. To establish whether this age-related reproductive failure results from diminished oocyte quality or uterine/endometrial inadequacy, Sauer and colleagues studied the efficacy of oocyte donation to older women between the ages of 40 and 44 years with ovarian failure[23]. This resulted in eight embryo transfers with five viable pregnancies, one with twins. A sixth pregnancy ended in miscarriage. Five normal infants were delivered by Cesarean section and one stillborn infant was delivered vaginally. The authors compared the outcome with those for women under the age of 40 with ovarian failure who also had oocyte donation and ovulating women 40 years or older who were undergoing standard IVF. They found no significant difference in the rate of implantation or ongoing pregnancy between older and younger women who received oocyte donation. These rates were significantly higher than those for infertile ovulating women of a similar age who were undergoing standard IVF. The authors concluded that the endometrium retains its ability to respond to gonadal steroids and provides a receptive environment for embryo implantation and gestation even in older women. Abdalla and co-workers, in a much bigger study analyzing the results of their first 100 cycles of oocyte donation, reported a decline in pregnancy rate with age, with a rate of only 9% in women above the age of 40 years. This was despite the fact that the age of the donor was not significantly different between older and younger patients[26]. This decline in the pregnancy rate was no longer true when they analyzed the results of their first 3 years' experience (371 cycles) with oocyte donation[29]. The same group of investigators has recently published results of a study in which they matched every recipient aged 39 years or less with a recipient aged between 40 and 52 years, with a minimum age difference of 5 years[30]. The matched recipients received oocytes from the same donor. A total of 52 transfer cycles was performed in each age group (young vs. old) and there were no differences in pregnancy (38.5% vs. 38.5%), delivery (25% vs. 23%) and miscarriage rates (35% vs. 40%). This is in contrast with the results of Borini and colleagues[31], who found that the pregnancy and implantation rates were higher in women under the age of 40 compared to those above the age of 40 and concluded that this difference is due to uterine factors. There was no significant difference in the miscarriage rate between the two groups. Although the situation is far from clear, on balance of evidence, it would appear that the age of the recipient does not have as large an influence on the outcome of ovum donation cycles, compared to autologous oocyte assisted conception cycles (Table 2).

RISK

The majority of reports on the outcome of pregnancies following oocyte donation have described the outcome for only a small number of women[34–36]. Pados and associates[36] found that pregnancy-induced hypertension occurred in one-third of women in their series, and that threatened miscarriage in the first trimester occurred in one-third of women also. In the largest series of deliveries following oocyte donation, comprising 232 pregnancies, Abdalla and colleagues[37] confirmed the finding of Pados of an increased incidence of pregnancy-induced hypertension in recipients of ovum donation. The overall incidence in that study was 23% and, in singleton pregnancies, 21%. There was no association between age of ovarian failure and risk of pregnancy-induced hypertension. Interestingly, multiparous women also had a high incidence of pregnancy-induced hypertension (19%); one-fifth of the multiparous women had married for a second time. Other findings were a high incidence of postpartum hemorrhage (11%), with 6% requiring a blood transfusion, and an increased incidence of small-for-gestational-age pregnancies, especially in those with ovarian failure. These complications are not associated with the age of the recipient, and younger and older women receiving oocyte donation should be considered at similar risk. The authors recommend, therefore, that all these women should be cared for by a consultant obstetrician and that cross-matched blood should be available throughout pregnancy, especially during the period following delivery[37].

MORAL AND ETHICAL ISSUES

A mother has previously been regarded as the woman who both produces the ova and carries the child. With the advent of oocyte donation and surrogacy, the terms 'genetic mother', 'carrying mother' and 'surrogate mother' have been added. To those undergoing infertility treatment, the definition of motherhood depends on their predicament. To the couple undergoing surrogacy, the genetic source of the oocytes is of paramount importance. On the other hand, couples on the receiving end of oocyte donation would have no hesitation in considering that the mother is the one who gives birth to the child. It is impossible to decide who is correct.

While patients anxious to achieve pregnancies are favorably disposed towards egg

Table 2 Pregnancy per cycle related to age of recipient*

Study	Group A (age ≤ 39 years)	Group B (age ≥ 40 years)
Navot et al., 1994[32]	11/51 (21.5%)	12/51 (23.5%)
Cano et al., 1995[33]	21/45 (46.7%)	25/45 (55.5%)
Borini et al., 1996[31]	27/57 (47.3%)	14/57 (24.5%)
Abdalla et al., 1997[30]	20/52 (38.5%)	20/52 (38.5%)
Total	79/205 (38.5%)	71/205 (34.6%)*

*Variance 0.513, degree of freedom 1, $p = 0.473$, not significant

donation, the existence of favorable attitudes in others and, thus, the amount of social support that such patients will receive depend upon the wider social environment. A survey of public opinion showed that more than half of the responders of both sexes were favorably disposed towards egg donation. Men exhibited significantly more positive attitudes towards oocyte donation by a sister, than did women[38]. In theory, the donation of oocytes should parallel the donation of semen, but there are important differences. Oocyte donation inevitably requires the donor to undergo the inconvenience and potential hazards of ovarian hyperstimulation and oocyte recovery[39].

Whether or not the parents plan to tell the child of his or her genetic origin is an important issue, and it is recognized that secrets can have a negative effect on the family unit by placing a lie at the center of the most basic of human relationships. Kirkland and associates, in 1992, found that patients who were receiving oocyte donation were equally divided with regard to the issue of telling the child[40]. Two-thirds of the donors thought that they would not want to know of their genetic origin had they developed from a donated egg[41]. As pointed out by Bertrand-Servais and colleagues[42], donor anonymity allows oocyte recipients to impose their own identity patterns onto the future child and to introduce him/her in an unbiased way to their own lives. It is tempting, however, to liken oocyte donation with adoption[43]. On the other hand, Robertson argues that egg donation is preferable to adoption because each rearing parent will have either a genetic or a gestational relationship to the offspring, and he believes that the separation of female genetic material and parenting that occurs in egg donation appears to pose the least risk of family conflict or psychological confusion for the offspring[44]. Whichever decision is made, couples should acknowledge the profound responsibility of following that decision.

COUNSELING

Although infertile couples are not sick, they have been patients as long as they have been on treatment. Their life revolves around their fertility problem, and sex becomes mechanical and occurs on demand. They incur intrusions into the most basic human relationship and, slowly, they lose the closeness that they once had. They become vulnerable because of the pressure they are under, and a gradual loss of confidence develops. Feelings of guilt and jealousy become most upsetting, and they have a profound feeling of grief. Although many of them may be critical of their medical care, when offered any opportunity to have a child, they will be highly susceptible to any suggestions. Gamete donation, although it may initially sound appealing, evokes a wide range of emotional, social and religious thoughts. When a couple feel desperate, they may accept such a suggestion without carefully thinking about the implications for their relationship and any future children. In some situations, apparent acceptance may result not from a positive attitude, but from a sense of weakness and failure. As Mahlsted and Greenfeld discussed, the most important component of preparation is time[43]. It is extremely important, therefore, that clinics performing such treatment provide extensive counseling, which will help the couple to discuss, identify with and accept the issues involved in donor conception. Counseling should also encourage the couple to resolve the way infertility has affected them individually and as a couple. Physicians should be aware that couples may begin treatment with donor gametes before they are emotionally prepared. They should encourage couples, therefore, to examine the implications of their choices and to discuss the issues of secrecy and anonymity.

DONORS

As the procedure becomes more available not only for the treatment of patients with premature ovarian failure but also for women with genetic problems and those who have had failed attempts at *in vitro* fertilization, the demand increases for oocyte donors.

Direct payment for ovum donation in the UK is considered unethical as it lowers human dignity. There is also the concept that the genetic material may result in a new individual who has been purchased. Indirect payment in the form of sharing the cost of IVF treatment between an infertile patient donor and an ovum donation recipient was also criticized, as it was felt that this was a payment in kind to the donors. Despite such criticism, egg sharing does seem to be working well, but Ahuja and colleagues warned that donors should be carefully selected, and that strict common-sense safeguards be applied[45] to avoid 'patient coersion'.

Voluntary, benevolent anonymous donors are by far the greatest potential source of ovum donation, but pose the greatest ethical problems. While not insignificant, the risks from ovarian hyperstimulation syndrome (OHSS) and surgical oocyte retrieval, however, appear to be small. It is vital, nevertheless, to emphasize that oocyte donation is primarily a way to help young women achieve pregnancy.

The need for donor anonymity is complex. Donors may fear contact with these children, and the couple may be vulnerable and confused about a child's feelings towards his/her identity. The Human Fertilisation and Embryology Authority (HFEA) guideline allows donation from known or anonymous origins. The attitudes of donors and recipients in relationship to anonymity were studied by Kirkland and associates, who found that most patients are not secretive, as 86% of donors and 71% of recipients told at least one person other than their partner about their efforts[40]. Donors and recipients differed when the relationship between them was examined. Sixty-three per cent of donors would still donate if the recipient was told their name, but only 23% of recipients would agree to receive oocytes if their name was made available to the donor. Likewise, 70% of donors would prefer to donate to a known person, while only 44% of recipients were prepared to take eggs from a known donor. Although 55% of donors had no objection to the children contacting them as adults, 90% of recipients were against the donor contacting the child later in life. Donors and recipients expressed a preference for anonymity (71% of donors and 86% of recipients). Finally, although 86% of voluntary donors would like to know the outcome of their donations, more than 80% of them denied any connection with that child. These figures indicate that both donors and recipients consider gestational parentage more important than genetic parentage. Khamsi and co-workers, in a smaller survey of 10 recipient couples and their known donors in Canada, found that anonymity was a primary concern for both the recipients and the donors, with 80% of the surveyed couples not planning to inform the child of his/her origins[46].

FUTURE

A new process that allows efficient harvesting from the intact murine ovary and maturation and fertilization *in vitro* of germinal vesicle oocytes has been described[47]. The implication of this study is that some patients from whom ovaries might have been removed surgically and who were destined to have ovarian failure could have their oocytes matured *in vitro*, fertilized and then frozen for future use. Recently, there have been more reports of successful *in vitro* maturation of immature oocytes, fertilization and even the birth of a child[48,49].

Another increasingly established area is 'oocyte self-donation'. This is a situation in which the woman undergoes ovulation induction and egg collection prior to treatment with radio- or chemotherapy that might destroy ovarian function. The collected oocytes will be fertilized by the partner's sperm and resulting embryos are to be cryo- preserved for future use following a successful bone marrow transplant. Ultimately, however, the future of oocyte donation lies with the refinement of oocyte cryopreservation which will solve the problems of synchronization and markedly reduce the need for oocyte donors.

Finally, other unsavory offerings in the future include cadaveric donation and fetal ovarian tissue donation but, in order not to become as disillusioned as one prominent professor in the United States[19], it is necessary, perhaps, to tread warily.

References

1. Jones JS, DeMoraes Rheusen M. A new syndrome of amenorrhoea with hypergonadotrophism and apparently normal follicular apparatus. *Am J Obstet Gynecol* 1969;104:597–600
2. Kinch R, Plunkett E, Sment M, *et al.* Primary ovarian failure: a clinicopathological and cytogenetic study. *Am J Obstet Gynecol* 1965;91:630–44
3. Jacobs H, Murray M. The premature menopause. In Campbell S, ed. *The Management of the Menopause and Postmenopausal Years.* Lancaster, UK: MTP 1976:359–67
4. Conway GS. Premature ovarian failure. *Curr Opin Obstet Gynecol* 1997;9:202–6
5. Aubard Y, Teissier MP, Grandjean MH, *et al.* Early menopause. *Gynecol Obstet Biol Reprod* 1997;26:231–7
6. Moraes M, Blizzard R, Garcia Bunuch R, *et al.* Autoimmunity and ovarian failure. *Am J Obstet Gynecol* 1972;112:693–6
7. Aiman J, Smentek C. Premature ovarian failure. *Obstet Gynecol* 1985;66:9–14
8. Baber R, Abdalla H, Studd J. The premature menopause. In Studd JWW, ed. *Progress in Obstetrics and Gynaecology,* Vol. 9. London: Churchill Livingstone, 1991:209–26
9. Alper M, Garner P. Premature ovarian failure: its relationship to autoimmune disease. *Obstet Gynecol* 1985;66:27–30
10. Rainbowe S, Ravnikar V, Dib S, *et al.* Premature menopause: monoclonal antibody defined T lymphocyte abnormalities and anti-ovarian antibodies. *Fertil Steril* 1989;5:450–4
11. Finegold WJ. *Artificial Insemination with Husband's Sperm.* Springfield, IL: Thomas, 1976:6
12. Trounson A, Leeton J, Besanko M, *et al.* Pregnancy established in an infertile patient after transfer of a donated embryo fertilised *in vitro. Br Med J* 1983;286:835–8
13. Lutjen P, Trounson A, Leeton J, *et al.* The establishment and maintenance of pregnancy using *in vitro* fertilization and embryo donation in a patient with primary ovarian failure. *Nature (London)* 1984;307:104–5
14. Yovich J, Blackledge D, Richardson P, *et al.* Pregnancies following pronuclear stage tubal transfer. *Fertil Steril* 1987;48:851
15. Asch R, Balmaceda J, Ord T, *et al.* Oocyte donation and gamete intrafallopian transfer in premature ovarian failure. *Fertil Steril* 1988;49:263
16. Abdalla H, Leonard T. Cryopreserved zygote intrafallopian transfer for anonymous oocyte donation. *Lancet* 1988;1:835
17. Younis JS, Simon A, Laufer N. Endometrial preparation: lessons from oocyte donation. *Fertil Steril* 1996;66:873–84
18. Sauer MV, Paulson RJ, Moyer DL. Assessing the importance of endometrial biopsy prior to oocyte donation. *J Assis Reprod Genet* 1997;14:125–7
19. Sauer MV. Oocyte donation: reflections on past work and future directions. *Hum Reprod* 1996;11:1149–50
20. de Ziegler D, Frydman R. Different implantation rates after transfer of cryopreserved embryos originating from donated oocytes or from regular *in vitro* fertilization. *Fertil Steril* 1990;54:682–8
21. Davies MC, Anderson MC, Mason B, *et al.* Oocyte donation: the role of endometrial receptivity. *Hum Reprod* 1990;5:862–9
22. Paulson RJ, Hatch IE, Lobo RA, *et al.* Cumulative conception and live birth rates after oocyte donation: implications regarding endometrial receptivity. *Hum Reprod* 1997;12:835–9
23. Sauer MV, Paulson RJ, Lobo RA. A preliminary report on oocyte donation extending reproductive potential to women over 40. *N Engl J Med* 1990;323:1157
24. Schwartz LB, Chiu AS, Courtney M, *et al.* The embryo versus endometrium controversy revisited as it relates to predicting pregnancy outcome in *in vitro* fertilization–embryo transfer cycles. *Hum Reprod* 1997;12:45–50
25. Borrero C, Remohi J, Ord T, *et al.* A program of oocyte donation and gamete intrafallopian transfer. *Hum Reprod* 1989;4:275
26. Abdalla H, Baber R, Kirkland A, *et al.* A report on 100 cycles of oocyte donation: factors affecting the outcome. *Hum Reprod* 1990;5:1018–22
27. Rotsztejn DA, Remhoi J, Weckstein LN, *et al.* Results of tubal embryo transfer in premature ovarian failure. *Fertil Steril* 1991;54:348–50
28. Rosenwaks Z, Davis OK, Damario MA. The role of maternal age in assisted reproduction. *Hum Reprod* 1995;10:165–73
29. Abdalla HI, Burton G, Kirkland A, *et al.* Age, pregnancy and miscarriage: uterine versus ovarian factors. *Hum Reprod* 1993;8:1512–17
30. Abdalla HI, Wren ME, Thomas A, *et al.* Age of the uterus does not affect pregnancy or implantation rates; a study of egg donation in women of different ages sharing oocytes from the same donor. *Hum Reprod* 1997;12:827–9
31. Borini A, Bianchi L, Violini F, *et al.* Oocyte donation program: pregnancy and implantation rates in women of different ages sharing oocytes from single donor. *Fertil Steril* 1996;65:94–7
32. Navot D, Drews MR, Bergh PA, *et al.* Age-related decline in female fertility is not due to diminished capacity of the uterus to sustain embryo implantation. *Fertil Steril* 1994;61:97–101

33. Cano F, Simon C, Remohi J, et al. Effect of aging on the female reproductive system: evidence for a role of uterine senescence in the decline in female fecundity. *Fertil Steril* 1995;64:584–9
34. Sauer MV, Paulson RJ, Lobo RA. Pregnancy in women 50 or more years of age: outcomes of 22 consecutively established pregnancies from oocyte donation. *Fertil Steril* 1995;64:111–15
35. Soderstrom-Anttila V, Hovatta O. An oocyte donation program with goserelin down-regulation of voluntary donors. *Acta Obstet Gynecol Scand* 1995;74:288–92
36. Pados G, Camus M, Van Steirteghem A, et al. The evolution and outcome of pregnancies from oocyte donation. *Hum Reprod* 1994;9:538–42
37. Abdalla HI, Billett A, Kan AKS, et al. Obstetric outcome in 232 ovum donation pregnancies. *Br J Obstet Gynaecol* 1998;105:in press
38. Lessor R, Reitz K, Balmaceda J, et al. Survey of public attitudes towards oocyte donation between sisters. *Hum Reprod* 1991;5:889–92
39. Bromwich P. Oocyte donation. *Br Med J* 1990;300:1671–2
40. Kirkland A, Power M, Burton G, et al. Comparison of attitudes of donors and recipients to oocyte donation. *Hum Reprod* 1992;7:355–7
41. Power M, Baber R, Abdalla H, et al. A comparison of the attitudes of volunteer donors and infertile patient donors on an ovum donation programme. *Hum Reprod* 1990;5:352–5
42. Bertrand-Servais M, Letur-Konirsch H, Raoul-Duval A, et al. Psychological considerations of anonymous oocyte donation. *Hum Reprod* 1993;8:874–9
43. Mahlsted PP, Greenfeld DA. Assisted reproductive technology with donor gametes: the need for patient preparation. *Fertil Steril* 1989;52:908–14
44. Robertson J. Ethical and legal issues in human egg donation. *Fertil Steril* 1989;52:353–63
45. Ahuja KK, Simons EG, Fiamanya W, et al. Egg-sharing in assisted conception: ethical and practical considerations. *Hum Reprod* 1996;11:1126–31
46. Khamsi F, Endman MW, Lacanna IC, et al. Some psychological aspects of oocyte donation from known donors on altruistic basis. *Fertil Steril* 1997;68:323–7
47. Randal GW, Awadalla SG, Shivers A. Isolation, *in vitro* maturation, and fertilization of germinal vesicle oocytes obtained from the intact murine ovary. *J In Vitro Fertil Embryo Transfer* 1990;7:314–20
48. Trounson A, Wood C, Kausche A. *In vitro* maturation and fertilization and developmental competence of oocytes recovered from untreated polycystic ovarian patients. *Fertil Steril* 1994;62:353–62
49. Barnes FL, Crombie A, Gardner DK, et al. Blastocyst development and birth after *in vitro* maturation of human primary oocytes, intracytoplasmatic sperm injection and assisted hatching. *Hum Reprod* 1995;10:3243–7

11
New delivery systems for hormone replacement therapy

I. S. Fraser and Y. Wang

INTRODUCTION

Definition and performance of delivery systems

Delivery systems are 'devices' designed to modify the release of a drug in some specific way, usually at a controlled rate over a specific period of time. They come in a wide range of forms for releasing drugs into different body compartments. The possible routes include slow-release oral tablets, and transdermal, subcutaneous, intramuscular, transvaginal and intrauterine administration. The systems can be designed to release various combinations of estrogens, progestogens and androgens at various dosages appropriate for hormone replacement (Figure 1).

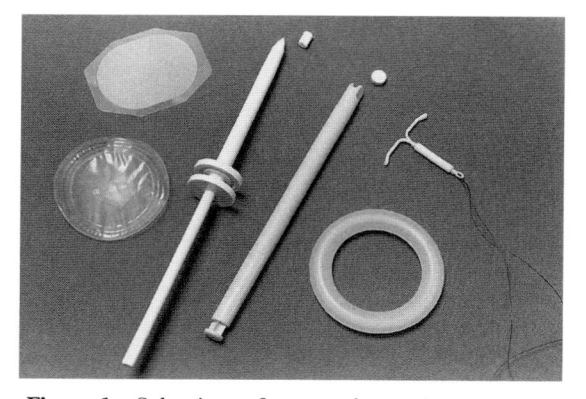

Figure 1 Selection of currently marketed delivery systems for hormone replacement therapy

The pharmacokinetic aim of most delivery systems for hormone replacement therapy (HRT) is to achieve release rates close to zero-order (steady state of release), and thus result in relatively constant blood levels over prolonged periods of time, leading to optimum symptom relief at minimum blood levels with minimal side-effects and metabolic effects. Unfortunately, no system is perfect and all available systems are capable of improved performance.

Need for improved delivery systems

Some women regard HRT as unnatural, unnecessary and even harmful for long-term use. However, from an evolutionary point of view, it could be said that it is 'unnatural' for a large number of women to spend around 30 years of their lives in the postmenopausal phase, for the body was not designed to cope with this. There is a high level of morbidity in the postmenopausal phase, with increased rates of bone loss, cardiovascular damage, central nervous system degeneration and urogenital and skin atrophy, all of which are exacerbated by the dramatic decline in estradiol production. Hormone replacement therapy is a potentially life-extending, bone-conserving, cardioprotective and neuroprotective intervention. Recent data clearly demonstrate that long-term HRT improves general health, reduces morbidity and mortality and increases the quality of life. There is a strong and increasing argument in favor of encouraging the majority of postmenopausal women to seriously consider lifelong HRT. As many women have problems with taking any medication on a long-term basis, one of the aims of delivery systems is to make compliance as easy as possible.

Advantages of delivery systems

Ideally, delivery of different dosage forms of HRT should avoid adverse effects, retain efficacy, and improve patient compliance and satisfaction. These systems should probably mimic the relative proportions of estrogens observed in premenopausal women and provide a serum estradiol (E_2)/estrone (E_1) ratio of greater than 1:1.

Non-oral delivery systems are designed to avoid the large 'first-pass' effect through the gastrointestinal tract, portal system and liver which is associated with metabolic alterations in hepatic protein synthesis, lipid profile and bile composition. Most HRT delivery systems provide long-term constant release of a physiological level of steroids without large fluctuations in E_2 levels, improve the convenience of administration and provide high efficacy, safety and ease of use.

CURRENTLY AVAILABLE SYSTEMS

Transdermal delivery systems

This is currently the most active field for HRT delivery system research and refinement. Several different systems are marketed and numerous systems are under development, utilizing various types of technology with various combinations of steroids over different device life spans and using different adhesives.

Skin-patch delivery systems are usually called transdermal as the drug reservoir remains outside the skin, while steroid-containing gels that are massaged into the skin are often referred to as percutaneous systems, whereby the skin itself acts as a partial, temporary reservoir. Transdermal delivery occurs mainly by passive diffusion of lipid-soluble substances through lipophilic spaces between keratinized cells of the stratum corneum[1,2].

Percutaneous estrogen gels

A number of percutaneous, alcohol-based steroid-delivering gel systems, which contain 0.06% 17β-E_2 (Oestrogel®; Piette International, Brussels, Belgium), or 0.1% 17β-E_2 (Estreva®; Theramex Laboratory, Monaco) have been developed and marketed over the past 5 years. The daily dosage is 2.5–5.0 g of gel which releases 1.5–3.0 mg of E_2. The gel is generally applied to the lower abdomen, arms or shoulder once a day. Unfortunately, considerable interindividual variation of serum E_2 concentration occurs. Absorption is proportional to the surface area of application, intensity of rubbing-in and extent of removal by clothing. Generally, absorption is rapid (within 2–5 min). When used correctly, these systems are effective in climacteric symptom relief and in modification of objective parameters such as vaginal smear maturation and bone mineral density. They have the disadvantage of requiring relatively frequent daily administration[3,4].

Transdermal skin patch systems

Five or six differently constructed skin patches have been studied, but only two types have found favor for steroid delivery: reservoir patches and matrix patches. The newest systems all utilize matrix technology.

Estraderm TTS® (Novartis, Basel, Switzerland) is a well-established transdermal reservoir patch (the first marketed E_2 patch) for the delivery of 25, 50 or 100 μg estradiol per day through a twice-weekly application. It comprises a reservoir which contains estradiol in a gel with a small amount of alcohol as a flux enhancer. Estradiol is released continuously through a rate-limiting membrane upon application of the system to intact skin. The system delivering 50 μg of estradiol per day has an active surface area of 10 cm^2.

In the matrix patches, the hormone is evenly dispersed as a micronized suspension in a very thin adhesive matrix containing, for example, 0.299 g of 17β-E_2 per cm^2. The adhesive containing the active constituent is protected during wear by a backing membrane of flexible trans-lucent polyurethane film. The rate of drug delivery is controlled by diffusion through the skin rather than by use of a rate-limiting membrane as in the reservoir patches. The side nearest the skin is protected before application by a semirigid translucent silicone-coated film. Increasing the surface area of the device results in an increase in the amount of steroid absorbed. Matrix patches have been developed in a range of doses based on patch size; for example, a patch containing 2.2 mg of 17β-E_2 in 7.15 cm^2 will release 25 µg per day; 3.3 mg in 11 cm^2 will release 37.5 µg per day; 4.4 mg in 14.5 cm^2 will release 50 µg per day; 6.7 mg in 22 cm^2 will release 75 µg per day; 8.8 mg in 29 cm^2 will release 100 µg per day. This range of patches will cover the needs of the great majority of HRT users.

In reservoir patches, the absorption process is influenced by the ethanol contained in the drug reservoir. In the immediate phase following its application, the flux of estradiol is proportional to the flux of alcohol which is transported across the skin much faster than the hormone. As a consequence, depletion of ethanol in the reservoir leads to a higher saturation of the drug, and finally leads to a decline in transdermal estradiol delivery. So, the twice weekly reservoir patches have a release profile which gives a very rapid initial rise within 3–4 h followed by a slower rise to a second peak at 48 h and then a gradual decline to low levels at 96 h[5–9].

In the matrix patches, the absence of ethanol results in a different pharmacokinetic behavior. The rate of drug delivery from the system is rather constant over the entire application period, resulting in less fluctuation of the plasma level. The extent of drug delivery depends solely on the E_2 content of the adhesive matrix per unit of area, and the size of the system. Mean serum levels of estradiol of around 90–120 pmol/l can be expected during the use of 50-µg patches, with approximately double the concentration (180–210 pmol/l) from the 100-µg patches. Serum estrone levels are very similar to those of estradiol, and are much lower than those seen after oral administration. The new 7-day matrix patches tend to maintain more constant blood hormone levels (Figure 2) than twice weekly patches or most other delivery systems.

Newer transdermal systems currently being explored include several combination estrogen–progestogen patches, both of sequential and continuous combined types. Sequential

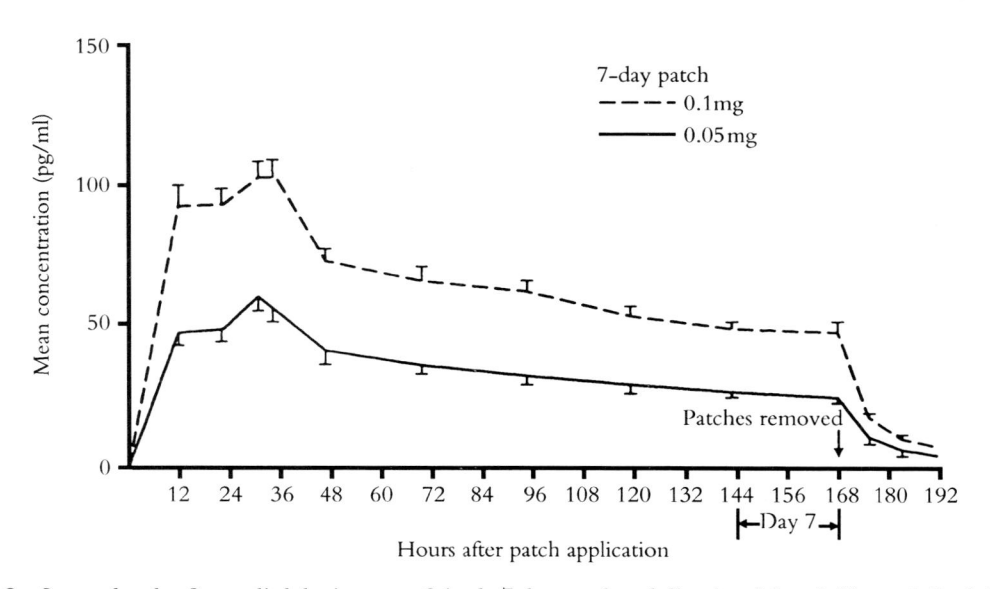

Figure 2 Serum levels of estradiol during use of single 7-day patches delivering 0.1 or 0.05 mg daily. Adapted from reference 8, with permission

'Combi patches' are marketed in several countries. The progestogen is usually norethisterone acetate, and the system generally works well. There is a need for a greater choice of dosage combinations.

Transdermal estradiol-releasing and combination systems are highly effective at relieving the full range of menopausal symptoms, and at prevention and treatment of osteoporosis at low and conventional doses through all post-menopausal ages[10–12]. They contribute to cardioprotection by way of a number of mechanisms including improvement in lipid and lipoprotein levels[10,13], even in women with hypercholesterolemia[14], increased ratio of prostacyclin to thromboxane A_2[15], increased levels of nitric oxide (endothelium-derived relaxing factor)[16], reduction of endothelin-1 (a strong vasoconstrictor)[17] and an apparently more physiological state of the hemostatic balance[18].

Side-effects are relatively minor, the most common adverse effect being skin irritation. This ranges from transient erythema or pruritus to severe contact dermatitis. The incidence is 15–40% in women with reservoir patches, and is less than 10% in the latest 7-day patches[8,19,20]. Some women react to either the adhesive or the alcohol in the reservoir, but not to the estradiol[10]. Occlusion of the skin by the impermeable plastic backing may block sweating, and may occasionally allow microbial proliferation in sweat which exacerbates skin inflammation, Premature detachment is another significant problem. Adhesion is approximately equal for these two kinds of patches in most studies[5], but some have suggested better adhesion in the matrix patches. Breast tenderness, headaches and nausea are generally minor and transient.

Androgen-releasing skin patches have been extensively explored for the delivery of testosterone in hypogonadal men[21], but testosterone does not easily cross the skin barrier and permeation enhancers are required. Unfortunately, these enhancers lead to a high incidence of local skin reactions[22]. It is not yet clear whether these systems will have a role for testosterone delivery in women.

Acceptability of transdermal systems is high in most cultures, and it appears that matrix patches have a number of advantages over reservoirs. The newer adhesives are more effective and less likely to cause local skin irritation.

Subdermal implants

Subcutaneous hormone implants have been in regular use for the control of menopausal symptoms since their first use by Bishop in London in 1938. Estradiol- and testosterone-releasing implants were extensively pioneered by Greenblatt in the 1940s and 1950s and more recently by Studd and colleagues[23]. These biodegradable implants consist of fused, crystalline steroid in a single compressed pellet which erodes very slowly at the surface following insertion, releasing the active hormone into the subcutaneous fat. The implants come in different sizes (e.g. 20, 50, 75 and 100 mg of estradiol), to provide different durations of action from 6 months to greater than 1 year. They have a number of advantages and disadvantages (Table 1).

Subdermal testosterone implants have been used extensively for androgen replacement in hypogonadal males, but their use in women has been more controversial. For some years, they have been used in the management of low libido in women with very low testosterone levels after surgical castration or natural menopause, who have not improved with estradiol alone. They should always be used in conjunction with adequate estrogen (often also given by implant), to reduce the incidence of androgenic side-effects associated with the high free testosterone levels which occur when serum estradiol and sex hormone-binding globulin levels are low[31].

Second-generation, non-biodegradable estradiol implants are now under development. Those studied to date consist of an estradiol-containing polydimethylsiloxane matrix covered with a thin polydimethylsiloxane rate-limiting membrane. Their major advantage is of providing much lower and more constant serum levels. The first silastic implants were 32 mm in length and 2.5 mm in thickness. A set of three implants was found to result in serum estradiol concentrations that were close to those achieved during Estraderm 50 transdermal therapy and led to successful relief of climacteric symptoms for more than a year[32,33]. It should be possible to design a single implant which could last 1–2 years.

The sustained release of estradiol by non-biodegradable silastic implants avoids the problems of symptom recurrence at high, but declining serum levels and tachyphylaxis. Much lower serum levels will also be more easily opposed by lower doses of progestogen. Easy removal of non-biodegradable implants also simplifies the timing of reinsertion.

Intramuscular injections

Injections of estrogenic preparations or combinations of estrogen and progestogen esters have been used for many years for the relief of postmenopausal symptoms, but most of the preparations suffer from a short duration of action and need frequent injections. They also result in very high early blood levels and a variable duration of action. A few combinations can be given at 6–8-week intervals. The progestogen-only preparation depot medroxyprogesterone acetate (DMPA) has been suggested to afford a suitable alternative to estrogen therapy for reducing vasomotor symptoms and may prevent bone resorption[34]. The estrogen–progestogen combination injections are not currently regarded as promising for future HRT systems, but DMPA could be combined effectively with oral, subcutaneous, transdermal or transvaginal estrogen.

Menopausal vaginal rings

Vaginal ring delivery systems for HRT are only in their infancy, although the only hormone-releasing vaginal ring which is currently marketed is an ultralow-dose menopausal ring. Numerous contraceptive vaginal rings are under development, but none has yet been marketed. Menopausal rings for systemic HRT are currently in clinical trial. Most vaginal rings

Table 1 Advantages and disadvantages of subcutaneous biodegradable estradiol implants

Advantages	Disadvantages
(1) Relatively constant estradiol levels, often followed by a slow decline over many months;	(1) Considerable variation in blood levels of estradiol and duration of effect between different women;
(2) Favorable E_2/E_1 ratios;	(2) With higher-dosage implants, especially 100 mg, a type of tachyphylaxis sometimes occurs[29,30];
(3) Excellent symptom relief, although the early recurrence of atypical vasomotor and headache symptoms with the onset of estradiol decline from its initial peak may be a problem in some women;	(3) Relatively short life span of the smaller implants (up to 6 months);
	(4) Cannot readily be removed after insertion if intolerable but rare side-effects supervene;
(4) Decrease in total serum cholesterol and LDL cholesterol and increase in HDL cholesterol[24];	(5) Need regular moderate-dosage progestogen exposure for women who still have a uterus;
(5) 75-mg E_2 implants significantly increase bone mineral density, reduce the rate of skeletal turnover and increase the collagen composition and cross-links in the bone and skin of osteoporotic postmenopausal women[25–27]. Bone mineral density appears to be greater than would be expected in users of conventional oral HRT[28].	(6) Breakthrough bleeding or menorrhagia may occur when progestogen dosage is inadequate[24];
	(7) Occasionally the implants may be spontaneously expelled shortly after insertion, usually because of insufficiently deep insertion (much more common with testosterone implants).

E_2, estradiol; E_1, estrone; LDL, low-density lipoprotein; HDL, high-density lipoprotein; HRT, hormone replacement therapy are designed with a steroid-containing core and outer polymer sheath and, thus, provide a diffusion-controlled release rate adjusted by the thickness of the outer sheath. After vaginal insertion, estradiol from the core is continuously transported across the outer sheath to the vaginal wall, where it enters the pelvic venous (systemic) circulation without first traversing the gut, portal blood system or liver (avoiding the 'first-pass' effect). The life span of the device is mainly controlled by the drug loading in the core.

Vaginal rings have a number of advantages which include:

(1) Provision of great flexibility of dosage, e.g. ranging between ultralow-dose systems and higher-dose systemic-effect rings;

(2) Easy insertion and removal, under the woman's control;

(3) Avoidance of the skin irritations sometimes associated with transdermal patches; nothing is visible as opposed to transdermal and subdermal delivery;

(4) Ready absorption of estrogen through the vaginal epithelium to yield serum steroid values with physiological $E_2 : E_1$ ratios;

(5) High acceptability for many women, provided that they are comfortable about touching their genitalia[35,36].

Ultralow-dose estradiol-releasing system

The only marketed ring is an ultralow-dose estradiol-releasing system (Estring®; Pharmacia, Sweden and Upjohn, USA) which releases estradiol at a constant rate of 5–10 µg/day (mean 8 µg/day) over a 3-month period. This ring is designed for use without an opposing progestogen, because the release rate is so low that, when tested with a progestogen for 7 days, it does not usually induce any withdrawal bleeding from the endometrium. Initially, there is a rapid absorption of estradiol through the very thin atrophic postmenopausal vaginal mucosa, but once estradiol-induced maturation and thickening of the vaginal epithelium has occurred, there is a corresponding reduction in absorption of estradiol[35] and subsequent endometrial proliferation is very uncommon.

This ring is capable of producing a high level of relief from hypo-estrogenic vaginal symptoms and from some urinary symptoms, such as vaginal dryness, dyspareunia, pruritus, dysuria and urgency. All objective signs of vaginal atrophy including vaginal mucosa pallor, petechiae, friability, dryness, mucosal maturation values and other indices of vaginal cytological maturation improve greatly. Progestogen exposure is not necessary[35–37] (Figure 3). Occasionally, women experience mild breakthrough bleeding or spotting, some superficial vaginal erythema and spontaneous expulsion, but endometrial proliferation is rarely recorded on biopsy. Most women express a clear preference for the convenience and efficacy of the ring (compared with estrogen creams), which was graded excellent or good by 84% of Estring users[38].

Higher-dose estradiol-releasing rings

Higher-dose estradiol-releasing rings have been designed to release between 50 and 200 µg of estradiol per day. Most preliminary testing has been carried out in hysterectomized women. Rings delivering approximately 100, 150 and 200 µg/day of estradiol have produced mean serum estradiol levels of between 60 and 140 pg/ml (180–400 pmol/l). These levels lead to excellent relief of postmenopausal symptoms, significant reduction of total and low-density

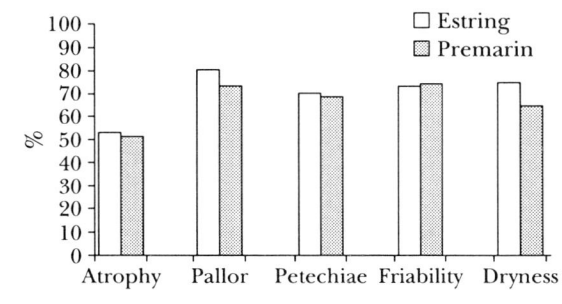

Figure 3 Percentages of women experiencing cure of atrophic vaginal mucosal signs after 3 months of treatment with Estring or Premarin vaginal cream. Adapted from reference 38, with permission

lipoprotein (LDL) cholesterol (no significant change or an increase of high-density lipoprotein, HDL), decrease of serum follicle-stimulating hormone (FSH) levels and increased maturation values of vaginal epithelial cells[39]. Vaginal discomfort, slippage or spontaneous expulsion can sometimes occur, but overall satisfaction with ring use is generally high.

Combination estradiol–progestogen menopausal vaginal rings are currently in the early stages of clinical development, and should provide a valuable addition to the range of vaginal delivery systems.

These systems are likely to fulfill an important role for HRT in most societies in the future, as the vaginal route becomes more widely recognized as an appropriate route for treatment delivery. Acceptability of the vaginal approach to hormone delivery is high in contraceptive trials, and preliminary indications suggest that this will also be true for HRT users (Figure 4).

Intrauterine systems

The levonorgestrel-releasing intrauterine system (LNG-IUS; Levonova/Mirena®; Leiras, Helsinki and Schering, Berlin) was designed as a long-acting contraceptive (5–7 years), but has also proven to be effective in the treatment of menorrhagia and dysmenorrhea, reduction of ectopic pregnancy rate, prevention of uterine fibroid growth, and possible partial protection against pelvic inflammatory disease. It is also a promising system for hormone replacement therapy, as the LNG-IUS can render the endometrium atrophic and insensitive to the proliferative effects of estradiol without causing some of the unwanted side-effects of systemic progestogen.

The release rate for levonorgestrel from the LNG-IUS is 20 µg daily. After its release into the uterine cavity, levonorgestrel is quickly absorbed in small quantities via the capillary network in the basal layer of the endometrium into the systemic circulation. Levonorgestrel can be detected in the serum a mere 15 min after insertion of the device, and maximal serum concentrations are achieved within a few hours. Serum levels remain fairly stable between 100 and 200 µg/l ('minipill' levels) with a gradual decline over time, but the concentrations maintained at up to 78 months after insertion are sufficient to provide effective contraception[40]. The concentration of levonorgestrel is very much higher in the endometrium than in the circulation and the major effects of this device are seen on the endometrium.

This system is highly effective at preventing endometrial proliferation in HRT users[3,33,36,37] and has substantially more effect on endometrial suppression than subdermal administration[41]. At the 20-µg dosage, lipid effects were similar to those seen with oral levonorgestrel[42] and oral norethisterone acetate[43]. It appears to have no significant effect on carbohydrate metabolism, coagulation parameters and liver enzymes.

It appears probable that equally effective endometrial HRT protection could be provided by 10- or even 5-µg daily release. At these dosages, when combined with oral estradiol valerate, the system remained highly effective at protecting the endometrium, inducing amenorrhea, relieving postmenopausal symptoms and producing beneficial changes in circulating lipids[44]. The 20-µg device is relatively wide for insertion through the postmenopausal cervix, and it is hoped that 5–10-µg release rates will allow a more slimline device to be manufactured. A disadvantage of the device is the initial breakthrough bleeding and spotting for the first 2–3 months after insertion, which is usually followed by amenorrhea.

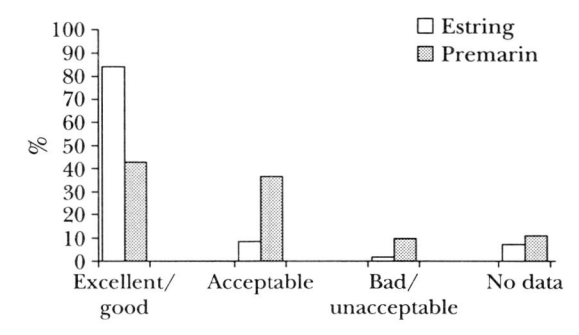

Figure 4 Percentages of women grading different levels of acceptability after 3 months of treatment with Estring or Premarin vaginal cream. Adapted from reference 38, with permission

NEW DELIVERY SYSTEMS

The present systems are still far from ideal and need further development. There are a substantial number of needs in further HRT delivery system development:

(1) The need for greater personal choice, flexibility and control of dosage;

(2) The need to maximize efficacy;

(3) The need to reduce or eliminate present disadvantages;

(4) The need to make really long-term use much easier.

A wide range of technologies needs to be explored further, to achieve acceptable solutions for the needs of widespread, long-term HRT usage in increasingly aging populations. There are likely to be particular benefits for the future development of non-biodegradable subdermal implants, menopausal vaginal rings and purpose-designed intrauterine systems. These 'high-tech' delivery system approaches have the potential for enormous benefit to mankind, but they need to be developed carefully, tested thoroughly and provided by well-trained health professionals to a well-informed public.

References

1. Balfour JA, Heel RC. Transdermal oestradiol: a review of its pharmacodynamic and pharmacokinetic properties, and therapeutic efficacy in the treatment of menopausal complaints. *Drugs* 1990;40:561–8
2. Kligman AM. Skin permeability: dermatological aspects of transdermal drug delivery. *Am Heart J* 1984;108:200–8
3. Suvanto-Luukkonen E, Sundström H, Penttinen J, *et al.* Percutaneous estradiol gel with an intrauterine levonorgestrel releasing device or natural progesterone in hormone replacement therapy. *Maturitas* 1997;26:211–7
4. Foidart JM, Beliard A, Hedon B, *et al.* Impact of percutaneous estradiol gels in postmenopausal hormone replacement therapy on clinical symptoms and endometrium. *Br J Obstet Gynaecol* 1997;104:305–10
5. Erianne JA, Winter L Jr. Comparison of the local tolerability and adhesion of a new matrix system (Menorest®) for estradiol delivery with an established transdermal membrane system (Estraderm TTS®). *Maturitas* 1997;26:95–101
6. Marty JP. Menorest®: technical development and pharmacokinetic profile. *Eur J Obstet Gynecol Reprod Biol* 1996;64(Suppl. 1):S29–33
7. Müller P, Botta L, Ezzet F. Bioavailability of estradiol from a new matrix and a conventional reservoir-type transdermal therapeutic system. *Eur J Clin Pharmacol* 1996;51:327–30
8. Gordon SF. Clinical experience with a seven-day estradiol transdermal system for estrogen replacement therapy. *Am J Obstet Gynecol* 1995;173:998–1004
9. Baracat E, Haidar M, Castelo A. *et al.* Comparative bioavailability study of a once-a-week matrix versus a twice-a-week reservoir transdermal estradiol delivery systems in postmenopausal women. *Maturitas* 1996;23:285–92
10. Jewelewicz R. New developments in topical estrogen therapy. *Fertil Steril* 1997;67:1–12
11. Cicenelli E, Cantatore FP, Galantino P, *et al.* Effects of continuous percutaneous estradiol administration on skeletal turnover in postmenopausal women: a 1-year prospective controlled study. *Eur J Obstet Gynecol Reprod Biol* 1996;69:109–13
12. Evans SF, Davie MWJ. Low and conventional dose transdermal oestradiol are equally effective at preventing bone loss in spine and femur at all post-menopausal ages. *Clin Endocrinol* 1996;44:79–84
13. Castelo-Branco C, Casals E, Sanllehy C, *et al.* Effects of progestogen on lipids, lipoproteins and apolipoproteins during transdermal estrogen replacement therapy with and without medroxyprogesterone acetate. *J Reprod Med* 1996;41:833–8
14. Perrone G, Stefanutti C, Galoppi P, *et al.* Effect of oral and transdermal hormone replacement therapy on lipid profile and lp(a) level in menopausal women with hypercholesterolemia. *Int J Fertil* 1996;41:509–15
15. Viinikka L, Orpana A, Puolakka J, *et al.* Different effects of oral and transdermal hormonal replacement on prostacyclin and thromboxane A_2. *Obstet Gynecol* 1997;89:104–7

16. Cicenelli E, Matteo G, Ignarro LJ, et al. Acute effects of transdermal estradiol administration on plasma levels of nitric oxide in postmenopausal women. *Fertil Steril* 1997:67:63–6
17. Wilcox JG, Stanczyk FZ, Hatch IE, et al. Endothelin levels decrease after oral and nonoral estrogen in postmenopausal women with increased cardiovascular risk factors. *Fertil Steril* 1997;67:273–7
18. The Writing Group for the Estradiol Clotting Factors Study. Effects on haemostasis of hormone replacement therapy with transdermal estradiol and oral sequential medroxyprogesterone acetate: a 1-year, double-blind, placebo-controlled study. *Thromb Haemostas* 1996;75:476–80
19. Speroff L, Whitcomb RW, Kempfert NJ, et al. Efficacy and local tolerance of a low-dose, 7-day matrix estradiol transdermal system in the treatment of menopausal vasomotor symptoms. *Obstet Gynecol* 1996;88:587–92
20. Utian W. Transdermal estradiol overall safety profile. *Am J Obstet Gynecol* 1987;156:1335–8
21. Arver S, Dobs AS, Meikle AW, et al. Improvement of sexual function in testosterone deficient men treated for 1 year with a permeation enhanced testosterone transdermal system. *J Urol* 1996;155:1604–8
22. Jordan WP Jr. Allergy and topical irritation associated with transdermal testosterone administration: a comparison of scrotal and nonscrotal transdermal systems. *Am J Contact Dermatitis* 1997;8:108–13
23. Thom M, Collins WP, Studd JWW. Hormonal profiles in postmenopausal women after therapy with subcutaneous implants. *Br J Obstet Gynaecol* 1981;88:426–33
24. Tzingounis VA, Perdikaris AG, Lioutas G, et al. Subcutaneous hormone replacement therapy. *Eur J Obstet Gynecol Reprod Biol*,1993;49:64–6
25. Holland EFN, Leather AT, Studd JWW. Increase in bone mass of older postmenopausal women with low mineral bone density after one year of percutaneous oestradiol implants. *Br J Obstet Gynaecol* 1995;102:238–42
26. Holland EFN, Chow JWM, Studd, JWW, et al. Histomorphometric changes in the skeleton of postmenopausal women with low bone mineral density treated with percutaneous estradiol implants. *Obstet Gynecol* 1994;83:387–91
27. Holland EFN, Studd JWW, Mansell JP, et al. Changes in collagen composition and cross-links in bone and skin of osteoporatic postmenopausal women treated with percutaneous estradiol implants. *Obstet Gynecol* 1994;83: 180–3
28. Savvas M, Studd JW, Norman S, et al. Increase in bone mass after one year of percutaneous oestradiol and testosterone implants in postmenopausal women who have previously received long-term oral oestrogens. *Br J Obstet Gynaecol* 1992;99:757–60
29. Gangar K, Cust M, Whitehead MI. Symptoms of oestrogen deficiency associated with supra-physiological plasma oestradiol concentrations in women with oestradiol implants. *Br Med J* 1989; 299:601–2
30. Garnett T, Studd JW, Henderson A, et al. Hormone implants and tachyphylaxis. *Br J Obstet. Gynaecol* 1990;97:17–21
31. Burger HG, Hailes J, Nelson J, et al. Effect of combined implants of oestradiol and testosterone on libido in postmenopausal women. *Br Med J* 1987;294:936–7
32. Suhonen SP, Allonen HO, Lähteenmäki P. Sustained-release subdermal estradiol implants: a new alternative in estrogen replacement therapy. *Am J Obstet Gynecol* 1993;169:1248–54
33. Suhonen SP, Allonen HO, Lähteenmäki P. Sustained-release estradiol implants and a levonorgestrel-releasing intrauterine device in hormone replacement therapy. *Am J Obstet Gynecol* 1995; 172:562–7
34. Lobo RA, McCormick W, Singer F, et al. Depo-medroxyprogesterone acetate compared with conjugated estrogens for the treatment of postmenopausal women. *Obstet Gynecol* 1984;63:1–5
35. Schmidt G, Andersson SB, Nordle Ö, et al. Release of 17-beta-oestradiol from a vaginal ring in postmenopausal women: pharmacokinetic evaluation. *Gynecol Obstet Invest* 1994;38:253–60
36. Kalogirou D, Antoniou G, Karakitsos P, et al. A comparative study of the effects of an estradiol-releasing vaginal ring combined with an oral gestagen versus transdermal estrogen combined with a levonorgestrel-releasing IUD: clinical findings and endometrial response. *Int J Fertil* 1996;41:522–7
37. Antoniou G, Kalogirou D, Karakitsos P, et al. Transdermal estrogen with a releasing intrauterine device for climacteric complaints versus estradiol-releasing vaginal ring with a vaginal progesterone suppository: clinical and endometrial responses. *Maturitas* 1997;26:103–11
38. Ayton RA, Darling GM, Murkies A, et al. A comparative study of safety and efficacy of continuous low-dose oestradiol released from an intravaginal ring versus conjugated equine oestrogen vaginal cream in the treatment of postmenopausal urogenital atrophy. *Br J Obstet Gynaecol* 1996;103:351–8
39. Nash HA, Brache V, Alvarez-Sanchez F, et al. Estradiol delivery by vaginal rings: potential for hormone replacement therapy. *Maturitas* 1997; 26:27–33

40. Sturridge F, Guillebaud J. A risk–benefit assessment of the levonorgestrel-releasing intrauterine system. *Drug Safety* 1996;15:430–40
41. Suhonen SP, Holmström T, Allonen HO, *et al.* Intrauterine and subdermal progestin administration in postmenopausal hormone replacement therapy. *Fertil Steril* 1995;63:336–42
42. Andersson K, Stadberg E, Mattsson LÅ, *et al.* Intrauterine or oral administration of levonorgestrel in combination with estradiol to perimenopausal women – effects in lipid metabolism during 12 months of treatment. *Int J Fertil* 1996;41:476–83
43. Raudaskoski TH, Thomás EI, Paakkari IA, *et al.* Serum lipids and lipoproteins in postmenopausal women receiving transdermal oestrogen in combination with a levonorgestrel-releasing intrauterine device. *Maturitas* 1995;22:47–53
44. Wolter-Svenson LP, Stadberg E, Andersson K, *et al.* Intrauterine administration of levonorgestrel in two low doses in HRT. A randomised clinical trial during one year: effects on lipid and lipoprotein metabolism. *Maturitas* 1995;22:199–205

12
Endometrial risks with hormone replacement therapy

J. H. Pickar

INTRODUCTION

Reports of the association of endogenous estrogens, produced by granulosa cell tumors of the ovary, and endometrial hyperplasia and carcinoma have appeared in the literature at least since the report of Stoeckel and Schröder in 1922[1]. Similarly, descriptions of the relationship of endometrial hyperplasia with endometrial carcinoma date back at least to 1936[2]. Case reports of an association between exogenous estrogens and endometrial hyperplasia and carcinoma have appeared at least since 1946[3]. However, it was not until 1975 that studies demonstrated an increased risk of endometrial cancer in women using unopposed estrogen[4,5]; approximately 4 years later, studies began reporting the reduced risk of endometrial cancer associated with the use of combined estrogen and progestin compared with estrogen alone[6,7].

RISK OF ENDOMETRIAL CARCINOMA

In 1975, the simultaneous reports by Ziel and Finkle[4] and Smith and colleagues[5] demonstrated an association between the use of unopposed estrogen and endometrial cancer. In the case–control study of Ziel and Finkle, the risk ratio for endometrial cancer with estrogen use was 5.6 for 1–4.9 years and increased to 13.9 for 7 or more years of use. In the case–control study of Smith and colleagues, the risk of endometrial cancer was 4.5 times greater among women receiving estrogen, and this effect was greatest for women without the known risk factors of obesity or hypertension.

Since the time of those initial reports, numerous epidemiological studies have been performed which have, in general, consistently demonstrated an increased risk of developing endometrial cancer in women with a uterus who

Table 1 Risk estimates from case–control studies of estrogen replacement therapy and endometrial cancer. Adapted from reference 8

Study		Relative risks (compared to never-users)	
Author	Year	Ever-users	Long-term users
Smith	1975	4.5	—
Ziel	1975	7.6	13.9
Mack	1976	5.6	8.8
Gray	1977	3.1	11.6
McDonald	1977	2.0	7.9
Wigle	1978	2.2	5.2
Horwitz	1978	12.0	—
Hoogerland	1978	2.2	6.7
Antunes	1979	6.0	15.0
Weiss	1979	7.5	8.2
Hulka	1980	—	4.2
Shapiro	1980	3.9	6.0
Jelovsek	1980	2.4	4.8
Spengler	1981	3.2	8.6
Stavraky	1981	4.2	14.4
Kelsey	1982	—	8.2
La Vecchia	1982	2.7	—
Henderson	1983	1.4	3.1

take unopposed estrogen (Table 1)[8]. A recent meta-analysis by Grady and co-workers reviewed the data[9]. Their analysis was based on English language studies published between 1970 and 1 April, 1994. The summary relative risk increased from 1.4 (95% confidence interval, CI 1.0–1.8) for less than 1 year of use to 9.5 (95% CI 7.4–12.3) for more than 10 years of use. The relative risk also increased from 3.4 (95% CI 2.0–5.6) for a conjugated estrogens dose of 0.625 mg to 5.8 (95% CI 4.5–7.5) for a dose ≥ 1.25 mg. However, there was no significant difference between intermittent and cyclical estrogen use (relative risk, RR 3.0; 95% CI 2.4–3.8) and continuous use (RR 2.9; 95% CI 2.2–3.8). This last finding is consistent with the work of Schiff and associates who had demonstrated over a decade earlier no difference in the incidence of endometrial hyperplasia regardless of whether the estrogen was given in a cyclical or continuous fashion[10].

Grady and colleagues also reported an increased incidence of endometrial cancer 5 or more years following the discontinuation of unopposed estrogen use (RR 2.3; 95% CI 1.8–3.1)[9]. This is consistent with the work of Shapiro and co-workers, who found rate ratios of 3.5 (95% CI 1.4–8.3) and 4.1 (95% CI 1.1–15) for women who had taken estrogen replacement for 1–4 and 5–9 years respectively and had ≥ 10 years since last use[11]. The report by Shapiro and co-workers also suggested an increase in not only localized (rate ratio 5.2; 95% CI 3.7–7.2) but also stage III and IV (rate ratio 3.1; 95% CI 1.5–6.4) endometrial cancer in women with ≥ 1 year of use. This is in agreement with the findings of Grady and colleagues of an increased risk of endometrial cancer death (RR 2.7; 95% CI 0.9–8.0) in 'ever users' of unopposed estrogen.

The use of combination estrogen and progestin therapy is more recent, and, as such, there are fewer reports on the incidence of endometrial cancer following combination therapy (Table 2)[12–15]. Additionally, the use of various durations and doses of progestins have made the data more difficult to interpret. Initially, progestins had been prescribed for 5–10 days each month and, more recently, they have been used for 12–14 days or more per cycle. Voigt and associates reported, based on a population-based case–control study, relative risks for developing endometrial cancer of 2.4 (95% CI 0.6–9.3) for progestin use of less than 10 days and 1.1 (95% CI 0.4–3.6) for progestin use of 10 or more days per month[12]. This is consistent with the subsequent report of McGonigle and co-workers that both the dosage and duration per cycle of progestin therapy may affect the risk for developing endometrial cancer[16].

Early reports from the Swedish community-based cohort in 1986 and 1989 did not demonstrate an increased risk of endometrial carcinoma following combination estrogen and progestin replacement therapy, relative risks being 0.6 (95% CI 0.2–1.4)[13] and 0.9 (95% CI 0.4–2.0)[14] respectively. Beresford and associates reported the results of a population-based case–control study on the risk of endometrial cancer associated with the use of combination estrogen and cyclical progestin treatment[15]. They reported that women using estrogen with cyclical progestin had a relative risk of 1.4 (95% CI 1.0–1.9), although with the use of progestin for less than 10 days per month the relative risk was 3.1 (95% CI 1.7–5.7). Grady and colleagues

Table 2 Risk of endometrial carcinoma with combination estrogen and progestin use.

Study	Year	Risk of endometrial carcinoma (95% CI)	Progestin use
Voigt et al.[12]	1991	2.4 (0.6–9.3)	< 10 days/month
		1.1 (0.4–3.6)	≥ 10 days/month
Persson et al.[13]	1986	0.6 (0.2–1.4)	—
Persson et al.[14]	1989	0.9 (0.4–2.0)	—
Beresford et al.[15]	1997	1.4 (1.0–1.9)	—
		3.1 (1.7–5.7)	< 10 days/month
		1.3 (0.8–2.2)	10–21 days/month

CI, confidence interval

reported in their meta-analysis a summary relative risk of endometrial cancer of 0.8 (95% CI 0.6–1.2) for estrogen and progestin use. However, they noted a difference in the results obtained from cohort studies (RR 0.4; 95% CI 0.2–0.6) and case–control studies (RR 1.8; 95% CI 1.1–3.1). The three cohort studies each showed a decreased risk in users of combination therapy while the three case–control studies each reported a non-significant increase in endometrial cancer risk[9]. When interpreting these results, the dose of estrogen, as well as the dose and duration per cycle of progestin, should be considered.

Clearly, the use of unopposed estrogen in women with a uterus is associated with an increased risk of endometrial cancer. This risk is both dose- and duration-dependent, and remains increased for a number of years following the discontinuation of therapy. The addition of a progestin for 12–14 or more days per month reduces this risk, but more data are needed to determine whether the risk is reduced to the level of risk for an untreated population. Additionally, the dose of progestin is important and must be matched to the estrogen dose.

ENDOMETRIAL HYPERPLASIA

One of the earliest reports on the association of endometrial hyperplasia and adenocarcinoma of the uterus is from the report in 1936 of Novak and Yui[2]. They reviewed 12 813 case specimens with 804 cases of endometrial hyperplasia and 104 of endometrial adenocarcinoma. They noted that 'one of the most surprising developments' of their study was finding typical and actively growing endometrial hyperplasia 'in women often far beyond the menopause'. They found 40 cases of hyperplasia in women 1–24 years after the menopause, of which 15 cases were in women 15 or more years after the last menstrual period. They also noted the 'surprisingly large proportion' of adenocarcinoma specimens having hyperplasia in the 'uninvolved endometrium'. In the 64 specimens in which both cancerous and non-cancerous mucosa were available, 39% had a co-existing hyperplasia. Novak and Yui concluded that there must be a relationship between endometrial hyperplasia and the development of adenocarcinoma of the endometrium. However, they also stated that the 'ordinary hyperplasia of the reproductive epoch' is frankly benign from the histological standpoint.

Morrow and Townsend summarized the reports of a number of investigators from the late 1950s to the late 1970s, indicating that the reported incidence of endometrial cancer following endometrial hyperplasia was less than 5% with cystic hyperplasia, 25% with adenomatous hyperplasia and 50% with atypical hyperplasia[17]. In 1985, Kurman and associates reported the results of their study, which has become one of the more often quoted references[18]. They evaluated endometrial curettings from 170 patients with endometrial hyperplasia which were accessioned at the US Armed Forces Institute of Pathology. These women did not have a hysterectomy performed for at least 1 year and none of the women received pelvic radiation. Follow-up was for 1–26.7 years (mean 13.4 years). It should be noted that the age range for the patients at the time of initial curettage was 17–71 years. Carcinoma occurred in 1% of 93 patients with simple hyperplasia, 3% of 29 patients with complex hyperplasia, 8% of 13 patients with simple atypical hyperplasia and 29% of 35 patients with complex atypical hyperplasia. Only 1.6% of patients with hyperplasia without atypia progressed to carcinoma while 23% of patients with atypical hyperplasia progressed ($p = 0.001$). The duration of progression in patients with hyperplasia to carcinoma was 9.5 years while it was 4.1 years in patients with atypical hyperplasia.

By definition, all endometrial hyperplasia is proliferative and the finding of an atypical hyperplasia in a postmenopausal woman is a reasonable risk factor for the subsequent occurrence of an endometrial carcinoma. The association of hyperplasia without atypia, particularly simple hyperplasia, with endometrial carcinoma is much weaker[19]. The finding of a proliferative endometrium without hyperplasia in this population has even less predictive value. In clinical trials, determination of the extent of development of endometrial hyperplasia has become the 'gold standard' for predicting the adequacy of the progestational component of hormone replacement therapy. Conversely, progestin doses resulting in complete secretory transformation of the endometrium may be excessive. Similarly, use of the day of onset of withdrawal bleeding may not be as reliable an indicator of risk to the endometrium as hyperplasia. Fortunately, data from both the Menopause Study Group and the Postmenopausal Estrogen/Progestin Interventions Trial (PEPI) confirm that, at the doses studied, in women taking hormone replacement therapy and developing hyperplasia, hyperplasia without atypia is seen far more commonly than atypical hyperplasia[19,20].

The report by Woodruff and Pickar for the Menopause Study Group was the first and, to date, the largest prospective, double–blind, randomized, clinical trial evaluating the endometrial effects of hormone replacement therapy[20]. The study enrolled 1724 postmenopausal women who had not undergone hysterectomy. The participants received either conjugated estrogens 0.625 mg daily or conjugated estrogens 0.625 mg per day plus one of four regimens of medroxyprogesterone acetate (MPA, 2.5 or 5.0 mg daily in continuous combined regimens or 5.0 or 10 mg daily for 14 days of each 28-day cycle). Patients participated for 1 year. Results demonstrated that, by the end of the study, 20% of the women taking estrogen alone had developed hyperplasia (55 cases of simple hyperplasia; two cases of complex hyperplasia); additionally, there was one case of endometrial carcinoma. In the groups taking combination therapy, only about 1% or less developed hyperplasia (all simple hyperplasia); there was also one case of endometrial carcinoma in the group receiving MPA 10 mg. In terms of preventing the development of endometrial hyperplasia, both the continuous combined and cyclical regimens were equally effective (Table 3).

More recently, the PEPI Trial reported results from their 3-year study of 875 postmenopausal women, of which 596 had not undergone hysterectomy (Table 4)[19]. Their findings were

Table 3 Menopause Study Group: incidence of endometrial hyperplasia at 12 months. Adapted from reference 20

Treatment group	n	Patients with positive biopsy specimens n	%
CE (0.625 mg)–MPA 2.5 mg, continuous combined	279	2	<1
CE (0.625 mg)–MPA 5.0 mg, continuous combined	274	0	0
CE (0.625 mg)–MPA 5.0 mg, days 15–28; cyclical	277	3	1
CE (0.625 mg)–MPA 10.0 mg, days 15–28; cyclical	272	0	0
CE, no MPA (placebo)	283	57	20

CE, conjugated estrogens (continuous daily use); MPA, medroxyprogesterone acetate

Table 4 PEPI Trial: endometrial biopsy changes. Adapted from reference 19

Result	Placebo	CE only	CE + MPA 10 mg (cyclical 12 days)	CE + MPA 2.5 mg (continuous combined)	CE + MP 200 mg (cyclical 12 days)
Normal	116	45	112	119	114
Simple (cystic) hyperplasia	1	33	4	1	5
Complex (adenomatous) hyperplasia	1	27	2	0	0
Atypia	0	14	0	0	1
Adenocarcinoma	1	0	0	0	0
Total	119	119	118	120	120

CE, conjugated estrogens (0.625 mg); MPA, medroxyprogesterone acetate; MP, micronized progesterone consistent with those of the Menopause Study Group. Participants received either conjugated estrogens 0.625 mg daily; conjugated estrogens 0.625 mg with MPA 2.5 mg daily; conjugated estrogens 0.625 mg with MPA 10 mg for 12 of each 28-day cycle or micronized progesterone 200 mg for 12 of each 28-day cycle, or placebo. By 3 years, the placebo group had two cases of hyperplasia without atypia and one adenocarcinoma. The estrogen-alone group had 60 cases of hyperplasia without atypia and 14 cases with atypia. The combination groups had 12 cases of hyperplasia without atypia and one with atypia (micronized progesterone group).

These studies provide a reminder that not all endometrial carcinomas which develop in postmenopausal women are hormonally related, and that with appropriate progestin doses matched to the estrogen dose, the risk of developing endometrial hyperplasia, and subsequently carcinoma, can be minimized. These findings are not unique to oral hormone replacement therapy (HRT) but have also been demonstrated with transdermal combinations. In an open-label non-comparative study in 136 postmenopausal women taking transdermal estradiol 50 µg for 2 weeks followed by the same estrogen dose combined with norethisterone acetate 0.25 mg for 2 weeks, after 12 cycles, Lindgren and colleagues found a 2% incidence of endometrial hyperplasia in the 110 women who completed the study, including one case of atypical hyperplasia[21].

A major consideration is the pathologist reporting the results of the endometrial biopsies. Recently, Whitehead and Pickar reported the results from one study in which there was significant disagreement among the pathologists[22]. This difference extended not only to the presence or absence of hyperplasia but also to the classifications given to the hyperplasia. Unfortunately, the current classification of endometrial hyperplasia does not prevent disagreement among those reporting the findings of endometrial biopsies. It is critical, therefore, that physicians be familiar with how their pathologists read biopsies and be willing to consider second blinded reviews of the biopsies when atypical hyperplasia is in question, as this diagnosis frequently results in hysterectomy in postmenopausal women.

BLEEDING PATTERNS

Archer and co-workers reported for the Menopause Study Group the findings regarding bleeding from their study of 1724 women[23]. Among women on the cyclical regimens, 16.1–18.8% of the cycles did not have bleeding. Withdrawal bleeding or spotting occurred in 77–81.3% of the cycles. The mean number of days of withdrawal bleeding was 6.5–7 and for withdrawal spotting 3.4–3.5. Irregular bleeding or spotting occurred in 16.8–19.3% of cycles. The incidence of bleeding was highest during the early cycles and then tended to decrease. The continuous combined regimens were associated with amenorrhea in 61.4–72.8% of the cycles. Among patients, between 40.4 and 52.6% experienced amenorrhea for at least cycles 7–13. Irregular bleeding and spotting occurred in 27.1–38.5% of the cycles. The percentage of patients experiencing amenorrhea increased and the incidence of irregular bleeding decreased with time. With estrogen alone, the incidence of breakthrough bleeding and spotting increased with time and occurred in 24.4% of cycles; amenorrhea occurred in 75.5% of cycles (Table 5).

In a recent report from Pickar and Archer for the Menopause Study Group, it was reported that, for women who had not had a hysterectomy and received unopposed estrogen, the 20% of patients who developed endometrial hyperplasia during the study had more bleeding days than women who did not develop hyperplasia ($p < 0.001$). The predictive value of amenorrhea in this treatment group to indicate a non-hyperplasia diagnosis was 95%. With combination estrogen and progestin regimens, either cyclical or continuous combined, irregular bleeding was not predictive of hyperplasia in this 1 year study[24]. Some irregular bleeding is anticipated as women acclimate to combination therapy. However, data from much longer studies will be necessary to examine the predictive value of irregular bleeding in women who experienced amenorrhea with continuous

Table 5 Menopause Study Group: bleeding patterns. Adapted from reference 23

Bleeding pattern	CE (0.625 mg)–MPA 2.5 mg (continuous combined)	CE (0.625 mg)–MPA 5.0 mg (continuous combined)	CE (0.625 mg)–MPA 5.0 mg (days 15–28: cyclical)	CE (0.625 mg)–MPA 10.0 mg (days 15–28: cyclical)	CE, no MPA (placebo)
Total number of cycles	3782	3726	3772	3732	3639
Amenorrhea incidence (% cycles)	61.4	72.8	16.1	18.8	75.5
Withdrawal bleeding*					
Incidence (% cycles)	—	—	68.4	62.6	—
Mean length (days)	—	—	6.5	7.0	—
SEM (days)	—	—	0.1	0.1	—
Withdrawal spotting**					
Incidence (% cycles)	—	—	12.9	14.4	—
Mean length (days)	—	—	3.4	3.5	—
SEM (days)	—	—	0.1	0.1	—
Irregular bleeding*					
Incidence (% cycles)	22.3	12.7	8.1	8.3	14.6
Mean length (days)	9.8	8.0	4.7	4.9	11.2
SEM (days)	0.2	0.2	0.2	0.2	0.3
Irregular spotting**					
Incidence (% cycles)	16.2	14.4	8.7	11.0	9.8
Mean length (days)	4.9	4.0	2.5	2.5	5.0
SEM (days)	0.2	0.1	0.1	0.1	0.3

CE, conjugated estrogens (continuous daily use); MPA, medroxyprogesterone acetate; *includes bleeding with or without spotting; **includes spotting only, no bleeding combined regimens or regular withdrawal bleeding with cyclical regimens. In an earlier report, Leather and colleagues reported two cases of adenocarcinoma of the endometrium in women who had taken continuous combined regimens for up to 10 years and reported episodes of breakthrough bleeding after achieving amenorrhea[25]. The carcinomas were diagnosed at 2 and 4.5 years of treatment. The first patient had previously been treated with a cyclical HRT regimen for 3 years. Her biopsy prior to starting continuous combined therapy was proliferative. At 1 year, an endometrial biopsy was reported as atypical hyperplasia, at 15 months as cystic hyperplasia, at 18 months as inadequate specimen, and at 24 months as adenocarcinoma. The other patient had received unopposed estrogen for 10 years, had developed vaginal bleeding prior to beginning continuous combined therapy, and her endometrial biopsy before beginning continuous combined HRT was reported as atypical hyperplasia. At 6 months her biopsy was reported as proliferative, at 18 and 28 months as inactive atrophic endometrium and at 54 months as adenocarcinoma. These two cases are instructive in at least three areas. First, consideration must be given to the patients' prior history, especially one which includes the use of unopposed estrogen in a woman who has not had a hysterectomy. Second, the presence of atypical endometrial hyperplasia on an earlier biopsy should be considered even when subsequent biopsies appear normal. Third, until additional data are available from large long-term studies, consideration should be given when bleeding develops in women who previously had amenorrhea on continuous combined therapy.

Other causes of abnormal uterine bleeding in addition to hyperplasia and malignancy must also be considered. Nagele and associates presented results of hysteroscopies performed on 157 women with abnormal uterine bleeding taking replacement therapy[26]. Five of the women failed to have a satisfactory hysteroscopy. Healthy functional endometrium was found in 46.1% of the women with a successful hysteroscopy. Focal lesions including submucous myomas and endometrial polyps were found in 42.7%. These findings are consistent with previous studies identifying structural abnormalities in significant numbers of patients having abnormal uterine bleeding while receiving replacement therapy. Downes and Al-Azzawi reported a 'high incidence' (47.6%) of structural lesions in women taking hormone replacement therapy and having irregular or heavy bleeding[27]. Townsend and colleagues reported reasonable outcomes in these patients following removal of the polyp or myoma[28].

LONG-CYCLE THERAPY

The role of long-cycle regimens of hormone replacement therapy, such as those with quarterly progestin, require additional study before drawing firm conclusions. The Scandinavian Long Cycle Study evaluated a regimen consisting of cycles of estradiol 2 mg daily for 68 days followed by estradiol 2 mg and norethindrone 1 mg for 10 days and then estradiol 1 mg for 6 days[29]. The study was discontinued after 3 years when 15 of 243 patients had either developed simple hyperplasia (8), complex hyperplasia (6, one with atypia) or endometrial cancer (1). The monthly cycle control group had one case each of simple and complex hyperplasia. This was principally an estradiol 2 mg regimen with a moderate progestin dose given for a reasonably short duration. In the study of Boerrigter and co-workers, 30 postmenopausal women were assigned to one of three groups. Both estradiol 1- and 2-mg regimens were studied along with a combination 1- and 2-mg or 'step-up' regimen[30]. In each cycle, the estrogen was taken for 84 days and gestodene 50 µg was also taken for the last 12 days. The study was two cycles in length. Endometrial biopsies were performed after the withdrawal bleeding in the beginning of cycle two (days 8–11), after the estrogen-only phase in cycle two (days 70–72) and then 8–11 days after stopping all medication. No hyperplasias were found in the first biopsy after the progestin. However, the estradiol 1-mg and estradiol 2-mg groups each had one hyperplasia, and the step-up regimen had two hyperplasias, at the second biopsy prior to the progestin phase (all cases were simple hyperplasia), although none of the patients had hyperplasia at the third biopsy following the progestin phase. With monthly cyclical regimens and continuous combined regimens, the objective has been to prevent excessive endometrial stimulation and the development of hyperplasia. It appears that, with long-cycle regimens, we may be routinely treating hyperplasias. If this is the case, significantly longer periods of follow-up than have been necessary for monthly cyclical or continuous combined regimens may be necessary to insure that the progestational treatment is adequate.

TRANSVAGINAL SONOGRAPHY

The measurement of endometrial thickness by transvaginal sonography (TVS) has become a useful tool for evaluating the endometria of postmenopausal women. Meuwissen and colleagues followed the endometrial responses of 184 non-hysterectomized women receiving unopposed estrogen for 4 weeks up to 24 months with TVS[31]. In part, these women were to have had amenorrhea for at least 3 months and a double layer endometrial thickness of 4 mm or less for inclusion in the study. Transvaginal sonography was repeated 4–6 weeks after initiation of therapy and, based on the endometrial thickness, at an interval of 4–16 weeks thereafter. Endometrial sampling was performed when the endometrial thickness by TVS was 8 mm or more, when there was vaginal bleeding and at 1 year. When the endometrial thickness reached 8 mm or more with unopposed estrogen, a progestin was given for 12 days and the estrogen was withheld for 3 weeks. Progestins were also given when there was vaginal bleeding and biopsy results suggested 'endometrial abnormality'. By the end of 2 years, all but 21 women had either discontinued the unopposed estrogen treatment or had episodes of progestin addition. Sixteen cases of endometrial hyperplasia were identified, five on the first on-treatment biopsy. The minimum endometrial thickness at which hyperplasia was found was 5 mm, and three cases were identified with a thickness of less than 8 mm. Eight cases of hyperplasia occurred within 4 months of initiating treatment and, in three of these cases, within 2 months and without apparent explanation. The finding of these early hyperplasias is consistent with that of Boerrigter and co-workers in their study of quarterly progestin regimens. The majority of atrophic endometria (43) occurred with a thickness of 7 mm or less, although, there were five in the 8–10-mm range and one in the ≥ 17-mm range. The authors concluded that, for women with a uterus receiving unopposed estrogen, TVS alone was of only limited value as the 4-mm cut-off for normal endometrial thickness was rapidly reached.

Granberg and associates reported the TVS findings from a Nordic multicenter study, for a group of 1110 women with postmenopausal bleeding scheduled for curettage, who had been receiving either combination estrogen and progestin (202), estrogen alone (149) or not receiving replacement therapy (759)[32]. Transvaginal sonography was performed either the same day as, or up to 3 days prior to, curettage. There were a total of 112 hyperplasias. Endometrial thickness was found to be 1–4 mm in six cases, 5–8 mm in 27 cases and > 8 mm in 79 cases. Additionally, there were 114 endometrial cancers. Endometrial thickness in nine cases was 5–8 mm, in 105 cases it was > 8 mm and there were no cases reported with 1–4-mm thickness. Endometrial polyps were found in 140 cases: six had an endometrial thickness of 1–4 mm, 29 had a thickness of 5–8 mm and 105 had a thickness of > 8 mm. They concluded that TVS is a valuable tool for excluding endometrial abnormalities in women regardless of whether they receive hormone replacement therapy. Additionally, the endometrial thickness cut-off should be < 4 mm, regardless of whether they receive hormone replacement therapy.

SUMMARY

In women with a uterus, unopposed estrogen replacement therapy is associated with an increased risk of endometrial hyperplasia and cancer. Combination estrogen and progestin replacement therapy with appropriately selected and matched doses significantly reduces this risk. The role of long-cycle regimens is, at this time, unclear. Endometrial biopsy or curettage continues to be the gold standard for evaluating the effects of hormone replacement therapy on endometrial histology. Familiarity with the way individual pathologists report endometrial findings is critical to the care of patients. Both hysteroscopy and transvaginal sonography are useful tools to aid in the evaluation of the endometrium.

Combination estrogen with cyclical progestin replacement is usually associated with regular withdrawal bleeding, while continuous combined regimens are associated with increasing amenorrhea with time. Estrogen alone, although initially associated with amenorrhea, is associated with an increasing incidence of breakthrough bleeding with time. Although amenorrhea with estrogen-alone regimens was 95% predictive of a non-hyperplasia diagnosis, irregular bleeding with combination estrogen and progestin therapy was not predictive of hyperplasia in a 1 year study. Nevertheless, persistent unexplained irregular bleeding should be appropriately evaluated, not only to rule out hyperplasia or malignancy, but also to identify other treatable causes such as endometrial polyps or myomas.

References

1. Stoeckel and Schröder. Nordwestdeutsch Gesellschaft für Gynakologie. *Zentralbl Gynakol* 1922;46:193–208
2. Novak E, Yui E. Relation of endometrial hyperplasia to adenocarcinoma of the uterus. *Am J Obstet Gynecol* 1936;32:674–98
3. Fremont-Smith M, Meigs JV, Graham RM, et al. Cancer of the endometrium and prolonged estrogen therapy. *J Am Med Assoc* 1946;131:805–8
4. Ziel HK, Finkle WD. Increased risk of endometrial carcinoma among users of conjugated estrogens. *N Engl J Med* 1975;293:1167–70
5. Smith DC, Prentice R, Thompson DJ, et al. Association of exogenous estrogen and endometrial carcinoma. *N Engl J Med* 1975;293:1164–7
6. Hammond CB, Jelovsek FR, Lee KL, et al. Effects of long-term estrogen replacement therapy. II. Neoplasia. *Am J Obstet Gynecol* 1979;133:537–47
7. Gambrell RD, Massey FM, Casteneda TA, et al. Reduced incidence of endometrial cancer among postmenopausal women treated with progestogens. *J Am Geriatr Soc* 1979;27:389–94
8. Peterson HB, et al. In Mishell DR, ed. Genital neoplasia. *Menopause: Physiology and Pharmacology*. Chicago: Yearbook Medical Publishers, 1987:275–98
9. Grady D, Gebretsadik T, Kerlikowske K, et al. Hormone replacement therapy and endometrial cancer risk: a meta-analysis. *Obstet Gynecol* 1995;85:304–13
10. Schiff I, Komarov Sela H, Cramer DM, et al. Endometrial hyperplasia in women on cyclic or continuous estrogen regimens. *Fertil Steril* 1982;37:79–82
11. Shapiro S, Kelly JP, Rosenberg L, et al. Risk of localized and widespread endometrial cancer in relation to recent and discontinued use of conjugated estrogens. *N Engl J Med* 1985;313:969–72
12. Voigt LF, Weiss NS, Chu J, et al. Progestagen supplementation of exogenous oestrogens and risk of endometrial cancer. *Lancet* 1991;338:274–7
13. Persson IR, Adami HO, Eklund G, et al. The risk of endometrial neoplasia and treatment with estrogens and estrogen–progestogen combinations. *Acta Obstes Gynecol Scand* 1986;65:211–17
14. Persson I, Adami HO, Bergkvist L, et al. Risk of endometrial cancer after treatment with oestrogens alone or in conjunction with progestogens: results of a prospective study. *Br Med J* 1989;298:147–51
15. Beresford SAA, Weiss NS, Voigt LF, et al. Risk of endometrial cancer in relation to use of oestrogen combined with cyclic progestagen therapy in postmenopausal women. *Lancet* 1997;349:458–61
16. McGonigle KF, Karlan BY, Barbuto DA. Development of endometrial cancer in women on estrogen and progestin hormone replacement therapy. *Gynecol Oncol* 1994;55:126–32
17. Morrow CP, Townsend DE. Cancer of the uterine corpus. Endometrial hyperplasia. In *Synopsis of Gynecologic Oncology*. New York: John Wiley, 1981:133–85
18. Kurman RJ, Kaminski PF, Norris RJ. The behavior of endometrial hyperplasia. A long-term study of untreated hyperplasia in 170 patients. *Cancer* 1985;56:403–12

19. The Writing Group for the PEPI Trial. Effects of hormone replacement therapy on endometrial histology in postmenopausal women. The Postmenopausal Estrogen/Progestin Interventions (PEPI) Trial. *J Am Med Assoc* 1996;275:370–5
20. Woodruff JD, Pickar JH for the Menopause Study Group. Incidence of endometrial hyperplasia in postmenopausal women taking conjugated estrogens (Premarin) with medroxyprogesterone acetate or conjugated estrogens alone. *Am J Obstet Gynecol* 1994;170:1213–23
21. Lindgren R, Risberg B, Hammar M, *et al.* Endometrial effects of transdermal estradiol/norethisterone acetate. *Maturitas* 1992;15:71–8
22. Whitehead MI, Pickar JH. Variation between pathologists in the reportings of endometrial histology with combination oestrogen/progestogen therapies. Presented at *British Medical Society Meeting*, Exeter, UK, July 1996
23. Archer DF, Pickar JH, Bottiglioni F for the Menopause Study Group. Bleeding patterns in postmenopausal women taking continuous combined or sequential regimens of conjugated estrogens with medroxyprogesterone acetate. *Obstet Gynecol* 1994;83:686–92
24. Pickar JH, Archer DF for the Menopause Study Group. Is bleeding a predictor of endometrial hyperplasia in postmenopausal women receiving hormone replacement therapy? *Am J Obstet Gynecol,* 1997;177:1178–83
25. Leather AT, Savvas M, Studd JWW. Endometrial histology and bleeding patterns after 8 years of continuous combined estrogen and progestogen therapy in postmenopausal women. *Obstet Gynecol* 1991;78:1008–10
26. Nagele F, O'Connor H, Baskett TF, *et al.* Hysteroscopy in women with abnormal uterine bleeding on hormone replacement therapy: a comparison with postmenopausal bleeding. *Fertil Steril* 1996;65:1145–50
27. Downes E, Al-Azzawi F. The predictive value of outpatient hysteroscopy in a menopause clinic. *Br J Obstet Gynaecol* 1993;100:1148–9
28. Townsend DE, Fields G, McCausland A, *et al.* Diagnostic and operative hysteroscopy in the management of persistent postmenopausal bleeding. *Obstet Gynecol* 1993;82:419–21
29. Cerin A, Heldaas K, Moeller B for the Scandinavian Long Cycle Study Group. Adverse endometrial effects of long-cycle estrogen and progestogen replacement therapy (letter). *N Engl J Med* 1996;334:668–9
30. Boerrigter PJ, van de Weijer PHM, Baak JPA, *et al.* Endometrial response in estrogen replacement therapy quarterly combined with a progestogen. *Maturitas* 1996;24:63–71
31. Meuwissen JHJM, Oddens BJ, Klinkhamer PJJM. Endometrial thickness assessed by transvaginal ultrasound insufficiently predicts occurrence of hyperplasia during unopposed oestrogen use. *Maturitas* 1996;24:21–30
32. Granberg S, Ylostalo P, Wikland M, *et al.* Endometrial sonographic and histologic findings in women with and without hormonal replacement therapy suffering from postmenopausal bleeding. *Maturitas* 1997;27:35–40

13
The clinical problem of treating osteoporosis with estrogens

E. F. Eriksen and M. Kassem

INTRODUCTION

The association of osteoporosis and estrogen deficiency has been appreciated for at least 50 years based on the original work of Albright and colleagues[1]. A large volume of information is available that documents the importance of estrogen in maintaining skeletal homeostasis in both humans and in various animal models. Recently, the use of cell culture models and molecular biology techniques have increased our understanding of the mechanistic basis of estrogen action on bone cells. Finally, the results of a large number of cohort and case–control studies and the initiation of large controlled trials that address the benefits and risks of long-term hormone replacement therapy in post-menopausal women are becoming available, and can help in guiding the individual patient considering hormone replacement therapy as an anti-osteoporosis and/or anti-aging treatment modality. The aim of the present review is to give an updated summary of estrogen action on the skeleton and the current status of hormone replacement therapy as a treatment option for the prevention and treatment of the osteoporotic syndrome.

The effect of estrogen on bone is best understood by considering the structural organization of the skeleton. The skeleton comprises discrete microscopic units named by Frost as basic multicellular units (BMUs)[2,3]. This arrangement, which is called the intermediate organization of the skeleton, is similar to the organization of kidney cells into nephrons[2]. The BMU consists of a group of bone resorbing cells (osteoclasts) and a group of bone forming cells (osteoblasts) and their respective precursors. It may also include other cell types present in the bone microenvironment and which are in continuous interaction with these cells. While the BMUs mediate all the skeletal activities involved in skeletal growth and fracture repair, their main function is to 'remodel' the skeleton. Bone remodeling is a replacement mechanism whereby the BMUs remove microscopic parts of the skeleton at discrete loci by osteoclasts and replace them with new bone formed by the osteoblasts. The aim of remodeling is to maintain the mechanical integrity of the skeleton by preventing fatigue damage, and it also serves metabolic functions by providing new bone of low bone mineral density[3]. Remodeling activation involves all parts of the skeleton, but it is more pronounced in the axial than the appendicular skeleton and it continues throughout the adult life of higher vertebrates. Imbalance between the amount of bone resorbed by osteoclasts and the subsequent amount of bone laid down by osteoblasts at remodeling sites forms the basis of the age-related and menopause-related bone loss. Estrogens have been shown to regulate different aspects of the remodeling process and their effects will be discussed at cell, tissue and organ levels of organization.

Estrogen synthesis and menopause

While the menopause is defined as the cessation of menstruation, its hormonal basis starts many years before this final event. During the menopause, levels of 17β-estradiol, which is the major estrogen during the reproductive period, decline dramatically. Similarly, estrone levels decline following the menopause, but it becomes the main circulating estrogen owing to the peripheral aromatization of both adrenal and ovarian androgens that takes place mainly in adipose tissues. The role of residual estrogens in skeletal homeostasis is not completely known. Postmenopausal serum estrogen levels were correlated with bone mass measurement in different skeletal sites, with rates of bone loss or with the presence of osteoporotic fractures in some but not all of the studies[4-6]. In a recent study where estrogen levels were suppressed to nearly undetectable levels in postmenopausal women by an aromatase inhibitor (Letrazole), increased serum levels of biochemical markers of bone resorption were observed, suggesting that even low levels of serum estrogen are important for bone homeostasis in the late postmenopausal period[7].

ESTROGEN EFFECTS ON BONE CELLS

General mechanism of estrogen action

Estrogen is a steroid hormone and its interaction with target cells is mediated through a specific receptor (estrogen receptor, ER), which is a member of a superfamily of ligand-dependent transcription factors. This family includes receptors of other steroid hormones, calcitriol and vitamin A. Two different isoforms of ER are currently characterized (ERα and ERβ). The isoform ERα is the most extensively studied and well known. The isoform ERβ has recently been cloned and its physiological role is under current investigation[8]. Upon binding to its ligand, ER dimerizes and this ER homodimer binds to specific DNA sequences termed estrogen responsive elements (EREs) located near the promoter sequences of target genes. Interaction of ERs with EREs leads to transcription activation and increased messenger mRNA and protein levels coded for these target genes. A cascade model for ovarian steroid action has been proposed to explain their observed effects on target tissues[9]. According to this model, sex steroids exert their effects first on regulatory genes or early response genes (e.g. c-fos, c-jun). Protein products of these genes subsequently stimulate transcription of structural genes or 'late genes' (e.g. growth factor genes). This cascade model is consistent with the observed effects of estrogen on osteoblasts, where estrogen treatment leads to the rapid increase in c-fos and c-jun levels which forms the AP-1 transcription factor. Several osteoblast-specific genes contain AP-1 binding sites and they show delayed increase in transcription following treatment with estrogen (e.g. induction of the transforming growth factor-β (TGF-β) gene following estrogen treatment *in vitro*)[9].

Estrogen receptors in bone

For many years, the detection of ERs and estrogen responses in osteoblast cultures and in bone organ cultures was elusive, and led to the conclusion that estrogen effects on the skeleton are indirect and probably mediated through changes in other calcitropic hormones. The use of more sensitive binding assays for detection of ERs and measurements of steady state levels of ER mRNA using molecular biology techniques led to the unequivocal identification of ERα in osteoblasts[10,11]. The number of ERα receptors found in the osteoblasts was low compared with that found in reproductive tissues (200–1600 binding sites/nucleus in osteoblasts vs. 10 000–20 000 in the uterus). However, these ERs could mediate the increase in osteoblast-specific proteins upon treatment with 17β-estradiol (see below). *In situ* reverse transcriptase–polymerase chain reaction (IS-RT–PCR) studies of normal human bone demonstrated that ERs were present at high concentrations in osteoblasts and to a lesser extent in osteocytes and osteoclasts[12]. In addition to in osteoblasts, ERs have been demonstrated in osteoclasts[13] and marrow stromal cells (osteoblast precursors)[14].

Effects of estrogen on osteoblasts

The discovery of ERs in osteoblasts prompted several investigators to examine the direct effects of estrogen treatment on osteoblast function. However, the results have been very inconsistent. For example, estrogen has been reported to increase[15], decrease[16] or have no effect[17] on osteoblast cell proliferation. Also, its effects on osteoblast function have been variable. Some authors found increased collagen type I production upon treatment with estrogen[15] while others were not able to detect these changes[17]. These discrepancies may reflect differences in the cell culture methods or the osteoblast cell model employed, or a variation of the number of estrogen receptors in different osteoblastic cell preparations[18]. To overcome these problems, several authors developed immortalized osteoblastic cell lines that are transfected with several copies of the ER gene and, therefore, possess a sufficient and stable number of ER binding sites[19,20]. Using these models, estrogen was found to inhibit osteoblast cell proliferation and osteocalcin production, to increase alkaline phosphatase production and to exert no effect on collagen type I production[21]. The inhibitory effect of estrogen on cell proliferation was further demonstrated to be the result of modulating the production and effects of insulin-like growth factors (IGFs) and IGF binding proteins (IGFBPs) on osteoblasts. Estrogen was found to increase production and gene expression of IGFBP-4, which blocks the effects of IGFs on their target cells and leads to inhibition of cell growth in a variety of cell types[22].

Effects of estrogen on osteoclasts

Both avian and human osteoclasts express ERα, and estrogen treatment leads to inhibition of bone resorption activity of osteoclasts in these models[13]. Estrogen treatment leads to increased production of TGF-β by osteoclasts[23], which in turn may act on the osteoclasts in an autocrine fashion to induce osteoclast cell death (apoptosis) and, thus, inhibit bone resorption[24].

The nature of bone resorption and bone formation during bone remodeling mentioned above necessitates a continuous interaction between the osteoblasts and osteoclasts and probably other cell types in the bone microenvironment. These interactions are mediated through a multitude of cytokine and growth factors that are found in the bone microenvironment. For a long time, it had been observed that the response of cultured osteoclasts to systemic hormones was dependent on the presence of osteoblasts. It was hypothesized, therefore, that systemic hormones exert their effects on osteoclasts indirectly by stimulating osteoblasts to produce factors that are capable of controlling osteoclast cell differentiation and function[25]. Thus, estrogen was shown, in addition to its direct effects on osteoblasts and osteoclasts, to exert profound effects on cytokine balance in the local milieu of bone. Estrogen has been found to inhibit production and gene expression of a number of osteoclast-stimulating cytokines (e.g. interleukin-6, IL-6) or to stimulate the production of osteoclast-inhibiting cytokines (e.g. TGF-β). In addition, *in vivo* studies demonstrated that ovariectomy was associated with increased production of a number of osteoclast-stimulating cytokines (IL-6, IL-1 and tumor necrosis factor-α, TNF-α) by bone marrow and stromal cells and by peripheral blood monocytes (which are putative osteoclast precursors)[14,26]. Blocking the release or the effects of these cytokines, either through estrogen replacement or through administration of a specific antagonist, was demonstrated to abolish the ovariectomy-related bone loss[26–28].

The role of bone resorbing cytokines in increased bone turnover and in mediating bone loss in the postmenopausal woman (Figure 1) is controversial, and contradictory results have been reported by different investigators[14,26,29]. In a recent study, a variety of cytokines in bone marrow plasma that should reflect the bone microenvironment were measured. No differences in the marrow plasma levels of IL-6, IL-6 soluble receptor, IL-1α, IL-1β or IL-1 receptor

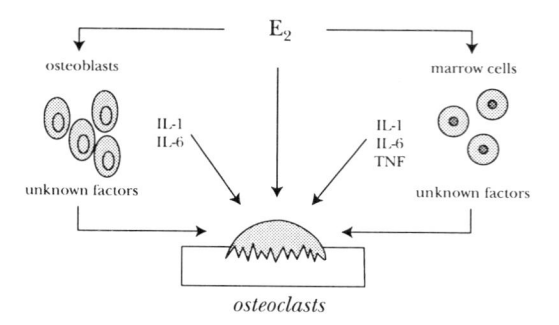

Figure 1 Cytokine secretion from marrow mononuclear cells and osteoblasts is regulated by estrogen: interleukin 1 and 6 (IL-1, IL-6) and tumor necrosis factor-α (TNF-α). Furthermore, estrogen may exert direct effects via binding to osteoclastic estrogen receptors or indirectly via binding to osteoblastic estrogen receptors

antagonist, were seen among a group of postmenopausal women, half of whom were taking estrogen replacement therapy[29]. It is plausible that part of the estrogen action on the skeleton is mediated through changes in cytokines and growth factors present in bone, and it seems that a large number of cytokines are affected. However, the relative contributions of each of them remain to be determined.

ESTROGEN EFFECTS AT THE TISSUE LEVEL

The organization of the skeleton into BMUs composed of groups of osteoclasts and osteoblasts makes it impossible to generalize directly from the findings of cell culture in relation to whole organisms. Techniques of quantitative histology (bone histomorphometry) allow detailed studies of the dynamics of bone remodeling and the activities of both osteoblasts and osteoclasts *in vivo*. In humans, this is mostly studied using iliac bone biopsies. A large number of studies have addressed effects of estrogen deficiency and estrogen replacement on the skeleton of growing and mature animals (mainly rats and mice). Few studies have addressed the effects of estrogen on the human skeleton. Estrogen is essential for the maintenance of normal bone mass and bone volume. Ovariectomy leads to a decline in bone mineral density and in bone ash weight in mature rats, and these effects can be prevented by estrogen treatment[30]. These effects are mediated by increased activation frequency and increase in bone resorption compared to bone formation[30]. To date, no anabolic effects of estrogen on bone have been observed. While some authors reported that estrogen can increase bone formation in the ovariectomized rat model[31], further analysis of these data suggests that the results are artefactual and related to decrease in bone resorption during estrogen treatment[32].

The histological studies in humans published to date have mainly studied women around the age of 65 with osteoporosis[33]. No evidence for a reversal of bone balance from negative to positive was demonstrable[33]. The only significant effect demonstrable was a 50% reduction of activation frequency (i.e. initiation rate of new remodeling cycles)[33]. We recently studied bone biopsies obtained in early postmenopausal women before and after 2 years of treatment with either sequential estrogen–progestogen or placebo. In this study, we found that the untreated women displayed an increase in resorptive activity and a progressively more negative bone balance at the level of individual remodeling units[34]. In the women treated with hormone replacement therapy (HRT), however, no such increase was observed, and bone balance was preserved, actually becoming slightly positive[34]. The osteoclastic resorption rate was more than halved in the women treated with HRT.

Thus, the main action of estrogen treatment at the tissue level is a reduction of bone turnover[33]. During the menopause, women develop increased bone turnover, and a lowering of turnover reduces bone loss. Furthermore, it reduces the risk of disintegration of the trabecular bone structure due to perforative resorption of trabeculae[3,12,33]. These are thought to be the main mechanism of action, and is also corroborated by the different responses seen between areas of the skeleton rich in cancellous bone and areas dominated by cortical bone.

The reduced resorption activity leads to a reduction in turnover, which has been demonstrated with almost all of the biochemical markers of bone remodeling available (e.g.

osteocalcin, alkaline phosphatase, procollagen peptides, hydroxyproline, collagen cross-links). Generally, a 50% reduction of bone turnover is seen[34-36].

TREATMENT REGIMENS

Estrogen is still given mainly in oral formulation, but dermal patches are gaining increased recognition. In non-hysterectomized women, progestogens have to be added to protect against endometrial cancer, while hysterectomized women can be treated with estrogen alone. Traditionally, the United States has used estrogens (equinolones) derived from the urine of pregnant mares, while Europe has used synthetic estradiol preparations. Subcutaneous estradiol implants with testosterone have also been shown to be effective.

In recent years, transdermal preparations have emerged that permit lower dosing of the hormone, because these formulations bypass the hepatic first-pass metabolism. Initially, only estradiol could be supplied transdermally, but recent formulations permit simultaneous administration of progestogens. As the transdermal route of administration bypasses the hepatic first-pass metabolism, changes in hepatic protein synthesis, commonly associated with the oral route, are avoided. Whether these changes are reflected in differences pertaining to side-effects remains to be established. Weissberger and colleagues[37] demonstrated that transdermal administration led to increases in circulating IGF-1 levels and suppression of circulating levels of growth hormone (GH), while oral administration caused opposite changes in the two peptides. Although both peptides exert pronounced effects on skeletal remodeling, there is no evidence to date that the differences demonstrated are reflected in different skeletal responses to transdermal and oral estrogen–progestogen formulations. Stevenson and co-workers compared Premarin and transdermal estrogen, and found similar increase in bone mass after 18 months of treatment (Figure 2)[38], but long-term studies are lacking. Some studies indicate that especially female smokers lose the protective effect of oral estrogens[39], and might benefit more from the transdermal route of administration, but the evidence is still disputed[40].

EFFECTS OF HRT ON BONE MASS

A multitude of studies have reported effects on estrogen deficiency or repletion on the overall skeletal homeostasis using techniques of bone mass measurement and biochemical markers of

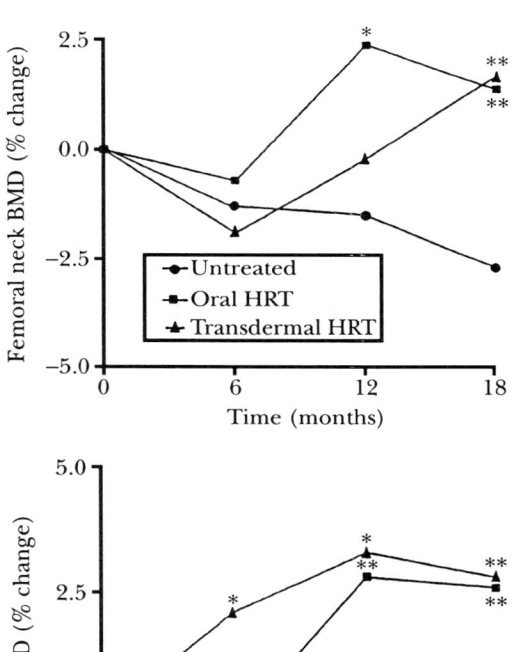

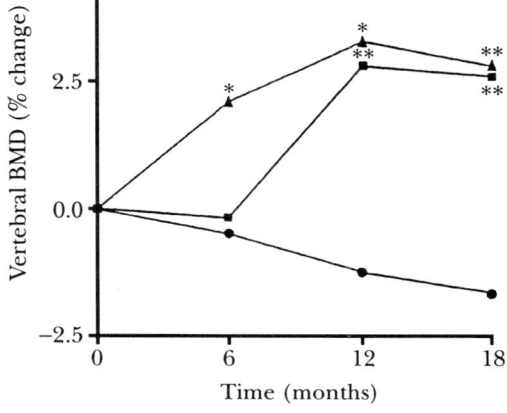

Figure 2 Changes in bone mineral density (BMD) after treatment with transdermal estrogen hormone replacement therapy (transdermal HRT), oral conjugated equine estrogens (oral HRT) and placebo: after 18 months, effects on bone mass were similar for transdermal and oral HRT groups, while placebo group lost bone. *$p < 0.01$, **$p < 0.001$ vs. untreated. Reproduced from reference 38, with permission

bone formation (alkaline phosphate, osteocalcin) and bone resorption (urine collagen cross-links). Estrogen deficiency is associated with increased serum levels of bone resorption and bone formation markers, and estrogen replacement therapy blocks these effects[41]. Increased bone turnover leads to bone loss, especially in the cancellous bone and to a lesser extent in cortical bone. Increased bone loss around the time of the menopause is superimposed on the age-related rate of bone loss (which is estimated to be around 1% per year) and is termed the accelerated phase of bone loss. It starts during the perimenopausal period and is clearly seen after surgical ovariectomy. Its rate has been estimated to be 8% per year for cancellous bone and 2% per year for cortical bone in the axial skeleton[42,43]. The accelerated phase of bone loss slows after 2–4 years in cancellous bone and 5–7 years in cortical bone. Similar results were obtained from radiocalcium kinetic and balance studies that showed menopausal increase in bone turnover and a relative increase in bone resorption compared to bone formation[44].

A vast number of studies have demonstrated similar increases in bone mass after 2–3 years of estrogen–progestogen treatment. The response seen in these studies is similar in both immediate postmenopausal and older women. Generally, a 5–7% increase in bone mass occurs within 12–18 months, followed by a plateau[45–50]. The subsequent changes in bone mass have been controversial: some studies have described a fall in bone mass, while others have described constant bone mass.

The response to estrogen differs between areas of the skeleton rich in cortical bone and areas of the skeleton rich in cancellous bone. The most pronounced increases in bone mass are seen in cancellous bone, while the data obtained from areas rich in cortical bone, such as the forearm, display only preservation of bone mass (Figure 3)[51]. Thus, forearm measurements are less well suited to monitor the HRT effects on bone mass. In a long-term study by Lindsay and Tohme where oophorectomized women were studied over a period of 10 years, the metacarpal index, which mainly reflects changes in cortical bone mass, also remained constant, while the values in controls decreased[52].

Recent data, however, suggest that a pronounced continuous increase in cancellous

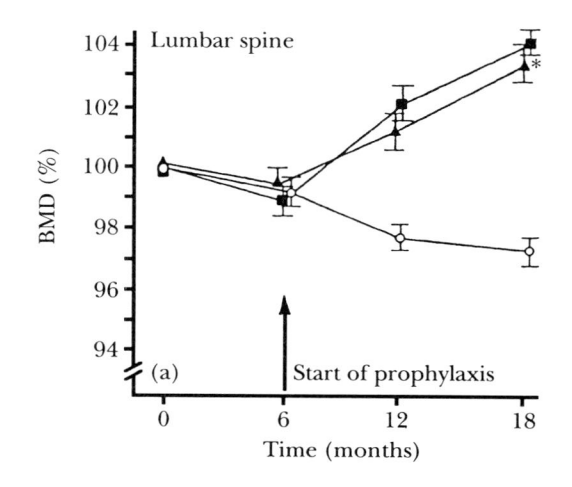

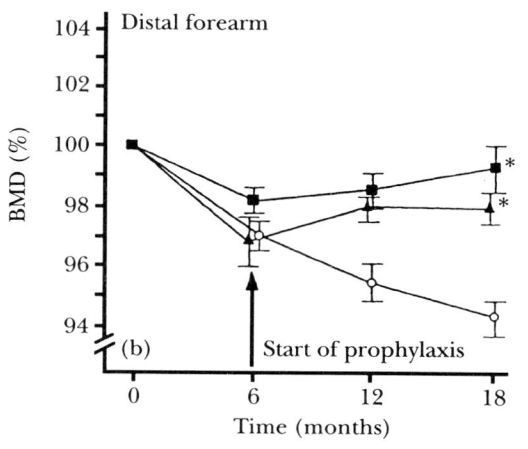

Figure 3 Changes in bone mineral density (BMD) in spine (a) and forearm (b) after 1½ years of estrogen replacement therapy (ERT) with either cyclical or continuous estradiol–norethisterone: note increase in vertebral bone mass compared with only preservation of bone mass in forearm. *$p < 0.01$, vs. placebo. Reproduced from reference 51, with permission

— ■ — Continuous combined estrogen and progestogen,
— ▲ — sequential estrogen and progestogen;
— ○ — placebo

bone mass can be achieved with long-term HRT. Pia Eiken and colleagues[53] recently presented data based on a randomized, prospective study of postmenopausal women treated with either cyclic or continuous combined estrogen–progestogen for 10 years. Estrogen-treated women exhibited 13.1% higher bone mass in the spine than controls. The most surprising finding was a continued increase in bone mass, even between years 5 and 8 of the study, suggesting slight anabolic properties of the treatment regimen. Bone mass in the forearm was preserved, but was 18% higher than in untreated women, who displayed a continuous decrease.

The role of progestogen in bone response is still unknown. One study by Lindsay and associates reported that two progestogens, gestronol and mestranol, also preserved bone mass[54]. Over a period of 1 year, the women treated with the two progestogens increased their metacarpal bone mineral content by 0.1–0.6%, which is less than most responses recorded in estrogen users. The placebo group lost 1.7%. No firm evidence for synergistic action of estrogens and progestogens has been provided to date, however. The vast majority of studies suggest no difference in bone mineral density (BMD) response between estrogen alone and combined estrogen–progestogen therapy[45–49]. In the study by Eiken and co-workers[53], no significant difference between cyclic and continuous combined treatment was demonstrable, except that BMD increased by 15.9% in the continuous combined group compared with 11.1% in the sequential group. However, there is still a great lack of knowledge regarding the action of progestogens on bone.

Thus, the long-term effects are still controversial, but newer studies suggest that impressions may have to be revised towards a slightly anabolic action of HRT (Figure 4). Further studies, however, are needed to further corroborate the few long-term studies available.

EFFECTS OF HRT ON FRACTURES

Numerous retrospective studies have demonstrated antifracture efficacy of HRT with a compound reduction in relative risk for hip fracture ranging between 0.5 and 0.75[55–58]. Only one randomized, prospective study on the antifracture efficacy of estrogen exists, namely the study by Lufkin and colleagues[59], showed significant reduction in vertebral fracture rates in women receiving transdermal estrogen plus oral cyclic progestogen for 1 year.

In a retrospective cohort study from the UK by Spector and associates, 1075 women exposed to opposed estrogen replacement therapy (ERT) were compared with 1741 non-exposed women attending a menopause clinic. For the most frequently observed fracture in this particular age group, the distal forearm fracture, the authors found a 30% risk reduction after exposure to estrogen[60].

The mean duration of estrogen treatment in many patients participating in most retrospective studies (3–5 years) is far below the time considered necessary to achieve significant effects on the skeleton (10 years or more). One of the few long-term studies was published by Ettinger and co-workers[61], who studied the antifracture efficacy of estrogen in women treated for a mean period of 17.6 years. They reported a 50% reduction in spinal fracture rate (Figure 5). Thus, in the few studies of women subjected to prolonged exposure to estrogen, pronounced reductions in fracture rates have been recorded. Therefore, the current large, randomized investigations under way in various

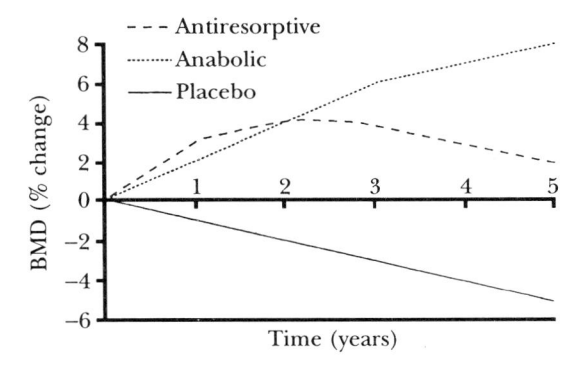

Figure 4 Changes in bone mineral density (BMD) over time as deduced from short-term estrogen replacement therapy (ERT) studies (antiresorptive: broken line), and from long-term studies (anabolic: dotted line): these curves are compared with typical curve describing bone loss in untreated women

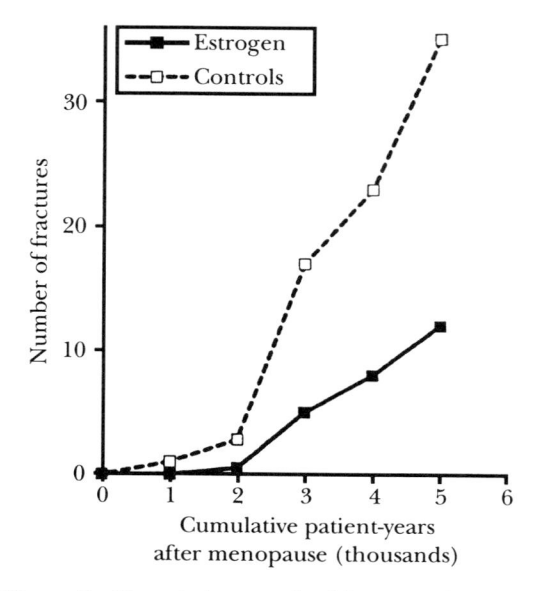

Figure 5 Cumulative vertebral fractures in women receiving long-term estrogen replacement therapy (ERT) compared with untreated controls: note significant reduction of fractures in women on ERT. Reproduced from reference 61, with permission

countries, which use longer treatment periods, will be of significant interest.

PROBLEMS ASSOCIATED WITH ERT

Although no long-term studies have dealt with this problem, current knowledge of ERT indicates that lasting skeletal benefit from ERT demands long treatment periods of 10 years or more. Adherence to such long treatment periods, however, is difficult to achieve for most women. Up to 75% of women who start HRT are reported to drop out within the first 6 months[62]. The main concerns among women starting ERT are fear of weight gain, breast and endometrial cancer and bleeding disturbances. Many also consider ERT 'unnatural'[62,63]. In a Danish prospective, placebo-controlled long-term study[64], 151 early-postmenopausal women were initially started on one of placebo, continuous combined or sequential estrogen–progestogen therapy. In this setting of a controlled clinical trial, 40% remained on ERT after 8 years, and a trend towards greater acceptance of continuous combined therapy was seen. Fear of osteoporosis seems to be a very important force driving women to take ERT[65–67]. In an Italian study, 70% of women considered osteoporosis to be the most important postmenopausal problem, but 67% were also afraid that long-term treatment might be harmful[67]. Furthermore, women with low bone mass and increased risk of osteoporosis show a 1-year compliance rate of 50%[65].

After termination of ERT, bone loss ensues. Most studies suggest that the loss rate is similar to that seen in untreated early-postmenopausal women[50], while others have suggested an initial phase of accelerated bone loss[68]. A significant part of any eventual acceleration of early bone loss rate may be caused by the increase in remodeling space following the increases in bone turnover that occur after termination of ERT. Thus, the shorter the treatment period, the shorter the duration of protection against fractures.

The loss of bone mass after ERT termination underscores the importance of long-term treatment to achieve significant protection against fractures. In a recent study based on the Framington cohort, Felson and colleagues reported significantly increased bone mass (11%) in 75-year-old women, who had taken hormones for 7 or more years, while women with shorter treatment durations only exhibited 3% higher bone mass than untreated women[69]. A recent Swedish study[70] demonstrated that current users of ERT revealed significantly lower odds ratios for hip fracture (0.37; 95% confidence interval 0.24–0.53), while previous users did not (odds ratio 0.76; 95% confidence interval 0.57–1.01). This study also suggested that early institution of ERT (within 8 years after the menopause) was more effective than later initiation of treatment. Furthermore, combined estrogen–progestogen seemed to offer more effective protection.

HOW DOES ERT COMPARE WITH OTHER OSTEOPOROSIS TREATMENTS?

In the past few years, several studies have demonstrated the efficacy of bisphosphonates for the treatment of osteoporosis. Storm and associates and Watts and co-workers[71,72] demonstrated increases in BMD of 4–5% in the spine after 3 years and significant antifracture efficacy of cyclical intermittent treatment with etidronate. Liberman and colleagues[73] and Black and associates[74] tested a newer bisphosphonate, alendronate, and reported an 8% increase in spinal BMD and 5% in hip BMD after 3 years. They also showed convincing antifracture efficacy with a 50% reduction in moderately affected osteoporotics (up to one fracture) and an 80% reduction in severely affected individuals (more than two fractures).

Tilyard and co-workers[75] reported significant antifracture protection with low-dose calcitriol in women with established spinal osteoporosis (i.e. vertebral fractures). Women receiving 0.5 µg of calcitriol per day exhibited a 66% reduction in spinal fractures after 3 years. Gallagher and Goldgar[76] reported a 2% increase in bone mass, but no antifracture efficacy of 0.62 µg per day of calcitriol. A larger French multicenter study, however, demonstrated a 40% reduction in hip fractures after 18 months of treatment with low-dose vitamin D and calcium[77].

Calcitonin increases bone mass by an average of 1–4% over a period of 3 years[78,79], but only one study has demonstrated significant antifracture efficacy[79]. Fluoride is able to increase bone mass at a rate of up to 10% per year, but is currently subject to discussion with respect to its antifracture efficacy[80,81]. In small studies, parathyroid hormone has been very effective, with increases in bone mass similar to those with fluoride[82], and larger controlled trials are currently evaluating the antifracture efficacy of parathyroid hormone as a treatment option.

When comparing these results with the results for estrogen therapy summarized above, it is obvious that estrogen is able to achieve similar increases in bone mass. Furthermore, in epidemiological studies, the antifracture efficacy at the hip is similar to that reported for vitamin D therapy, and in the spine similar to that reported for bisphosphonate therapy. Thus, ERT compares well with other antiresorptive regimens, although the documentation is lacking for large-scale prospective clinical trials that have been performed with vitamin D and bisphosphonates. Whether newer anabolic treatment options will be more effective remains to be established.

MONITORING ESTROGEN THERAPY

Various biochemical markers of bone turnover have been suggested for monitoring responses to therapy. In numerous clinical studies, formative markers such as osteocalcin and bone alkaline phosphatase, and resorption markers such as hydroxyproline and collagen cross-links in urine have been found to decrease within a few months after institution of estrogen therapy[35,36]. Changes in bone marker levels also correlate with changes in bone mass (i.e. the more pronounced the reduction, the higher the gain in bone mass)[35]. As the main determinant of bone changes in patients treated with HRT is the reduction in remodeling space (i.e. the amount of bone currently undergoing remodeling), this correlation is hardly surprising. It has to be remembered that such correlations have been obtained in large groups of patients. Their use in individual patients, however, is hampered by the large intraindividual variations of these markers. When repeated measurements are performed in the same individual, the day-to-day variation ranges between 25 and 40%[83]. This means that quite pronounced changes in bone turnover have to take place before a reduction can be demonstrated with certainty in an individual. Therefore, useful as these markers may be for monitoring bone remodeling in groups, it is still premature to use them for monitoring therapy in individual patients. More specific and/or less variable markers have to be characterized before this strategy can be said to be cost-effective. Repeated measurements of biochemical markers would reduce the variation, of course, but are unrealistic to perform in the large populations currently treated with HRT.

Repeated BMD measurements in the spine and hip currently constitute the best way to monitor the response to estrogen therapy. However, with the error for BMD measurements ranging between 1% in the spine and 1–3% in the hip, and changes in bone mass after HRT varying between 1 and 3% per year, the interval between measurements should be at least 2 years to detect a significant response[84,85]. Bone mineral density values obtained at shorter intervals will be difficult to interpret with certainty. Based on the results summarized above pertaining to compliance, regular controls have to be instituted. The demonstration of a significant skeletal response to treatment, in the present authors' opinion, certainly increases adherence to long-term treatment. Whether continued repeated measurements of BMD at 2-year intervals are necessary is still debatable. If a positive response is demonstrated after the first 2 years, new BMD measurements seem superfluous. This single measurement should be sufficient to detect the minute proportion of women not responding to ERT[86].

It seems wise, however, to monitor plasma estradiol levels after institution of ERT. In recent studies by Studd and colleagues[87,88], a significant correlation between plasma estradiol and bone mass increments was demonstrated (Table 1). This is logical, keeping the well-known dose-dependent relationship between estrogen dose and bone mass in mind. It has not been shown that repeated measurements during the course of ERT treatment are of use, but a single control after 3 months is indicated to determine the women with increased first-pass metabolism or poor absorption of the hormone. Furthermore, potentially troubling side-effects can be dealt with, before they lead the women to discontinue ERT.

FUTURE PROSPECTS

After initial animal experiments showed preservation of bone mass in ovariectomized rats treated with anti-estrogens such as tamoxifen, this field has expanded widely in recent years. Currently, large multicenter phase-3 studies are under way with the anti-estrogens raloxifene and levormeloxifene. The hope is that these compounds will be able to exert positive effects on bone, cardiovascular system and brain, without causing putative serious estrogen-related side-effects such as endometrial cancer and breast cancer, eliminating the need for concomitant progestogen administration. These regimens may also permit the treatment of women with previous breast cancer, who are currently faced with very different messages depending on whether they see a gynecologist or an oncologist.

Table 1 Percentage change in bone density on three different doses of hormone implants after 1 year. Reproduced from reference 88, with permission

	Estradiol implant			
	25 mg	50 mg	75 mg	Controls
Lumbar spine	5.56*	6.45*	10**	−0.63
Femoral neck	4.16*	4.10*	6.13*	−1.82

*, $p < 0.05$ compared with controls; **, $p < 0.01$ compared with 25 mg estradiol

The place for these new treatment regimens in the future treatment of osteoporosis remains to be established. Until then, traditional estrogen–progestogen treatment remains the drug of choice for the treatment of postmenopausal osteoporosis.

The biggest clinical problem in relation to HRT is still the pronounced lack of compliance owing to bleeding disturbances, breast tenderness, weight gain and, last but not least, fear of breast cancer. It is important, therefore, to take time with every woman to discuss these issues thoroughly, including the expected duration of each. The putative risk for breast cancer has to be put into perspective with regard to the risk for other diseases, especially cardiovascular disease. Furthermore, it is important to emphasize that most initial side-effects such as bleeding disturbances or breast tenderness subside within a few months in most women. If possible, a woman should try to stay on estrogen therapy for at least 6 months before she makes a decision on whether to discontinue. Finally, it is important to discuss the duration of therapy, which has to be prolonged (exceeding 10 years) to achieve optimal bone protection. The message will probably be much clearer and more specific in years to come when the results of several long-term, randomized studies of estrogen effects will be in hand.

References

1. Albright F, Smith PH, Richardson AM. Postmenopausal osteoporosis. *J Am Med Assoc* 1941;116:2465–474
2. Hattner R, Epker BN, Frost HM. Suggested sequential mode of control of changes in cell behaviour in adult bone remodelling. *Nature (London)* 1965;206:489–90
3. Parfitt AM. Bone remodeling: relationship to the amount and structure of bone, and the pathogenesis and prevention of fractures. In Riggs BL, Melton LJ, eds. *Osteoporosis: Etiology, Diagnosis, and Management*. New York: Raven Press, 1988: 45–93
4. Riggs BL, Jowsey J, Kelly PJ, et al. Effect of sex hormones on bone in primary osteoporosis. *J Clin Invest* 1969;48:1065–72
5. Van Hemert AM, Birkenhager JC, De Jong FH. Sex hormone binding globulin in postmenopausal women: a predictor of osteoporosis superior to endogenous oestrogens. *Clin Endocrinol* 1989;31:499–509
6. Slemenda C, Hui SL, Longcope C. Sex steroids and bone mass: a study of changes about the time of menopause. *J Clin Invest* 1987;80:1261–9
7. Heshmati HM, Khosla S, Robins SP, et al. Endogenous residual estrogen levels determine bone resorption even in late postmenopausal women. *J Bone Miner Res* 1997;12(Suppl 1):S121
8. Kuiper C, Enmark E, Pelto-Huikko M, et al. Cloning of a novel estrogen receptor expressed in rat prostate and ovary. *Proc Natl Acad Sci USA* 1996; 93:5925–30
9. Turner RT, Riggs BL, Spelsberg TC. Skeletal effects of estrogen. *Endocr Rev* 1994;16:275–300
10. Eriksen EF, Colvard DS, Berg NJ, et al. Evidence of estrogen receptors in normal human osteoblast-like cells. *Science* 1988;241:84–6
11. Komm BS, Terpening CM, Benz DJ, et al. Estrogen binding, receptor mRNA and biologic response in osteoblast-like osteocarcoma cell. *Science* 1988;241:81–4
12. Hoyland JA, Mee AP, Baird P, et al. *Bone* 1997;20:87–92
13. Oursler MJ, Pederson L, Fitzpatrick L, et al. Human giant cell tumors of the bone (osteoclastomas) as estrogen target cells. *Proc Natl Acad Sci USA* 1994;91:5227–31
14. Girasole G, Jilka RL, Passeri G, et al. 17 beta-estradiol inhibits interleukin-6 production by bone marrow-derived stromal cells and osteoblasts *in vitro*: a potential mechanism for the antiosteoporotic effect of estrogens. *J Clin Invest* 1992;89:883–91
15. Ernst M, Heath JK, Rodan GA. Estradiol effects on proliferation, messenger ribonucleic acid for collagen and insulin-like growth factor-I, and parathyroid hormone-stimulated adenylate cyclase activity in osteoblastic cells from calvariae and long bones. *Endocrinology* 1989;125:825–33
16. Gray TK, Flynn TC, Gray KM, et al. 17β-estradiol acts directly on the clonal osteoblastic cell line UMR 106. *Proc Natl Acad Sci USA* 1987;88: 6267–71
17. Keeting PE, Scott RE, Colvard DS, et al. Lack of a direct effect of estrogen on proliferation and differentiation of normal human osteoblast-like cells. *J Bone Miner Res* 1991;6:297–304
18. Davis VL, Couse JF, Gray TK, et al. Correlation between low levels of estrogen receptors and estrogen responsiveness in two rat osteoblast-like cell lines. *J Bone Miner Res* 1994;9:983–91
19. Harris SA, Tau KR, Enger RJ, et al. Estrogen response in the hFOB 1.19 human fetal osteoblastic cell line stably transfected with the human estrogen receptor gene. *J Cell Biochem* 1995;59:193–201
20. Migliaccio S, Davis VL, Gibson MK, et al. Estrogens modulate the responsiveness of osteoblast-like cells (ROS 17/2.8) stably transfected with estrogen-receptor. *Endocrinology* 130:2617–24
21. Robinson JA, Harris SA, Riggs BL, et al. Estrogen regulation of human osteoblastic cell proliferation and differentiation. *Endocrinology* 1997;138: 2919–27
22. Kassem M, Okazaki R, DeLeon D, et al. Potential mechanism of estrogen-mediated decrease in bone formation: estrogen increases production of inhibitory insulin-like growth factor-binding protein-4 in a human osteoblastic cell line with high levels of estrogen receptors. *Proc Assoc Am Physicians* 1996;108:155–61
23. Robinson JA, Riggs BL, Spelsberg TC, et al. Osteoclasts and transforming growth factor-β: estrogen-mediated isoform-specific regulation of production. *Endocrinology* 1996;137:615–21
24. Hughes DE, Dai A, TiHee JC, et al. Estrogen promotes apoptosis of murine osteoclasts mediated by TGF-β. *Nat Med* 1996;2:1132–6
25. Rodan GA, Martin TJ. Role of osteoblasts in hormonal control of bone resorption – a hypothesis. *Calcif Tissue Int* 1981;33:344–51
26. Jilka RL, Hangoc G, Griasole G, et al. Increased osteoclast development after estrogen loss: mediation by interleukin-6. *Science* 1992;257: 88–91
27. Kimble RB, Vannice JL, Blowdow DC, et al. Interleukin-1 receptor antagonist decreases bone loss

and bone resorption in ovariectomized rats. *J Clin Invest* 1994;93:1959–67
28. Kitazawa R, Kimble RB, Vannice JL, *et al.* Interleukin-1 receptor antagonist and tumor necrosis factor binding protein decrease osteoclast formation and bone resorption in ovariectomized mice. *J Clin Invest* 1994;2397–406
29. Kassem M, Khosla S, Spelsberg TC, *et al.* Cytokine production in the bone marrow microenvironment: failure to demonstrate estrogen regulation in early postmenopausal women. *J Clin Endocrinol Metab* 1996;81:513–18
30. Turner RT, Evans GL, Wakley GK. Mechanism of action of estrogen on cancellous bone balance in tibiae of ovariectomized growing rats: inhibition of indices of formation and resorption. *J Bone Miner Res* 1993;8:359–66
31. Chow J, Tobias JH, Colston KW, *et al.* Estrogen maintains trabecular bone volume in rats not only by suppression of bone resorption but also by stimulation of bone formation. *J Clin Invest* 1992;89:74–8
32. Turner CH. Do estrogens increase bone formation? (editorial). *Bone* 1991;12:305–6
33. Steiniche T, Hasling C, Charles P, *et al.* A randomized study on the effects of estrogen/gestagen or high dose oral calcium on trabecular bone remodeling in postmenopausal osteoporosis. *Bone* 1989;10:313–20
34. Eriksen EF, Langdahl B, Glerup H, *et al.* Hormone replacement therapy (HRT) preserves bone balance by preventing osteoclastic hyperactivity in postmenopausal women: a randomized prospective histomorphometric study. *J Bone Miner Res* 1996;11(Suppl 1):S449
35. Hasling C, Eriksen EF, Melkko J, *et al.* Effects of a combined estrogen–progestogen regimen on serum levels of the carboxy-terminal propetide of human type I procollagen in osteoporosis. *J Bone Miner Res* 1992;6:1295–9
36. Riis BJ, Overgaard K, Christiansen C. Biochemical markers of bone turnover to monitor the bone response to postmenopausal hormone replacement therapy. *Osteoporosis Int* 1995;5:276–80
37. Weissberger AJ, Ho KK, Lazarus L. Contrasting effects of oral and transdermal routes of oestrogen replacement therapy on 24-hour growth hormone (GH) secretion, insulin-like growth factor I and GH-binding protein in postmenopausal women. *J Clin Endocrinol Metab* 1991;72:374–81
38. Stevenson JC, Cust MP, Gangar KF, *et al.* Effects of transdermal versus oral hormone replacement therapy on bone density in spine and proximal femur in postmenopausal women. *Lancet* 1990;336:265–9
39. Kiel DP, Baron JA, Anderson JJ, *et al.* Smoking eliminates the protective effect of oral oestrogens on the risk for hip fracture among women. *Ann Int Med* 1992;116:716–21
40. Naessén T, Persson I, Thor L, *et al.* Maintained bone density at advanced ages after long term treatment with low dose oestradiol implants. *Br J Obstet Gynaecol* 1993;100:454–9
41. Garnero P, Sornay Rendu E, Chapuy MC, *et al.* Increased bone turnover in late postmenopausal women is a major determinant of osteoporosis. *J Bone Miner Res* 1996;11:337–49
42. Riggs BL, Wahner HW, Dann WL, *et al.* Differential changes in bone mineral density of the appendicular and axial skeleton with aging. *J Clin Invest* 1981;67:328–35
43. Richelson LS, Wahner HW, Melton LJ, *et al.* Relative contributions of aging and estrogen deficiency to postmenopausal bone loss. *N Engl J Med* 1984;311:1273–5
44. Heaney RP, Recker RR, Saville PD. Menopausal changes in bone remodeling. *J Lab Clin Med* 1978;92:964–70
45. Ettinger B, Genant HK, Cann CE. Postmenopausal bone loss is prevented by treatment with low-dose oestrogen with calcium. *Ann Intern Med* 1987;106:40–3
46. Christiansen C, Christensen MS, Transbøl I. Bone mass in postmenopausal women after withdrawal of oestrogen/progestogen replacement therapy. *Lancet* 1981;1:459–61
47. Christiansen C, Riis BJ. 17-beta-estradiol and continuous norethisterone: a unique treatment for established osteoporosis in elderly women. *J Clin Endocrinol Metab* 1990;71:836–41
48. Lindsay R, Tohme JF. Oestrogen treatment of patients with established postmenopausal osteoporosis. *Obstet Gynecol* 1990;76:290–5
49. Prince RL, Smith M, Dick IM. Prevention of postmenopausal osteoporosis. A comparative study of exercise, calcium supplementation, and hormone-replacement therapy. *N Engl J Med* 1991;325:1189–95
50. Christiansen C, Christensen MS, McNair P, *et al.* Prevention of early postmenopausal bone loss: controlled 2-year study in 315 normal females. *Eur J Clin Invest* 1980;10:273–9
51. Munk Jensen N, Nielsen SP, Obel EB, *et al.* Reversal of postmenopausal vertebral bone loss by oestrogen and progestogen: a double blind placebo controlled study. *Br Med J* 1988;296:1150–2
52. Lindsay R, Tohme JF. Oestrogen treatment of patients with established postmenopausal osteoporosis. *Obstet Gynecol* 1990;76:290–5
53. Eiken P, Pors Nielsen S, Kolthoff N. Effects on bone mass after eight years of hormonal

replacement therapy. *Br J Obstet Gynaecol* 1997; 104:702–7
54. Lindsay R, Hart DM, Purdie D, *et al.* Comparative effects of oestrogen and a progestogen on bone loss in postmenopausal women. *Clin Sci Mol Med* 1978;54:193–5
55. Hutchinson TA, Polansky SM, Feinstein AR. Postmenopausal oestrogens protect against fractures of hip and distal radius. *Lancet* 1979; 2:705–7
56. Johnson RE, Specht EE. The risk of hip fracture in postmenopausal females with and without oestrogen exposure. *Am J Publ Health* 1981; 71:139–44
57. Paganini-Hill A, Ross RK, Gerkins VR, *et al.* Menopausal oestrogen therapy and hip fractures. *Ann Intern Med* 1981;95:28–31
58. Khoyi AA, Middleton RK. Oral contraceptives in osteoporosis. *Ann Pharmacother* 1992;26:1094–5
59. Lufkin EG, Wahner HW, O'Fallon WM *et al.* Treatment of postmenopausal osteoporosis with transdermal oestrogen. *Ann Intern Med* 1992; 117:1–9
60. Spector TD, Brennan B, Harris PA, *et al.* Do current regimes of hormone replacement therapy protect against subsequent fractures? *Osteoporosis Int* 1992;2:219–24
61. Ettinger B, Genant HK, Cann CE. Long term oestrogen replacement therapy prevents bone loss and fractures. *Ann Intern Med* 1985;102:319–24
62. Studd JJ, Panay N, Zamblera D, *et al.* HRT and long term compliance: the efficacy and safety of menorest. *Int J Gynaecol Obstet* 1996;52:S21–5
63. Rozenberg S, Vandromme J, Kroll M, *et al.* Compliance to hormone replacement therapy. *Int J Fertil Menopausal Stud* 1995;40:23–32
64. Eiken P, Kolthoff N. Compliance with long term oral hormonal replacement therapy. *Maturitas* 1995;22:97–103
65. Torgerson, DJ, Donaldsson, C, Russell IT, *et al.* Hormone replacement therapy: compliance and cost after screening for osteoporosis. *Eur J Obstet Gynecol Reprod Biol* 1995;59:57–60
66. Ringa V, Ledesert B, Breart G. Determinants of hormone replacement therapy among postmenopausal women in the French Gasel cohort. *Osteoporosis Int* 1994;4:16–20
67. Perrone G, Capri O, Borrello M, *et al.* Attitudes towards estrogen replacement therapy. Study conducted on a sample of women attending an ambulatory care center for the treatment of menopause. *Mineva Ginecol* 1993;45:603–8
68. Trémolliéres F, Pouilles JM, Ribot C. Cessation of estrogen replacement therapy is associated with a significant vertebral bone loss: a longitudinal study. *J Bone Miner Res* 1997;12:S103

69. Felson DT, Zhang Y, Hannan MT, *et al.* The effect of postmenopausal estrogen therapy on bone density in elderly women. *N Engl J Med* 1993; 329:1141–6
70. Michaelson K, Baron JA, Fahramand BY, *et al.* The effect of opposed and unopposed hormone replacement therapy on hip fracture risk. *J Bone Miner Res* 1997;12:S104
71. Storm T, Thamsborg G, Steiniche T, *et al.* Effect of intermittent cyclical etidronate therapy on bone mass and fracture rate in women with postmenopausal osteoporosis. *N Engl J Med* 1990; 322:1265–71
72. Watts NB, Harris ST, Genant KH, *et al.* Intermittent cyclical etidronate treatment of postmenopausal osteoporosis. *N Engl J Med* 1990;323:73–9
73. Liberman UA, Weiss SR, Broll J, *et al.* Effect of oral alendronate on bone mineral density and incidence of fractures in postmenopausal osteoporosis. *N Engl J Med* 1995;333:1437–43
74. Black DM, Cummings SR, Karpf DB, *et al.* Randomised trial of effect of alendronate on risk of fracture in women with existing vertebral osteoporosis. *Lancet* 1996;348:1535–41
75. Tilyard MW, Spears GF, Thomson J, *et al.* Treatment of postmenopause osteoporosis with calcitriol or calcium. *N Engl J Med* 1992;326:357–62
76. Gallagher JC, Goldgar D. Treatment of postmenopausal osteoporosis with high doses of synthetic calcitriol. A randomized controlled study. *Ann Intern Med.* 1990;113:649–55
77. Chapuy MC, Arlot ME, Duboeuf F, *et al.* Vitamin D and calcium to prevent hip fractures in elderly women. *N Engl J Med* 1992;327:1637–42
78. Haas HG, Liebrich BM, Schaffner W. Calcitonin and osteoporosis – a critical review of the literature 1980–1989. *Klin Wochenschr* 1990;68:359–71
79. Overgaard K, Hansen MA, Jensen SB, *et al.* Effect of salcatonin given intranasally on bone mass and fracture rates in established osteoporosis: a dose-response study. *Br Med J* 1992;305:556–61
80. Riggs BL, Hodgson SF, O'Fallon WM, *et al.* Effect of fluoride treatment on the fracture rate in postmenopausal women with osteoporosis. *N Engl J Med* 1990;322:802–9
81. Pak CY, Sakhaee K, Zerwekh JE. Effect of intermittent therapy with a slow-release fluoride preparation. *J Bone Miner Res* 1990;5(Suppl.1): S149–55
82. Reeve J, Davies UM, Hesp R, *et al.* Treatment of osteoporosis with human parathyroid peptide and observations on effect of sodium fluoride. *Br Med J* 1990;301:314–18, 477
83. Blumsohn A, Eastell R. Prediction of bone loss in postmenopausal women. *Eur J Clin Invest* 1992;22:764–6

84. Genant HK, Block JE, Steiger P, *et al.* Appropriate use of bone densitometry. *Radiology* 1989;170:817–22
85. Pouilles JM, Trémolliéres F, Ribot C. Spine and femur densitometry at the menopause: are both sites necessary in the assessment of the risk of osteoporosis? *Calcif Tissue Int* 1993;52:344–7
86. Stevenson JC, Hillard TC, Lees B, *et al.* Postmenopausal bone loss: does HRT always work? *Int J Fertil Menopausal Stud* 1993;38:88–91
87. Studd J, Savvas M, Waston N, *et al.* The relationship between plasma estradiol and the increase in bone density in postmenopausal women after treatment with subcutaneous hormone implants. *Am J Obstet Gynecol* 1990;163:1474–9
88. Studd J, Holland EFN, Leather A, *et al.* The dose–response of percutaneous oestradiol implants on the skeletons of postmenopausal women. *Br J Obstet Gynaecol* 1994;101:787–91

14

Timing of postmenopausal estrogen for optimal bone mineral density

D. L. Schneider and D. J. Morton

INTRODUCTION

Estrogen therapy has been the mainstay for the prevention and treatment of osteoporosis in postmenopausal women[1,2]. A large body of data shows that estrogen either maintains bone or slows bone loss, and thereby prevents osteoporotic fractures[3–12]. In addition, recent studies suggested that lifetime estrogen replacement would be necessary to prevent osteoporosis. However, the majority of women who begin estrogen therapy discontinue use after an average of 5 years[13].

For many years, the standard recommendation has been that estrogen therapy should begin at the time of menopause, when rapid bone loss is known to occur. It was thought that estrogen taken for the first 10 years after the menopause would delay bone loss sufficiently to reduce a woman's risk of osteoporotic fractures in old age. Estrogen therapy initiated at older ages (more than 10 years postmenopause) was not expected to be effective as the rapid bone loss 'window of opportunity' would be past, and bone loss in older women was thought to be due to age, not estrogen deficiency[14,15].

Recent studies have challenged these assumptions. This paper will review the evidence that (1) estrogen therapy begun after age 60 can preserve and even increase bone density[16–23]; (2) estrogen therapy discontinued 5–10 years after the menopause carries no long-term benefit in term of bone density in old age[24–29]; and (3) estrogen begun after age 60 may be as effective in preserving bone as estrogen begun at the time of menopause and continued into late life[30]. These data are shown to be compatible with the estimated bone density model described by Ettinger and Grady[31].

SHORT-TERM STUDIES

Studies of women who began estrogen therapy at age 60 and older have shown significant increases in bone density after 1 or 2 years of use (Table 1)[16–23]. After 1 year of therapy, increase in bone mass ranged from 4.5 to 9.9% at the spine, 1.4 to 3.2% at the femoral neck and 3.1 to 11.7% at the ultradistal radius. In those studies that extended to a second year, there were further increases in bone mass at all sites with total changes from baseline ranging from 3.6 to 13.1%. The two studies[22,23] utilizing the newer bone mass measurement technique, dual energy X-ray absorptiometry (DXA), demonstrate results similar to those of the earlier studies.

During the first 1 or 2 years of estrogen therapy, the increases in bone mass in women who are late starters are thought to be due to the decrease of bone resorption more than bone formation, and a reduction in activation frequency of new bone remodeling cycles. Beyond 2 years of estrogen therapy, there is thought to be stabilization of bone mass followed by a slow decline.

Table 1 Summary of selected skeletal studies of bone mineral density in women who began estrogen therapy at age 60 and older

First author (year)	Study design and subject source	Subject number and estrogen type	Mean age (years)	Years of use	Bone density method	Sites	% bone mass increase at 1 year
Steiniche (1989)[16]	RCT: osteoporosis patients with fractures	n = 14, 17βE$_2$ + NETA; n = 14, calcium	66	1	DPA	spine	5.6
Christiansen (1990)[17]	RCT: osteoporosis patients	n = 16, 17βE$_2$ + NETA; n = 15, calcium	63.6	1 (2 for n = 7 on ERT)	DPA; SPA	spine ultradistal radius proximal radius	4.5 11.7 2.0
Lindsay (1990)[18]	RCT: osteoporosis patients	n = 22, CEE 0.625; n = 18, calcium	62.3	2	DPA	spine femoral neck	10.6* 5.5*
Birkenhager (1992)[19]	randomized matched pairs; osteoporosis patients with fractures	n = 18, 17βE$_2$ + MPA; n = 18, 17βE$_2$ + MPA + ND	60.7	2	DPA; SPA	spine ultradistal radius proximal radius	9.9 3.1 2.2
Lufkin (1992)[20]	RCT: osteoporosis patients with fractures	n = 36, 17βE$_2$ patch + MPA; n = 39, placebo	65.5	1	DPA; SPA	spine trochanter femoral neck mid-radius	5.3 7.6 2.6 1.0
Szejnfeld (1994)[21]	retrospective chart review; osteoporosis patients	n = 24, CEE 0.625 + MPA; n = 18, control	62	1	DPA	spine trochanter Ward's area femoral neck	4.7 4.9 3.6 1.4
Grey (1994)[22]	retrospective chart review; estrogen therapy patients	n = 44, CEE 0.625 + MPA; n = 19, control	64	1	DXA	spine femoral neck	7.0 3.0
Kohrt (1995)[23]	prospective case–control; osteopenic patients	n = 12, CEE 0.625 + MPA; n = 12, control	66	1	DXA	spine femoral neck trochanter Ward's area	5.0 3.2 3.2 6.6

*increase over 2 years; 17βE$_2$-estradiol; CEE, conjugated equine estrogens; DXA, dual energy X-ray absorptiometry; DPA, dual photon absorptiometry; ERT, estrogen replacement therapy; MPA, medroxyprogesterone acetate; ND, nandrolone decanoate; NETA, norethisterone acetate; RCT, randomized controlled trial; SPA, single photon absorptiometry

These short-term studies clearly and consistently show that women who start estrogen therapy 10 or more years after the menopause can maintain or increase bone density. Therefore, estrogen therapy can be considered for prevention as well as treatment of osteoporosis in older women who have been postmenopausal for many years.

STOPPING ESTROGEN THERAPY

Accelerated rates of bone loss have been observed after estrogen treatment has been discontinued, which is known as 'catch-up loss'. Erdtsieck and associates[24] observed rapid loss of bone mineral density (BMD) at the ultradistal radius and lumbar spine, 1 year following cessation of estrogen treatment that had been given for 3 years. Trémollieres and colleagues[25] observed a rapid phase of vertebral bone loss averaging 2.4% in the first 2 years after withdrawal of estrogen treatment (mean duration 4.4 years) that was similar to bone loss in untreated women during the first 2 years of menopause. The rate of bone loss was not related to the duration of estrogen therapy. A similar rate of 2.6% bone loss at the distal forearm was reported by Quigley and co-workers[26] for estrogen users who stopped estrogen after age 65 and lost bone more rapidly than women of similar age who had never taken estrogen. Moreover, Christiansen and colleagues[27] observed an annual decrease of 2.3% in bone mineral content at the distal forearm after withdrawal of estrogen treatment, a rate identical to the bone loss of untreated women.

Women who start estrogen at menopause then stop after 7 or 8 years may lose all bone benefit by age 75 because of this 'catch-up loss' phenomenon. Large population-based studies have demonstrated that discontinuing estrogen therapy may not preserve bone density late in life nor protect against osteoporotic fractures. In the Framingham study, Felson and associates[28] found preservation of bone density in women less than 75 years old who had taken estrogen for 7 years or more, but little residual effect on bone density in women 75 years and older. In the Study of Osteoporotic Fractures, Cauley and co-workers[29] observed no decreased risk for hip, wrist or non-spinal fractures in past users of estrogen (mean duration of use 4.8 years).

LATE START OF ESTROGEN THERAPY

We examined the past and current use of estrogen in 740 community-dwelling older white, postmenopausal women (Rancho Bernardo, California), over two-thirds of whom had used oral estrogen at some time[30]. Estrogen use was classified as never, past or current and stratified by time of initiation, either early after the menopause or after age 60. Age 60 was chosen to reflect the usual recommendation to take estrogen at or soon after the menopause for no more than 10 years. Five patterns of estrogen use were identified:

(1) Never-users;
(2) Past early-users (started before age 60 with no current use);
(3) Past late-users (started age 60 or older with no current use);
(4) Current late-users (started age 60 or older with current use);
(5) Current continuous-users (started before age 60 with current use).

Current continuous-users began estrogen an average of 2 years after the menopause and had used estrogen for an average of 20 years. Current late-users began estrogen 18 years after the menopause for an average of 9 years of use. As shown in Figure 1, current continuous-users had the highest BMD levels at all four sites, independent of duration of use. However, current late-users who had started estrogen after age 60 had BMD levels that were not statistically significantly different from those of current continuous-users. The BMD levels of the past early-users, who had taken estrogen for an average of 10 years and had discontinued it 17 years previously, were similar to those of never-users.

Ettinger and Grady[31] estimated the effect on BMD of rates of bone loss in women who did and

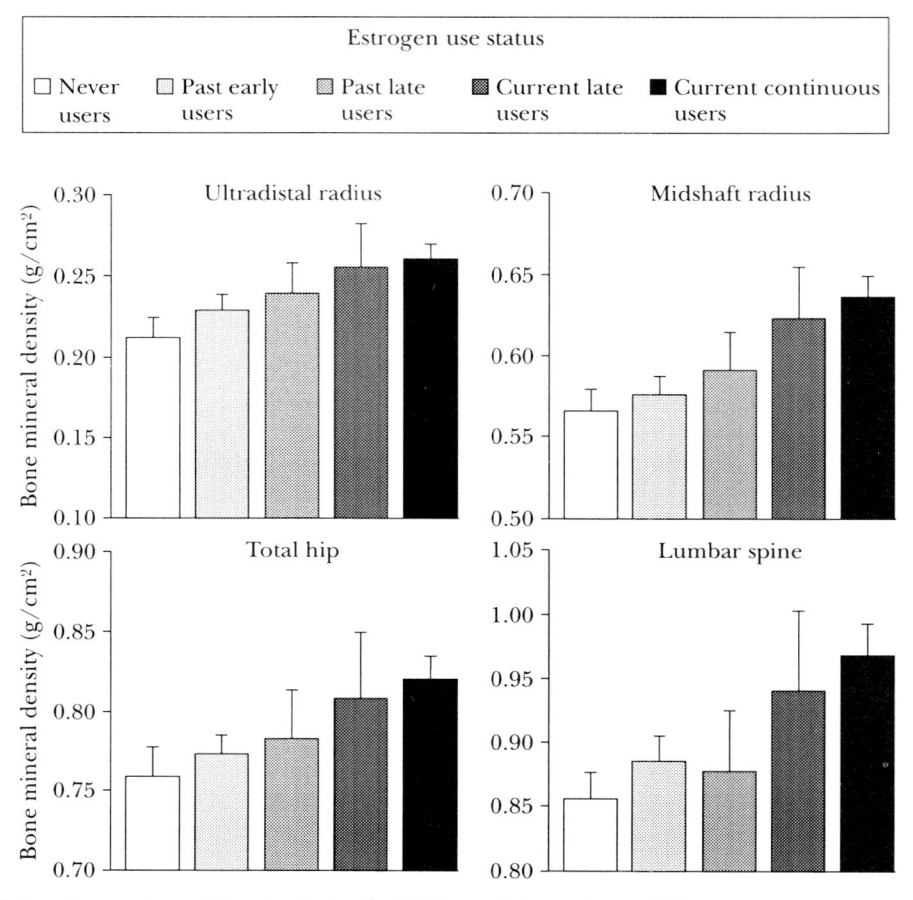

Figure 1 Mean bone mineral density (g/cm^2) (95% confidence interval) by estrogen use groups adjusted for age, body mass index, total calcium intake, bilateral oophorectomy, current smoking, alcohol use, exercise, and current use of thiazide diuretics, thyroid hormone and oral contraceptives. Reproduced from reference 30 with permission. Copyright 1997, American Medical Association

did not use estrogen. Assuming that all skeletal sites had similar rates of bone density change, the following estimates were made:

(1) An untreated woman loses 2% of bone density per year for the first 5 years after the menopause and 1% per year thereafter;

(2) A woman treated with long-term estrogen therapy loses 0.5% of bone density per year;

(3) A woman who stops taking estrogen loses 2% of bone density per year for 5 years and 1% per year thereafter;

(4) An older postmenopausal woman starting estrogen gains an additional 5–10% of bone density during the first 2 years of therapy and then loses 0.5% per year.

These estimates were used to predict the bone mineral density between ages 50 and 85 for four possible scenarios:

(1) Never-users of estrogen;

(2) Continuous-users (starting estrogen at menopause and continuing indefinitely);

(3) Early-users (starting estrogen at menopause and stopping at age 65);

(4) Late-users (starting estrogen at age 65 and continuing indefinitely).

As shown in Figures 2 and 3, at age 85 the estimated BMD was highest for continuous-users with only a small difference in comparison with late-users (2% assuming a 10% gain or 6% assuming a 5% gain). The estimated BMD difference was also small between never- users and early-users who had stopped after 15 years of use. The estimated BMD levels predicted by this model are similar to those BMD levels at four skeletal sites observed in the Rancho Bernardo cohort.

LIMITATIONS

The number of studies available for the present review is small and the available data have limitations. The prospective studies of starting estrogen therapy after age 60 are of short duration (1 to 2 years). The Rancho Bernardo study is cross-sectional; however it did substantiate the estimated BMD predicted by Ettinger and Grady's model. In addition, the present review encompassed the effect of timing of estrogen use on BMD levels not osteoporotic fractures, although BMD is considered the best predictor of fracture risk. To the knowledge of the present authors, there has been only one study of duration and timing of estrogen use in relation to fractures. Cauley and associates[29] found current estrogen use begun at any age reduced the risk of hip, wrist and all non-spinal fractures, but estrogen was most effective if initiated within 5 years of the menopause and used for longer than 10 years.

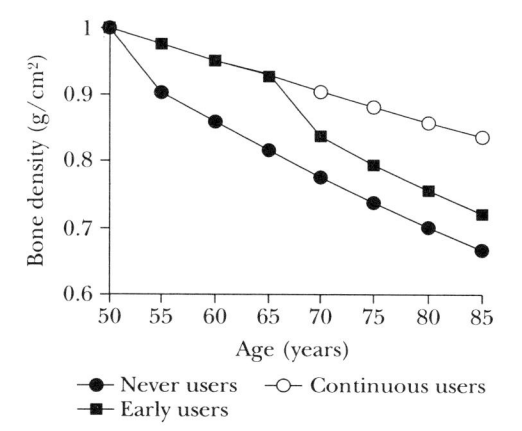

Figure 2 Estimated bone density by age in women who never used estrogen (never users), those who used continuously beginning at menopause (presumed to occur at age 50) (continuous users), and those who began at menopause and stopped at age 65 (early users). Reproduced from reference 31 with permission

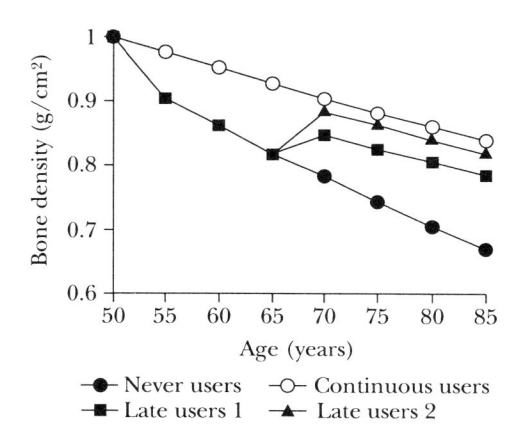

Figure 3 Estimated bone density by age in women who never used estrogen (never users), those who used continuously beginning at menopause (presumed to occur at age 50) (continuous users), and those who began at age 65 (late users). Calculations assume a 5% (late users, 1) or a 10% (late users, 2) increase in bone density at the time estrogen was started. Reproduced from reference 31 with permission

OTHER CONSIDERATIONS

In addition to the positive effects on bone, other benefits and risks of short- and long-term estrogen therapy need to be considered in helping to make the decision when to start and whether or not to stop estrogen therapy. Unfortunately, the studies of the major potential risk of estrogen therapy, that of breast cancer, and the major potential benefit, to coronary heart disease, are inconclusive. Women needing treatment for menopausal symptoms should not wait until later, while others who are asymptomatic may be able to delay initiation of therapy. However, women at high risk for osteoporosis or heart disease should consider estrogen therapy at the time of the menopause. On the other hand, women who are not at high risk for osteoporosis or heart disease may want to wait for 10 or 15 years beyond the menopause before making a decision to start estrogen therapy.

CONCLUSIONS

Based on the evidence that (1) women aged 60 and older demonstrate significant increases in bone mass after 1 or 2 years of estrogen use, (2) past use provides no long-term bone effects, and (3) women who start taking estrogen after age 60 or 65 have similar bone density to that of women who start immediately after the menopause, starting estrogen early may not be necessary and it may never be too late to achieve beneficial effects on bone.

Use of estrogen has been the mainstay for prevention of bone loss in postmenopausal women. Estrogen therapy has clearly been shown to maintain bone mass and to reduce postmenopausal bone loss, thereby lowering the risk of osteoporotic fractures. The studies reviewed confirm what clinicians have believed for several years: (1) current estrogen use is better than past use for maintenance of bone density; and (2) current estrogen therapy begun 10 or more years after the menopause might be as beneficial as continuous treatment begun at the time of menopause.

KEY POINTS FOR CLINICAL PRACTICE

(1) Women who had started taking estrogen at the menopause and continued into late life had the highest bone mineral density. Therefore, when a woman starts estrogen therapy at the menopause it should be continued indefinitely.

(2) Women who started taking estrogen after age 60 and continued taking it had surprisingly similar bone levels to those of women who had started estrogen at the menopause. Therefore, it may never be too late to start estrogen therapy for the beneficial bone effects. If a women has reached age 60 without estrogen therapy, she should be considered for starting estrogen.

(3) Women who started taking estrogen at the menopause and then stopped after an average of 10 years of use had only slightly better bone mineral density than those who had never taken it. Therefore, past use provides little or no long-term benefit for bone density. Once estrogen therapy is begun it should be continued indefinitely.

(4) If a woman is at high risk for osteoporosis or heart disease when she reaches the menopause, estrogen therapy should be considered immediately.

(5) If a woman is not experiencing vasomotor symptoms and is not at high risk for osteoporosis or heart disease, she may wait beyond early menopause before making a decision to start estrogen therapy.

(6) If a woman is known to be at high risk for breast cancer, it may be prudent for her to wait 10 years or more after the menopause before initiating estrogen therapy.

ACKNOWLEDGEMENT

The study of the Rancho Bernardo Cohort was supported by grant AG 07181 from the National Institute on Aging.

References

1. Christiansen C. Hormone replacement therapy and osteoporosis. *Maturitas* 1996;23:S71–6
2. Rosen CJ, Kessenich CR. The pathophysiology and treatment of postmenopausal osteoporosis. An evidence-based approach to estrogen replacement therapy. *Endocrinol Metab Clin North Am* 1997;26:295–311
3. Lindsay R, Hart DM, Aitken JM, *et al*. Long-term prevention of postmenopausal osteoporosis by oestrogen. Evidence for an increased bone mass

after delayed onset of oestrogen treatment. *Lancet* 1976;1:1038–41
4. Aitken JM, Hart DM, Lindsay R. Oestrogen replacement therapy for prevention of osteoporosis after oophorectomy. *Br Med J* 1973;3:515–18
5. Nachtigall LE, Nachtigall RH, Nachtigall RD, et al. Estrogen replacement therapy I: a 10-year prospective study in the relationship to osteoporosis. *Obstet Gynecol* 1979;53:277–81
6. Hutchinson TA, Polansky SM, Feinstein AR. Post-menopausal oestrogens protect against fractures of hip and distal radius. A case–control study. *Lancet* 1979;2:705–9
7. Lindsay R, Hart DM, Forrest C, et al. Prevention of spinal osteoporosis in oophorectomised women. *Lancet* 1980;2:1151–4
8. Weiss NS, Ure CL, Ballad JH, et al. Decreased risk of fractures of the hip and lower forearm with postmenopausal use of estrogen. *N Engl J Med* 1980;303:1195–8
9. Kreiger N, Kelsey JL, Holford TR, et al. An epidemiologic study of hip fracture in post-menopausal women. *Am J Epidemiol* 1982;116:141–8
10. Ettinger B, Benant HK, Cann CE. Long-term estrogen replacement therapy prevents bone loss and fractures. *Ann Intern Med* 1985;102:319–34
11. Maxim P, Ettinger B, Spitalny GM. Fracture protection provided by long-term estrogen therapy. *Osteoporosis Int* 1995;5:23–9
12. Kiel DP, Felson DT, Anderson JJ, et al. Hip fracture and the use of estrogens in postmenopausal women: the Framingham study. *N Engl J Med* 1987;317:1169–74
13. Utian WH, Schiff I. NAMS–Gallup survey on women's knowledge, information sources, and attitudes to menopause and hormone therapy. *Menopause* 1994;1:39–48
14. Riggs BL, Wahner HW, Seeman E, et al. Changes in bone mineral density of the proximal femur and spine with aging: differences between post-menopausal and osteoporotic syndromes. *J Clin Invest* 1982;70:716–23
15. Richelson LS, Wahner HW, Melton LJ III, et al. Relative contributions of aging and estrogen deficiency to postmenopausal bone loss. *N Engl J Med* 1984;311:1273–5
16. Steiniche T, Hasling C, Charles P, et al. A randomized study on the effects of estrogen/gestagen or high dose oral calcium on trabecular bone remodeling in postmenopausal osteoporosis. *Bone* 1989;10:313–20
17. Christiansen C, Riis BJ. 17β-estradiol and continuous norethisterone: a unique treatment for established osteoporosis in elderly women. *J Clin Endocrinol Metab* 1990;71:836–41
18. Lindsay R, Tohme JF. Estrogen treatment of patients with established postmenopausal osteoporosis. *Obstet Gynecol* 1990;76:290–5
19. Birkenhager JC, Erdtsieck RJ, Zeelenberg J, et al. Can nandrolone add to the effect of hormonal replacement therapy in postmenopausal osteoporosis? *Bone Miner* 1992;18:251–65
20. Lufkin EG, Wahner HW, O'Fallon WM, et al. Treatment of postmenopausal osteoporosis with transdermal estrogen. *Ann Intern Med* 1992;117:1–9
21. Szejnfeld VL, Souen JS, Baracat EC, et al. Do estrogens improve bone mass in osteoporotic women over ten years of menopause? *São Paulo Med J* 1994;112:517–20
22. Grey AB, Cundy TF, Reid IR. Continuous combined oestrogen/progestin therapy is well tolerated and increases bone density at the hip and spine in post-menopausal osteoporosis. *Clin Endocrinol* 1994;40:671–7
23. Kohrt WM, Birge SJ. Differential effects of estrogen treatment on bone mineral density of the spine, hip, wrist and total body in late post-menopausal women. *Osteoporosis Int* 1995;5:150–5
24. Erdtsieck RJ, Pols HAP, Van Kuijk C, et al. Course of bone mass during and after hormonal replacement therapy with and without addition of nadronlone decanoate. *J Bone Miner Res* 1994;9:277–283
25. Trémollieres F, Pouilles J-M, Ribot C. Cessation of estrogen replacement therapy is associated with a significant vertebral bone loss. *J Bone Miner Res* 1997;12:S103
26. Quigley MET, Martin PL, Burnier AM, et al. Estrogen therapy arrests bone loss in elderly women. *Am J Obstet Gynecol* 1987;156:1516–23
27. Christiansen C, Christensen MS, Transbol I. Bone mass in postmenopausal women after withdrawal of oestrogen/gestagen replacement therapy. *Lancet* 1981;1:459–61
28. Felson DT, Zhang Y, Hannan MT, et al. The effect of postmenopausal estrogen therapy on bone density in elderly women. *N Engl J Med* 1993;329:1141–6
29. Cauley JA, Seeley DG, Ensrud K, et al. Estrogen replacement therapy and fractures in older women. *Ann Intern Med* 1995;122:9–16
30. Schneider DL, Barrett-Connor EL, Morton DJ. Timing of postmenopausal estrogen for optimal bone mineral density. The Rancho Bernardo Study. *J Am Med Assoc* 1997; 277:543–7
31. Ettinger B, Grady D. Maximizing the benefit of estrogen therapy for prevention of osteoporosis. *Menopause* 1994;1:19–24

15
Value of bone markers in osteoporosis and related diseases

M. Bonde and C. Christiansen

INTRODUCTION

As bone is renewed in a continuous metabolic sequence, the underlying processes of bone resorption and bone formation are reflected in body fluids by the presence of various biochemical molecules. These are released from either the bone matrix or from the cells actively involved in the bone resorption. The molecules, which are usually named biochemical markers, can be measured in urine and serum and, thus, constitute an estimate of the turnover of bone[1].

Research in the field of biochemical markers of bone turnover has increased significantly over the past few years. This increase is related to several factors. First, the significance of early identification of the women at risk of osteoporosis is gaining acceptance. Therefore, it is important to develop diagnostic tools which can identify the women at highest risk. Moreover, new and improved drugs for osteoporosis have emerged for prevention of bone loss as well as for treatment of established osteoporosis[2–4]. Therefore, tools for monitoring the efficacy of the therapy are needed to optimize treatment.

There are three main factors for determining the risk of postmenopausal osteoporosis: peak bone mass, rate of bone loss and length of time during which bone is lost[5,6]. As a consequence, an important diagnostic tool for the assessment of risk of osteoporosis is the measurement of bone mass by dual energy X-ray absorptiometry (DEXA). Information about skeletal status, together with other clinical information, is important for medical decision making. Individuals with bone mass below a certain threshold could be offered therapy, to prevent further loss of bone.

By its very nature, determination of bone mass is a static measure and, therefore, is not a convenient tool to assess the rate of bone loss. It may be done by performing repetitive measurements but, as the change in bone mass is usually 1–3% per year and the precision of the DEXA methodology is in the same range, at least 2 years must pass between measurements[7]. Several studies have demonstrated, however, that biochemical bone markers are highly correlated to the rate of bone loss[8–10]. Thus, by measuring one marker or combining values from several markers, it has been possible to identify women at increased risk of osteoporosis.

For monitoring the efficacy of therapy, biochemical markers of bone turnover have proved to be helpful as they respond within just weeks after initiation of therapy[9,11,12]. The availability of preventive osteoporosis therapies, in which a woman is supposed to take medication from the onset of the menopause for the rest of her life, calls for a diagnostic tool, such as the measurement of a biochemical marker, assuring the woman that the therapy is efficient and that it is worthwhile to continue. A decrease in a bone marker value to a premenopausal level may give this assurance to the individual.

To substantiate existing data showing the usefulness of bone markers as risk assessment and monitoring tools, a large number of clinical studies are currently being performed. To enable a more widespread use of the biochemical markers, research aimed at identifying new more sensitive and specific markers is ongoing, as is the development of assays which are convenient and automated[13–19]. These combined efforts are necessary to generate the body of data needed for the establishment of biochemical markers of bone turnover as a routine tool in the daily management of osteoporosis and other bone diseases.

BONE FORMATION MARKERS

The bone formation process is mediated by the osteoblasts and involves synthesis of, for example, type I collagen, osteocalcin and alkaline phosphatase. For a molecule to be useful as a formation marker, it must be found in the blood circulation or excreted into urine. The above-mentioned molecules or, for collagen, the precursor (procollagen type I C-terminal propeptide, PICP), are all found in the circulation and, thus, can be measured in a serum or plasma sample. Today, these three markers are the most promising and the most well-documented of the bone formation markers.

Osteocalcin

Osteocalcin, or bone Gla protein, is a small non-collagenous protein with a molecular weight of 5800 g/mol[20,21]. Osteocalcin is found exclusively in bone and is the most abundant non-collagenous protein in bone. The synthesis of human osteocalcin by osteoblasts involves vitamin K for the formation of the γ-carboxylated glutamic acids (Gla) and vitamin D for the stimulation of its production. Osteocalcin has a high affinity for calcium and exhibits a compact calcium-dependent α-helical conformation, in which the Gla residues promote absorption to hydroxyapatite in the bone matrix[22–24]. Freshly synthesized osteocalcin is partly secreted into the bloodstream and partly incorporated into the bone matrix. Thus, circulating osteocalcin is associated with changes in the rate of bone formation in a number of metabolic bone diseases such as osteoporosis, primary hyperparathyroidism, hyperthyroidism, Paget's disease and renal osteodystrophy[25–27].

Osteocalcin was first suggested as a marker of bone formation in the early 1980s. The widespread use of this marker, however, is not yet established. Despite a large body of clinical data, the instability of intact osteocalcin in serum and plasma has limited its use as a routine marker. The intact osteocalcin is only stable for a few hours at room temperature, which is not feasible in clinical practice[18].

The instability of the osteocalcin is primarily caused by a labile six amino-acid COOH-terminal sequence which is easily cleaved off, resulting in the formation of a large NH_2-terminal mid-fragment (see Figure 1). This N-Mid fragment (amino acids 1–44), however, is significantly more stable than the intact molecule (Figure 2). Therefore, osteocalcin assays measuring the N-Mid fragment are the best candidates to gain acceptance for routine use. This is further illustrated by Figure 3 which shows

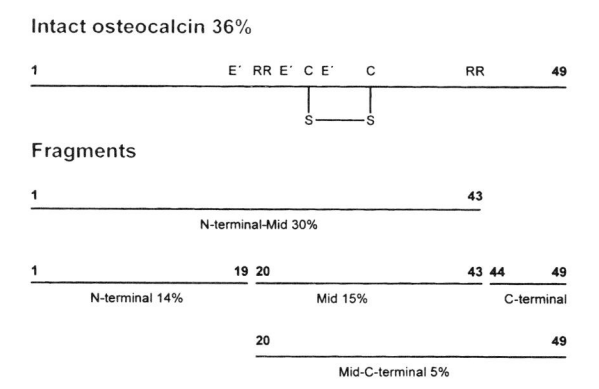

Figure 1 Circulating immunoreactive forms of human osteocalcin. Fragments shown on diagram can be released *in vitro* by trypsin digestion because of Arg–Arg bonds in positions 19–20 and 43–44. *In vivo* studies using specific monoclonal antibodies recognizing different epitopes on osteocalcin molecule have confirmed existence of such fragments in serum. However, C-terminal fragment has not been detected, probably because of rapid *in vivo* degradation and clearance from circulation[11]

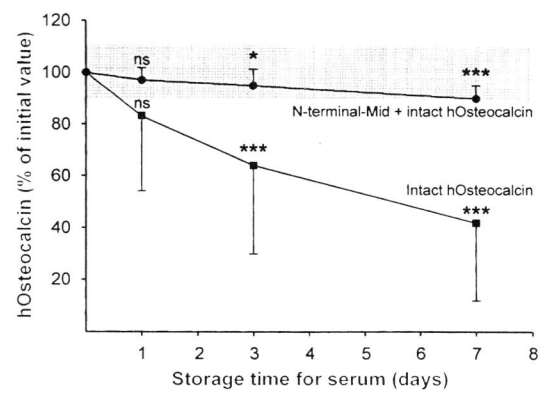

Figure 2 Stability of osteocalcin during storage of serum samples. Blood from 10 volunteers was allowed to stand at room temperature for 1 h before serum was collected. Stability of serum human osteocalcin (hOsteocalcin) during storage at 4 °C was then examined. Samples were frozen at −20 °C after 0, 1, 3 and 7 days. Serum concentrations were measured by N-Mid human osteocalcin enzyme-linked immunosorbent assay (ELISA) (●) and by ELSA-NAT-OST IRMA measuring intact human calcitonin only, (■) and expressed as percentages (± 1 SD) of initial values, *$p < 0.05$; ***$p < 0.001$; ns, not significant[18]

osteocalcin levels in a set of serum samples which has been stored at −20 °C[18]. As can be seen, results from measurement of intact osteocalcin in such samples from women receiving antiresorptive therapy do not relate to the actual changes known to occur in bone metabolism. On the contrary, the changes are reflected by measurement of the N-Mid fragment. Two immunoassays measuring the N-Mid fragment have been commercially available for the past 2–3 years: ELSA OSTEO IRMA (CIS, Paris, France) and N-MID™ Osteocalcin enzyme-linked immunosorbent assay (ELISA) (Osteometer BioTech, Herlev, Denmark). Moreover, measurement of the N-Mid osteocalcin has very recently become available using automated analyzers from Hoffmann La-Roche Diagnostics, Basel, Switzerland and Boehringer Mannheim (Mannheim, Germany).

Bone-specific alkaline phosphatase

Alkaline phosphatase is expressed by osteoblasts and, therefore, has been studied intensively as a marker of bone formation. The so-called 'bone-

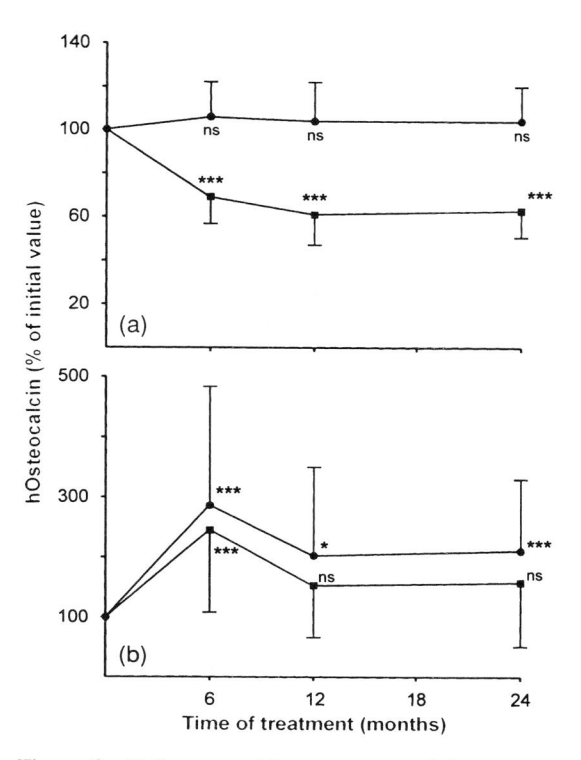

Figure 3 Follow-up of human osteocalcin concentrations after hormone replacement therapy in retrospective study. Blood samples were obtained from women receiving estrogen-like steroid ($n = 10$) (●) or placebo ($n = 10$) treatment (■) for 24 months. Serum samples were collected at day 0 (t_0) and after 6 (t_6), 12 (t_{12}) and 24 months (t_{24}). Serum concentrations of human osteocalcin (hOsteocalcin) were measured by N-Mid enzyme-linked immunosorbent assay (ELISA) (a) and by ELSA-NAT-OST IRMA (b). Results are expressed as percentages (± 1 SD) of pretreatment value. *$p < 0.05$; ***$p < 0.001$; ns, not significant[18]

specific' alkaline phosphatase is a product of the same gene as liver and kidney alkaline phosphatase[17,28]. The various alkaline phosphatases only differ in their tissue-related post-translational modifications. These modifications, primarily leading to differences in the carbohydrate side chains, have been used to develop assays which were meant to be 'bone-specific'. One such commercial assay is based on differences in the lectin-binding properties of liver and bone alkaline phosphatases (Boehringer Mannheim, Mannheim, Germany). Another commercial assay is based on quantifying bone alkaline phosphatase in a direct radioimmunometric assay (Ostase®; Hybritech, San Diego, USA). This assay, however, has been reported to have a cross-reactivity of 16% to the liver isoenzyme[17]. Bone alkaline phosphatase has been shown to be a promising marker in the assessment of disease activity in Paget's disease patients, and several studies have suggested its use to follow the efficacy of osteoporosis therapy. This is illustrated by Figure 4, in which the effect of a bisphosphonate (Fosamax™, Merck) on the serum level of bone-specific alkaline phosphatase is shown. The marker reflects the expected decrease in the rate of the bone formation following an antiresorptive therapy[29].

Procollagen type I carboxyl-terminal propeptide

Type I collagen accounts for more than 90% of the non-mineral component of bone. It is synthesized intracellularly as a large molecule, type I procollagen, which contains amino- and carboxyl-terminal globular extentions (propeptides)[30]. Before mature collagen fibrils are formed, these propeptides are cleaved from type I procollagen. Procollagen type I carboxyl-terminal propeptide (PICP) is a trimeric globular glycoprotein with a molecular weight of about 100 000 g/mol[31,32]. The PICP is released as an intact subunit of procollagen which is stabilized by interchain disulfide bridges. For each collagen molecule incorporated into a collagen fibril, one PICP molecule is released.

Owing to the close link with the incorporation of collagen type I into bone, PICP was suggested as a marker of bone formation several years ago[31]. A number of immunoassays have been developed for the measurement of the molecule, and a substantial body of data exists showing the usefulness of PICP as a marker of type I collagen biosynthesis. Especially, the use of PICP as a marker to monitor the effect of bisphosphonate therapy is promising[33]. The use of PICP as a marker of bone formation, however, has been called into question, as PICP by nature is not specific to bone and also comes from other tissues containing type I collagen. Studies have shown that PICP levels in postmenopausal women are only slightly elevated or not elevated at all above those of premenopausal controls[32,34]. As the formation of bone is known to increase after the menopause, as reflected in markers such as N-Mid osteocalcin and bone-specific alkaline phosphatase, these PICP results may indicate that PICP is not *in sensu strictu* a marker of bone formation, but more correctly is a marker of type I collagen synthesis.

BONE RESORPTION MARKERS

Osteoclasts mediate the bone resorption process. This process leads to degradation of the organic matrix resulting in the release of a large number of degradation products. These degradation products originating from the osteoclastic degradation of bone are generally fragments containing post-translational modifications of collagen, which makes them impossible for the body to reutilize. Examples of such modifications are fragments containing a collagen cross-linking molecule (e.g. pyridinoline, pyrrole) or fragments containing a modification in the bonds between the amino acids, as is seen in the C-telopeptides of type I collagen where EKAHD-β-GGR fragments are formed post-translationally[35–37].

A number of biochemical compounds have been suggested as markers of the bone resorption process. The most convincing data come

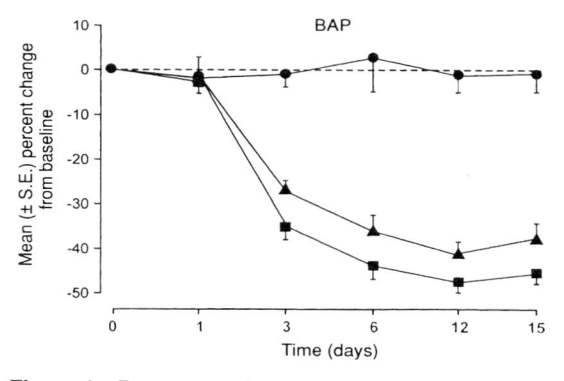

Figure 4 Response of bone-specific alkaline phosphatase (BAP) to treatment with alendronate 5 (▲) or 10 (■) mg/day or placebo (●) in 84 elderly osteoporotic women. Data are mean ± SEM[29]

from three of these: the pyridinolines[13,38,39], N-telopeptide degradation products of type I collagen (NTX) measured by the Osteomark® assay, Osteometer BioTech, Herlev, Denmark[15,40] and C-telopeptide degradation products (CTX) measured by CrossLaps™, Osteometer BioTech, Herlev, Denmark[16,41,42]. Whereas the two first markers are available only for urinary measurements, Cross Laps now can be measured in serum as well as in urine[19].

Pyridinolines

Pyridinoline (Pyr) and deoxypyridinoline (D-Pyr) are both mature, non-reducible cross-links of collagen: D-Pyr is only found in significant amounts in type I collagen in bone, whereas Pyr is a general cross-linker of collagen, i.e. Pyr is a major cross-linker in type II collagen[43,44]. Figure 5 shows a schematic illustration of the type I collagen molecule which forms the basis for the bone resorption markers mentioned above. The pyridinolines are excreted in urine in a so-called free form and a peptide-bound form, where telopeptides from the various collagen molecules are bound to Pyr or D-Pyr. The total excretion of both Pyr and D-Pyr has been shown to correlate well with radioisotopic measurement of bone resorption. It has been shown to be a promising marker in various metabolic bone diseases characterized by increased bone turnover, such as osteoporosis, Paget's disease, primary hyperparathyroidism and hyperthyroidism[45–48].

Measurement of the total urinary excretion of the pyridinolines has been used as an index of bone resorption for more than a decade. It is usually measured by reversed phase high-performance liquid chromatography (HPLC) of the cellulose-bound extract of hydrolyzed urine[49,50]. The HPLC methodology, however, is cumbersome and time-consuming and limits a widespread clinical use of the marker. Therefore, immunoassays were developed for direct determination of Pyr and D-Pyr. These assays measure a fraction (the free form) of the total

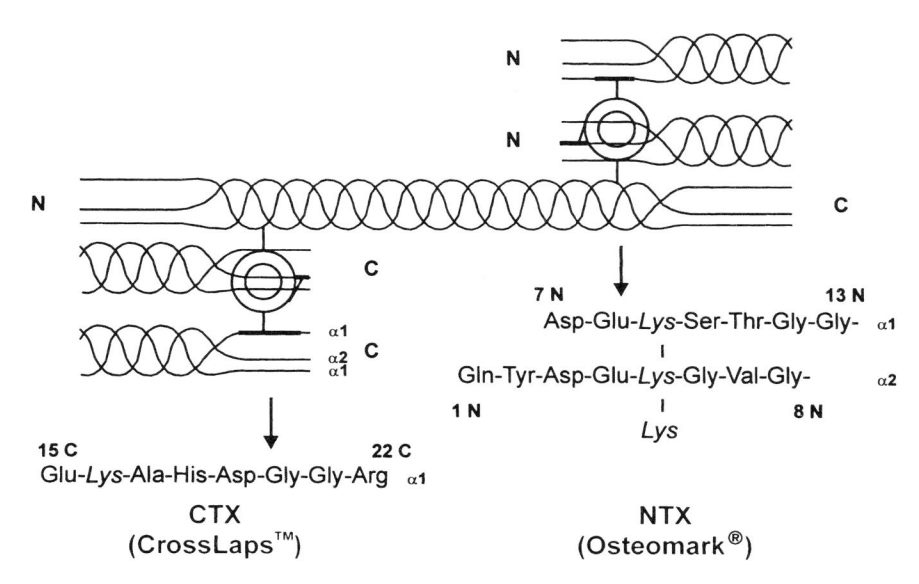

Figure 5 Type I collagen cross-linked peptides. Type I collagen molecules in bone matrix are linked by pyridinoline cross-links (pyridinoline or deoxypyridinoline) in region of N- and C-telopeptides. In CrossLaps™ assay, eight amino-acid sequence from C-telopeptide of α-1 chain is used as immunogen and standard. Thus, CrossLaps assay recognizes in urine type I collagen breakdown products (CTX) containing full or part of this sequence, whether linked or not linked with pyridinoline cross-link. Osteomark® immunoassay detects in urine cross-linked peptides (NTX) originating from degradation of N-telopeptides and presence of pyridinoline is required for antigenicity[11]

excretion of the Pyr or D-Pyr. Kits are commercially supplied by Metra Biosystems (Sunny Vale, CA, USA).

Studies have been performed to show that the free form, especially of deoxypyridinoline, correlates with the bone resorption process[14]. Some studies, however, have revealed that the free form of the deoxypyridinoline is not a good marker of the changes in bone resorption which take place during bisphosphonate therapy[29,51]. This is illustrated in Figure 6. As it is well established that bisphosphonates act exclusively on mineralized tissue (bone), it is notable that the decrease in bone resorption taking place following bisphosphonate therapy is not reflected in the excretion levels of the free form of deoxypyridinoline. Researchers also observed that, even after 2 years of bisphosphonate therapy (Fosamax), the free form of pyridinoline only decreased by about 15%, which was not significantly different from the placebo group[29]. These observations call for careful continued examination of the role of free pyridinolines as markers of bone resorption.

N-telopeptide degradation products

As mentioned above, a wide variety of products are released into circulation and excreted into urine as type I collagen is broken down. Some of the N-telopeptide degradation products of type I collagen (NTX) are quantitated by ELISA in the so-called Osteomark assay[15,40]. This assay is based on a monoclonal antibody raised against the N-telopeptide region shown in Figure 5. The assay, thus, reacts with fragments which contain a cross-linker and telopeptide elements from two peptide chains[40,52]. The advantage of the telopeptide assays (Osteomark and CrossLaps) over the pyridinoline assays is that the fragments measured in the telopeptide assays contain information of the collagen type from which they are derived. Thus, peptides derived from type II collagen (i.e. in rheumatoid arthritis and osteoarthritis) should not cross-react in the Osteomark or the CrossLaps assay. This is unlike the pyridinoline assays, where it is well established that a major part of the pyridinoline excreted in urine in the

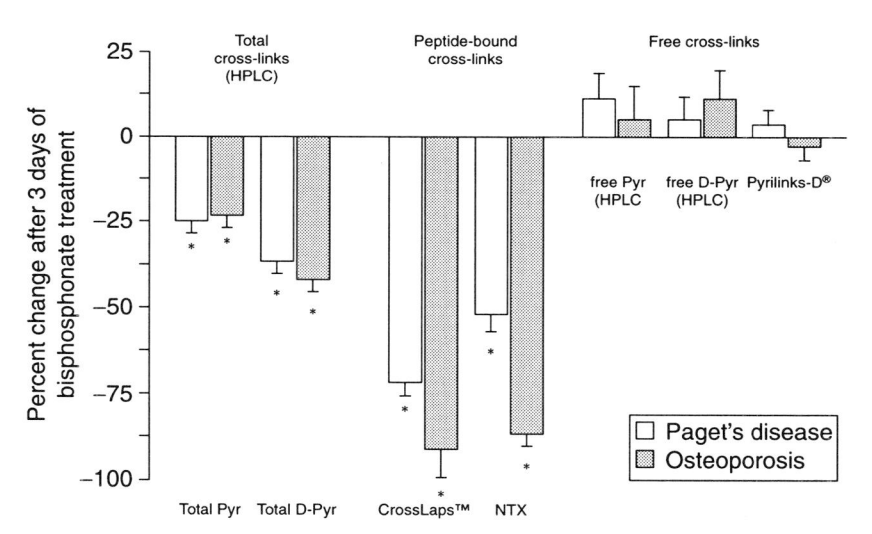

Figure 6 Percentage change in total, peptide-bound and free cross-link excretions in 14 Pagetic patients and in seven patients with osteoporosis after 3 days of intravenous treatment with bisphosphonate pamidronate (180 mg total dose). Total pyridinoline (Pyr) and total deoxypyridinoline (D-Pyr) are measured by high-performance liquid chromatography (HPLC) after urine hydrolysis. Peptide-bound cross-links are measured by two enzyme-linked immunosorbent assays (ELISAs) recognizing type I collagen peptides in C-telopeptide (CrossLaps™) and N-telopeptide (NTX) regions. Free cross-links are measured either with HPLC before urine hydrolysis (free Pyr and free D-Pyr) or with ELISA specific for free D-Pyr (Pyrilinks®-D). Results are expressed as mean ± 1 SEM. *$p < 0.001$ vs. pretreatment[51]

above-mentioned diseases comes from type II collagen found in cartilage[49,53].

Values measured in the Osteomark assay are elevated in postmenopausal women compared to premenopausal women[40,54]. Data obtained regarding the use of Osteomark for monitoring antiresorptive therapies such as hormone replacement and bisphosphonate therapies suggest that Osteomark is a sensitive index of bone resorption measurement in the postmenopausal population[29,51,55].

C-telopeptide degradation products

A large number of cross-linkers contribute to the variety of compounds released into the circulation and later excreted into urine. The more important cross-linkers are the pyridinolines and the pyrroles, but several others contribute to the cross-linking of type I collagen[56,57]. Figure 7 shows the biochemical structure of some of the cross-linkers of type I collagen. Aiming at an assay which should measure this pool of C-telopeptide fragments independently of the nature of the cross-linkers, the so-called CrossLaps assay was developed[41]. The assay is based on the use of antibodies which react with a peptide sequence of the α1 chain of the C-telopeptides of type I collagen (Glu-Lys-Ala-His-Asp-Gly-Gly-Arg). Furthermore, it has been shown that a variety of fragments of C-telopeptide degradation products of type I collagen are measured by ELISA, and that these fragments indeed contain different cross-linkers, thus showing that fragments do react and are recognized in the assay independently of the nature of the cross-linker[37].

Additionally, it has been found that the peptide sequence mentioned above can be isomerized at the aspartate (Asp) residue (i.e. there can be bonds to glycine (Gly) through the β- and α-carbonyl groups of the aspartate residue)[37,58,59]. As the isomerization apparently is a process which occurs as the tissue ages, measurement of the isomerized fragments, or β-fragments, is suggested to be an index of degradation of aged bone, whereas measurement of non-isomerized fragments, or α-fragments, is an index of degradation of more newly formed bone[59,60]. Immunoassays for measurement of the α-fragments as well as the β-fragments are commercially available (CrossLaps™ ELISA (β-fragments); α-CrossLaps™ RIA (α-fragments); Osteometer BioTech, Herlev, Denmark).

Values measured in the CrossLaps assays are elevated in postmenopausal compared to premenopausal women[9,16]. Data obtained regarding the use of CrossLaps assays for monitoring antiresorptive therapies such as hormone replacement and bisphosphonate therapies suggest that the marker is a sensitive and specific index of the bone resorption process[42,51,61]. In urine samples from a postmenopausal population, values from the CrossLaps ELISA and the α-CrossLaps radioimmunoassay (RIA) are highly correlated ($r = 0.94$)[59]. However, in patients with Paget's disease, there is a more pronounced increase over the reference group in the α-CrossLaps RIA than is seen in the CrossLaps ELISA[60]. This difference indicates that, when assessing the disease activity in Paget's disease, the measurement of α-fragments may be the more sensitive marker.

Recently, a CrossLaps assay measuring bone resorption in serum has become commercially available (Serum CrossLaps™ One Step ELISA; Osteometer BioTech, Herlev, Denmark). This assay is based on the fact that the C-telopeptide degradation products released from the bone

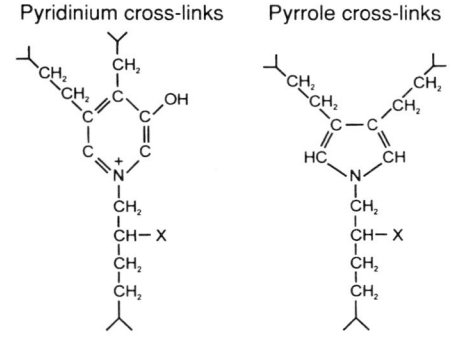

Figure 7 Structure of pyridinium cross-links, pyrrole cross-links (Erlich chromogens) and their glycosylated derivatives. Pyridinoline (Pyr) and deoxypyridinoline (D-Pyr) contain –OH and –H, respectively, at position X. Glycosylated derivatives of molecules contain groups O-Gal-Glu and O-Gal at position X. Structure of pyrrole cross-link was suggested by Kuypers et al.[57]

resorption process apparently exist as modified dipeptides[37]. These modified dipeptides contain a cross-linker and two modified peptide strings derived from the EKAHDGGR-region of type I collagen (Figure 8). By raising monoclonal antibodies to a modified synthetic peptide (EKAHD-β-GGR), a sandwich ELISA was developed.

CLINICAL VALUE OF BONE MARKERS

The need for careful and cost-effective management of osteoporosis calls for tools which allow valid prognosis and precise monitoring of the disease. Attempts to evaluate biochemical bone markers in this context and the possibility of combining results from the markers with other tools such as bone mass measurement, therefore, is of interest. The clinical research carried out has had two distinct and different focuses, namely (1) the potential use of the bone markers to follow-up therapy and (2) the potential use of the bone markers as prognostic tools to assess the risk of osteoporotic fractures.

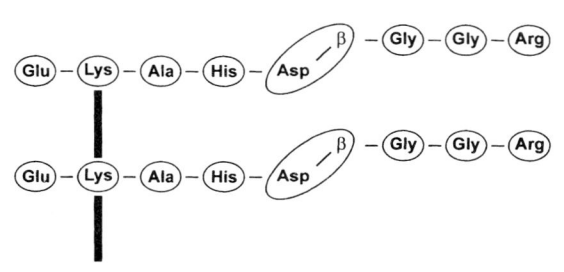

Figure 8 Modified dipeptide structure derived from osteoclastic degradation of C-telopeptides of type I collagen

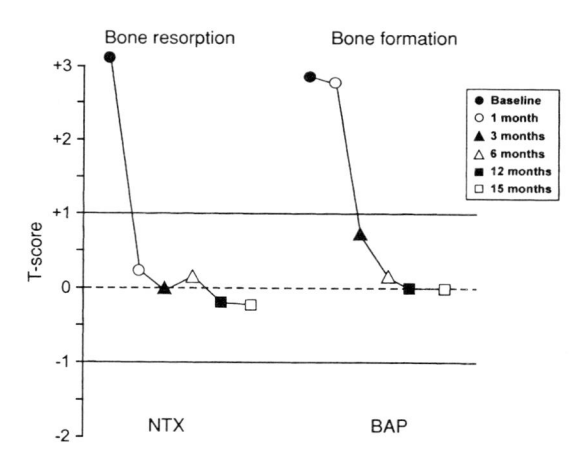

Figure 9 Mean T-score values for N-telopeptide degradation products (NTX) and bone-specific alkaline phosphatase (BAP) in elderly osteoporotic women at baseline and after 1, 3, 6, 12 and 15 months of treatment with alendronate (10 mg/day). T-scores are number of SDs from mean of 46 premenopausal women[29]

Therapy follow-up

Institution of efficient antiresorptive therapy introduces large changes in markers of bone turnover within a short period of time. Markers of bone resorption will decrease up to 80% within days, depending on the actual therapy administered[51]. Owing to the coupling between bone resorption and bone formation processes, levels of bone formation markers will usually start to decline 6–8 weeks after therapy has been initiated. After 3–6 months of continued therapy, the decrease in the level of the bone formation marker stops and a plateau is reached. In Figure 9, the effects of initiating bisphosphonate therapy on the levels of bone resorption and formation markers are shown.

Recently, a serum bone resorption marker has become commercially available (Serum CrossLaps™ One Step ELISA, Osteometer BioTech, Herlev, Denmark). This marker is the first of the bone resorption markers to be measured in serum (all other markers use urine specimens). Compared to urine, measurement of any biochemical marker in serum (or plasma) has distinct advantages: the serum marker does not need correction for creatinine and the diurnal variation in serum is usually considerably lower, leading to a smaller day-to-day variation. In particular, the influence of the day-to-day variation of urinary markers on the conclusions to be drawn has been discussed in the research community. Variations of 15–30% have been reported[11,29]. Under well-controlled circumstances, such as those existing in clinical investigations, it is probably possible to maintain an acceptable day-to-day variation in the range of 15–20% but, for use in daily practice, the day-to-day variation in urinary markers represents a potential problem. Therefore, the new serum bone resorption marker has great potential as the day-to-day variation is reported to be 13%[62]. The body of data from this serum assay is yet limited. However, the use of the marker to monitor antiresorptive therapies (hormone replacement and bisphosphonate) is shown in Figure 10.

Prevention of bone loss and new or further fractures requires relatively long-term therapy. Because the benefit of such therapy only occurs after many years and because of potential long-term adverse effects, compliance to osteoporosis therapy is a major problem. Rapid information, obtained from bone markers, relating to the apparent efficacy of the therapy, therefore, is of importance to increase the compliance. It has to be born in mind that, for example, in the case of preventive osteoporosis therapies, a woman may, in principle, need to take medication from the day she enters the menopause for 5 or 10 years, or even longer.

Prediction of skeletal response

Over the past few years, the main focus of clinical research into biochemical bone markers has been to evaluate their use as monitoring tools during antiresorptive therapies. More recently, papers have been presented which report the use of the markers as a tool which is not only able to monitor that the level of the bone marker has decreased after therapy has been instituted, but indeed finds a strong correlation between a change (decrease) in the bone marker from baseline to, for example, 3 months and the actual loss of bone over a 2-year period[55]. Thereby, the measurement of the bone marker becomes a predictive tool in the sense that, by use of results obtained with the biochemical marker, it can be predicted which women will benefit the most in terms of skeletal increase from the therapy administered. In Figure 11, the skeletal response to calcitonin therapy is shown when stratified according to short-term changes in the bone marker (CrossLaps). As can be seen, the group of women who exhibit the largest

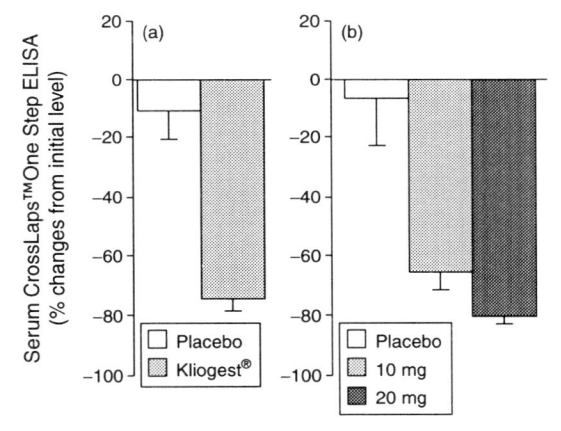

Figure 10 (a) Follow-up of serum CrossLaps™ values after hormone replacement therapy. Blood samples were obtained from postmenopausal women receiving hormone replacement therapy (Kliogest®) or placebo treatment. Serum samples were collected at baseline and 12 months. Results are expressed in percentage change (mean ± SEM) from pretreatment values. T-tests for unpaired data showed significant difference between placebo group and treated group ($p < 0.001$). (b) Follow-up of serum CrossLaps™ values after treatment with bisphosphonate Fosamax™. Blood samples were obtained from postmenopausal women receiving Fosamax™ or placebo treatment. Serum samples were collected at baseline and 12 months. Results are expressed in percentage change (mean ± SEM) from pretreatment values. T-tests for unpaired data showed significant difference between placebo group and each of treated groups ($p < 0.001$). There was also significant difference between two treated groups ($p = 0.03$). ELISA, enzyme-linked immunosorbent assay

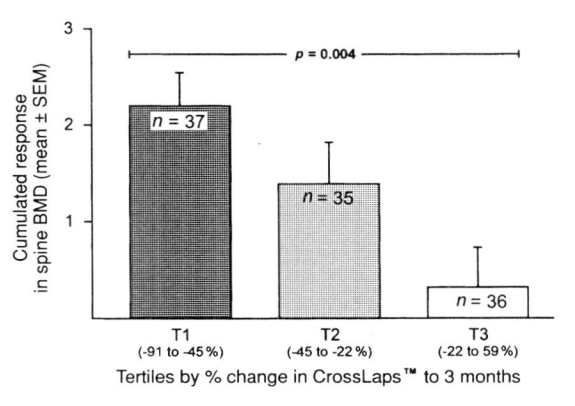

Figure 11 Skeletal response to calcitonin therapy after 2 years. Groups were stratified according to short-term changes (3 months) in CrossLaps™ values. BMD, bone mineral density

changes after 3 months (largest decrease in the bone marker value) is the group of women who gain most bone mass. These data strongly suggest that important information can be given to the woman concerning the likely influence of the instituted therapy on her bone mass. Such information derived from the use of a bone resorption marker can be given only a few months after the therapy has been instituted.

Risk assessment using biochemical markers

Research into the potential use of the biochemical markers of bone turnover as prognostic tools started more than a decade ago. Today, a number of studies demonstrate a close link between the level of biochemical markers and the rate of bone loss[8,63–65].

In a major study initiated in 1977, several hundred women had been followed without intervention. State-of-the-art biochemical markers were measured and bone mass was measured accordingly[8]. Data from this study demonstrates that, despite identical bone mass, a group of women who initially had been classified as 'fast bone losers' based on biochemical markers over a period of 12 years lost 50% more bone mass than women classified as 'slow bone losers' (total bone loss 26.6% vs. 16.6%, $p < 0.001$)[64]. Figure 12 shows the correlation between the bone mass actually measured after 12 years (in 1989) and the predicted bone mass which was based on one baseline bone mass measurement and baseline biochemical markers measured in serum and urine samples (serum alkaline phosphatase, serum osteocalcin, urinary calcium and urinary hydroxyproline)[64]. (Baseline was in 1977 when all women were 6 months to 3 years post-menopause). These results strongly suggest a general link between a bone marker index and the rate of bone loss.

The use of a combination of biochemical markers has been demonstrated to have the ability to predict the bone loss over a shorter period of time. Again, using a panel of four biochemical markers of bone turnover (urinary calcium, urinary hydroxyproline, serum alkaline phosphatase and serum osteocalcin),

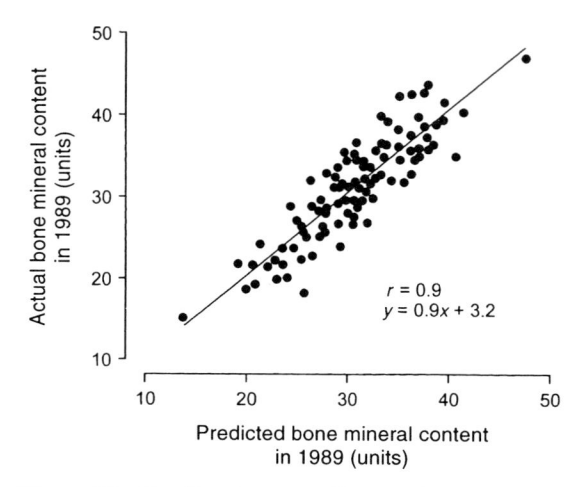

Figure 12 Predicted vs. actual bone mineral content in 1989 (predicted value from baseline bone mass and estimated bone loss). Multiple regression analysis: bone mineral content $p < 0.001$; estimated rate of bone loss $p < 0.005$[64]

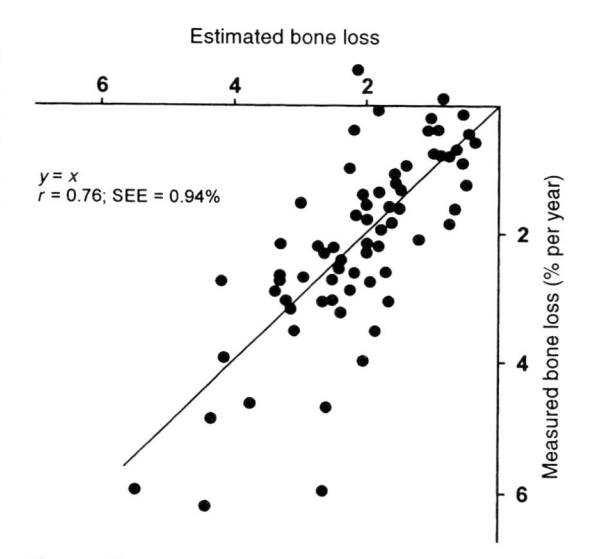

Figure 13 Relation between measured bone loss (%/year) and estimated bone loss using osteocalcin, alkaline phosphatase, urinary calcium and urinary hydroxyproline[63]

Christiansen and colleagues found a correlation of $r = 0.76$ with bone loss, as assessed by repetitive bone mass measurement over 2 years[63]. Results are shown in Figure 13. A number of other studies have demonstrated similar correlations, although using different biochemical markers. Uebelhart and co-workers found a correlation of $r = 0.77$ between change in bone mass over 2 years and a panel of biochemical markers (serum osteocalcin, urinary total excretion of D-Pyr and urinary hydroxyproline)[65]. Even on the basis of measurement of a single bone marker, strong correlations with change in bone mass have been reported ($r = 0.5-0.6$)[9,10].

Thus, the body of data supporting the existence of a close link between the rate of bone loss and values obtained from a bone marker index is large. However, the practical use of the ability of bone markers to assess the rate of bone loss has not yet gained widespread acceptance. A major reason for this may be that the investigations have primarily been initiated to show the existence of the correlation and not the practical use of the results. Only recently, Chesnut and associates have suggested an interpretation of the results arising from an investigation of bone markers and change in bone loss[55]. In this study, the bone marker value was used to stratify the women. Thus, the bone marker value will place a woman in a certain quartile and, for each quartile, a certain risk profile for losing bone can be determined. These data are shown in Figure 14.

Using this presentation of the results, the biochemical marker gains value as a tool which has the potential of identifying women at increased risk of losing bone. Such practical information is of major importance in the guidance of menopausal women and could be used in conjunction with a bone mass measurement to determine the optimal management of osteoporosis.

Fracture prediction using biochemical markers

Over the past few years, large clinical studies primarily addressing the link between the bone marker value and the risk of fracture have been initiated. These major studies obviously attract much attention, as osteoporotic fractures have severe individual and socioeconomic consequences. The inherent problems involved in the design of such studies are obvious; to obtain a significant number of fractures which allow for some generalization in the conclusions, either a large cohort of individuals (up to 10 000 women) could be followed for a few years, or a smaller cohort (200–400 women) could be followed over decades. The latter study design is not possible in 1997 as it is not acceptable from an ethical point of view to follow women for 10 or 15 years without intervening, knowing that efficient therapies exist and should be offered

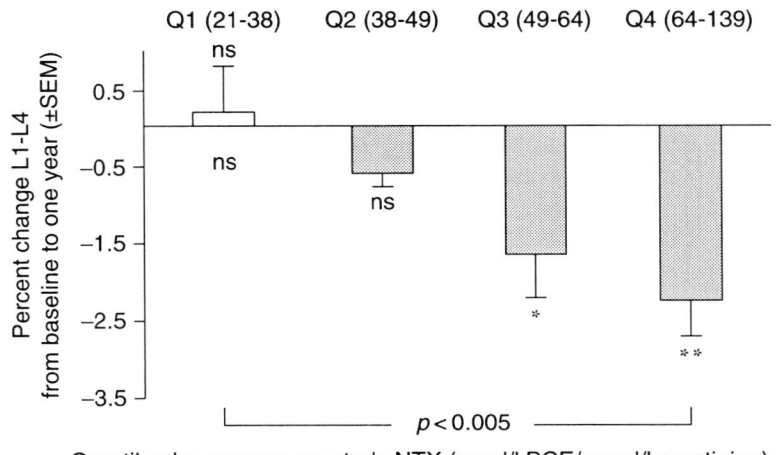

Figure 14 Response to calcium at spine by quartiles of N-telopeptide degradation products of type I collagen (NTX, average on study). ns, not significantly different from baseline; *significantly different ($p < 0.05$) from baseline; **significantly different ($p < 0.001$) from baseline; BCE, bone collagen equivalents[55]

to the women losing the most bone. Therefore, in 1997, the only feasible way of designing fracture studies is to include thousands of women and follow these over a few years.

Nevertheless, data about the relationship between bone markers and fracture incidence exist from a 15-year study[66]. In this study, it had been possible to follow 182 women for 15 years as the study was initiated in 1977 when no established therapy for arresting bone loss existed. In 1977, the women had undergone a natural menopause 6 months to 3 years previously, and they were between 45 and 54 years old. The main conclusions from this paper are that a group of women defined on the basis of biochemical bone markers as 'fast bone losers' had a two-fold higher risk of vertebral and peripheral fractures compared to the group of 'normal' or 'slow' bone losers. The risk factors low bone mass and high bone turnover were independent. Thus, women with both a low bone mass and a high rate of bone turnover immediately following the menopause had a higher risk of subsequent fractures than women with only one of the risk factors (odds ratio 3.0).

Results in accordance with the observation that low bone mass and fast bone loss are independent risk factors have recently been generated from a large prospective study of hip fractures in elderly healthy women in France (the EPIDOS study)[67]. These women were around the age of 70 years and were followed for 2 years. In those women who had a hip fracture during the 2-year follow up, baseline measurements of urinary CTX (CrossLaps ELISA) or free D-Pyr (Pyrilinks®-D ELISA) were significantly higher than in non-fractured controls (Table 1). A value of either of the markers which was increased above the normal range for premenopausal women was associated with a 90% (Pyrilinks-D) or a 120% (CrossLaps) increase in the risk of hip fractures. These observations were still significant after correction for bone mass, indicating that the information about future risk generated using biochemical markers is additive to the information about future risk generated by measurement of bone mass. Indeed, women having a high CrossLaps value and at the same time a low bone mass were shown to have an increased risk of 300%. Results are shown in Figure 15. These findings show that the combination of bone mass and bone turnover measurements should be useful to improve the risk assessment of osteoporotic fractures.

Several other studies have reported results which are supportive to the above-mentioned conclusions. Overgaard and Christiansen have shown that, in women who participated in a

Table 1 Increased bone marker levels as predictors of hip fracture in elderly women[67]

Bone markers (predictors)	Odds ratio (95% confidence interval)	
	Highest quartile of elderly	Above upper limit of premenopausal range
Osteocalcin	1.1 (0.7–1.9)	1.0 (0.6–1.6)
BAP	0.9 (0.6–1.4)	1.1 (0.7–1.7)
NTX	1.1 (0.7–1.9)	1.4 (0.9–2.2)
CTX	2.1 (1.3–3.3)	2.2 (1.3–3.6)
Free D-Pyr	1.5 (0.9–2.5)	1.9 (1.1–3.2)

BAP, bone-specific alkaline phosphatase; NTX, N-telopeptide degradation products; CTX, C-telopeptide degradation products; D-Pyr, deoxypyridinoline

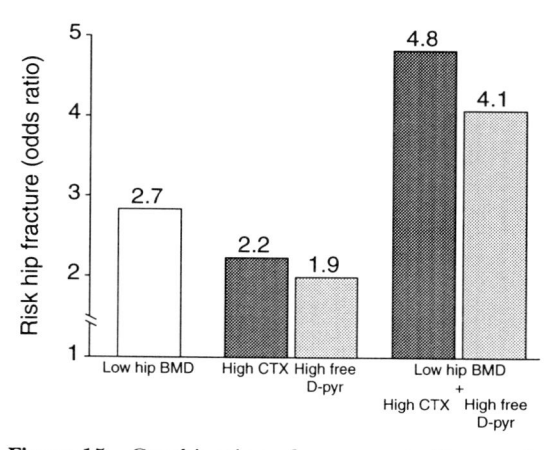

Figure 15 Combination of assessment of bone mineral density (BMD) and bone resorption rate to predict hip fracture risk in elderly. Low BMD was defined according to WHO guidelines, i.e. value lower than 2.5 SD below young adult mean (*T*-score ≤ 2.5) High bone resorption was defined by C-telopeptide degradation products (CTX) or free deoxypyridinoline (D-Pyr) values higher than upper limit (mean + 2 SD) of premenopausal range. Women with both low hip BMD and high bone resorption were at higher risk of hip fracture than women with either low hip BMD or high bone resorption[67]

double-blind placebo-controlled calcitonin study, those who experienced fractures had significantly higher levels of the bone marker (CrossLaps) than women who did not experience a fracture[61]. Conclusions from a recent study by Cummings and colleagues[68] as well as a study by a Dutch group[69] have reported concordant results about the link between an increased level of a bone marker and increased risk of osteoporotic fractures. Very recently, it was demonstrated by Ross and colleagues that, in a cohort of 512 Hawaiian women, elevated CrossLaps values as well as Ostase values were predictive of vertebral fracture[70].

Future outlook

Future use of biochemical bone markers as a routine tool in the daily management of postmenopausal osteoporosis is dependent on a number of different factors. Above all, the markers must prove to provide the general physician with information that can help to make optimal decisions together with the patient. It must be established that correct use of information from biochemical markers is necessary for an optimal management of osteoporosis, the final goal of such management being to reduce fracture incidence. Such use of biochemical markers requires high standards of these markers; some standards are met by the bone markers and already accepted, others need to be further substantiated. These standards relate to the technical performance of the assays to be used as well as to the supporting clinical data.

The occurrence of particular serum bone resorption markers, however, raises confidence that the above-mentioned standards will be met. Thus, it is to be expected within future years that biochemical bone markers will become established routine tools for following osteoporosis therapy as well as for assessing the future risk of osteoporotic fractures.

References

1. Delmas PD. Biochemical markers of bone turnover. *J Bone Miner Res* 1993;8:S549–55
2. Isenbarger DW, Chapin BL. Osteoporosis. Current pharmacologic options for prevention and treatment. *Postgrad Med* 1997;101:129–42
3. Compston JE. Prevention and management of osteoporosis. Current trends and future prospects. *Drugs* 1997;53:727–35
4. Sankaran SK. Osteoporosis prevention and treatment. Pharmacological management and treatment implications. *Drugs Aging* 1996;9:472–77
5. Christiansen C. What should be done at the time of menopause? *Am J Med* 1995;98:56S–9S
6. Christiansen C. Osteoporosis: diagnosis and management today and tomorrow. *Bone* 1995;17:513S–16S
7. Bjarnason NH, Bjarnason K, Haarbo J, *et al.* Tibolone: prevention of bone loss in late postmenopausal women. *J Clin Endocrinol Metab* 1996;81:2419–22
8. Christiansen C, Riis BJ, Rødbro P. Prediction of rapid bone loss in postmenopausal women. *Lancet* 1987;1:1105–8
9. Bonde M, Qvist P, Fledelius C, *et al.* Applications of an enzyme immunoassay for a new marker of bone resorption (CrossLaps™): follow-up on hormone replacement therapy and osteoporosis risk assessment. *J Clin Endocrinol Metab* 1995;80:864–8
10. Garnero P, Sornay-Rendu E, Chapuy M-C, *et al.* Increased bone turnover in late postmenopausal women is a major determinant of osteoporosis. *J Bone Miner Res* 1996;11:337–49
11. Garnero P, Delmas PD. Measurements of biochemical markers: methods and limitations. In Bilezikian JP, *et al.*, eds. *Principles of Bone Biology*. New York: Academic Press, 1996;1277–91
12. Bailey AJ, Ranta MH, Nicholls AC, *et al.* Isolation of α-amino adipic acid from mature dermal collagen and elastin. Evidence for an oxidative pathway in the maturation of collagen and elastin. *Biochem Biophys Res Comm* 1977;78:1403–10
13. Seyedin SM, Kung VT, Daniloff YN, *et al.* Immunoassay for urinary pyridinoline: the new marker of bone resorption. *J Bone Miner Res* 1993;8:635–41
14. Robins SP, Seibel MJ. Biochemical markers of bone metabolism: a critical evaluation. *Clin Lab* 1995;41:987–9

15. Hanson DA, Weis MA, Bollen A-M, et al. A specific immunoassay for monitoring human bone resorption: quantitation of type I collagen cross-linked N-telopeptides in urine. *J Bone Miner Res* 1992;7:1251–8
16. Garnero P, Gineyts E, Riou JP, et al. Assessment of bone resorption with a new marker of collagen degradation in patients with metabolic bone disease. *J Clin Endocrinol Metab* 1994;79:780–5
17. Garnero P, Delmas PD. Assessment of the serum levels of bone alkaline phosphatase with a new immunoradiometric assay in patients with metabolic bone disease. *J Clin Endocrinol Metab* 1993;77:1–8
18. Rosenquist C, Qvist P, Bjarnason NH, et al. Measurement of a more stable region of osteocalcin in serum by ELISA with two monoclonal antibodies. *Clin Chem* 1995;41:1439–45
19. Bonde M, Garnero P, Fledelius C, et al. Measurement of bone degradation products in serum using antibodies reactive with an isomerized form of an 8 amino acid sequence of the C-telopeptide of type I collagen. *J Bone Miner Res* 1997;12:1028–34
20. Price PA, Poser JW, Raman N. Primary structure of the γ-carboxyglutamic acid-containing protein from bovine bone. *Proc Natl Acad Sci USA* 1976;73:3374–5
21. Price PA, Nishimoto SK. Radioimmunoassay for the vitamin K-dependent protein of bone and its discovery in plasma. *Proc Natl Acad Sci USA* 1980;77:2234–8
22. Price PA, Williamson MK, Lothringer JW. Origin of the vitamin K-dependent bone protein found in plasma and its clearance by kidney and bone. *J Biol Chem* 1981;256:12760–6
23. Gundberg CM, Hauschka PV, Lian JB, et al. Osteocalcin: isolation, characterization and detection. *Meth Enzymol* 1984;107:516–44
24. Hauschka PV, Lian JB, Cole DE, et al. Osteocalcin and matrix Gla protein: vitamin K-dependent proteins in bone. *Phys Rev* 1989;69:990–1047
25. Pødenphant J, Christiansen C, Catherwood BD, et al. Serum bone Gla protein variations during estrogen and calcium prophylaxis of postmenopausal women. *Calcif Tissue Int* 1984;36: 536–40
26. Brown JP, Delmas PD, Malaval L, et al. Serum bone Gla protein: a specific marker for bone formation in postmenopausal osteoporosis. *Lancet* 1984;1:1091–3
27. Garnero P, Grimaux M, Demiaux B, et al. Measurement of serum osteocalcin with a human-specific two-site immunoradiometric assay. *J Bone Miner Res* 1992;7:1389–98
28. England TE, Samsoondar J, Maw G. Evaluation of the Hybritech Tandem-R Ostase immunoradiometric assay for skeletal alkaline phosphatase. *Clin Biochem* 1994;27:187–9
29. Garnero P, Shih WJ, Gineyts E, et al. Comparison of new biochemical markers of bone turnover in late postmenopausal osteoporotic women in response to alendronate treatment. *J Clin Endocrinol Metab* 1994;79:1693–700
30. Burgeson RE. The classical collagens: types I, II and III. In Mayne R, et al., eds. *Structure and Function of Collagen Types*. Orlando: Academic Press, 1987:1–23
31. Melkko J, Niemi S, Risteli L, et al. Radioimmunoassay of the carboxyterminal propeptide of human type I procollagen. *Clin Chem* 1990;36: 1328–32
32. Pedersen BJ, Bonde M. Purification of human procollagen type I carboxy-terminal propeptide cleaved as *in vivo* from procollagen and used to calibrate a radioimmunoassay of the propeptide. *Clin Chem* 1994;40:811–16
33. Christgau S, Qvist P, Bonde M. Effect of bisphosphonate treatment on the serum concentration of two collagen derived biochemical markers of bone metabolism. *Bone* 1995;17:48
34. Hassager C, Fabbri-Mabelli G, Christiansen C. The effect of the menopause and hormone replacement therapy on serum carboxyterminal propeptide of type I collagen. *Osteoporosis Int* 1993;3:50–2
35. Calvo MS, Eyre DR, Gundberg CM. Molecular basis and clinical application of biological markers of bone turnover. *Endocr Rev* 1996;17:333–68
36. Robins SP. Collagen crosslinks in metabolic bone disease. *Acta Orthop Scand* 1995;66:171–5
37. Fledelius C, Johnsen AH, Cloos PAC, et al. Characterization of urinary degradation products derived from type I collagen. Identification of a β-isomerized Asp-Gly sequence within the C-terminal telopeptide (α) region. *J Biol Chem* 1997; 272:9755–63
38. Robins SP. An enzyme-linked immunoassay for the collagen cross-link pyridinoline. *Biochem J* 1982;207:617–20
39. Black D, Duncan A, Robins SP. Quantitative analysis of the pyridinium crosslinks of collagen in urine using ion-paired reversed-phase high-performance liquid chromatography. *Anal Biochem* 1988;169:197–203
40. Gertz BJ, Shao P, Hanson DA, et al. Monitoring bone resorption in early postmenopausal women by an immunoassay for cross linked collagen peptides in urine. *J Bone Miner Res* 1994; 9:135–42
41. Bonde M, Qvist P, Fledelius C, et al. Immunoassay for quantifying type I collagen degradation products in urine evaluated. *Clin Chem* 1994;40: 2022–5
42. Ravn P, Clemmesen B, Riis BJ, et al. The effect on bone mass and bone markers of different doses of ibandronate: a new bisphosphonate for

prevention and treatment of postmenopausal osteoporosis: a 1-year, randomized, double-blind, placebo-controlled dose-finding study. *Bone* 1996;19:527–33
43. Eyre DR, Wu J-J, Woods PE. The cartilage collagens: structural and metabolic studies. *J Rheumatol* 1991;18:49–51
44. Eyre DR, Wu J-J, Niyibizi C, et al. The cartilage collagens – analysis of their cross-linking interactions and matrix organisation. In Smith DJ, et al., eds. *Methods of Cartilage Research* 1990: 28–33
45. Uebelhart D, Gineyts E, Chapuy M-C, et al. Urinary excretion of pyridinium crosslinks: a new marker of bone resorption in metabolic bone disease. *Bone Miner* 1990;8:87–96
46. Delmas PD, Schlemmer A, Gineyts E, et al. Urinary excretion of pyridinoline crosslinks correlates with bone turnover measured on iliac biopsy in patients with vertebral osteoporosis. *J Bone Miner Res* 1991;6:639–44
47. Delmas PD. Biochemical markers for the assessment of bone turnover. In Riggs BL, Melton III LJ, eds. *Osteoporosis: Etiology, Diagnosis, and Management*, 2nd edn. Philadelphia: Lippincott-Raven Publishers, 1995:319–33
48. Seibel MJ, Gartenberg F, Silverberg SJ, et al. Urinary hydroxypyridinium cross-links of collagen in primary hyperparathyroidism. *J Clin Endocrinol Metab* 1992;74:481–6
49. Fujimoto D, Suzuki M, Uchiyama A, et al. Analysis of pyridinoline, a cross-linking compound of collagen fibers, in human urine. *J Biochem* 1983; 94:1133–6
50. Pratt DA, Daniloff YN, Duncan A, et al. Automated analysis of the pyridinium crosslinks of collagen in tissue and urine using solid-phase extraction and reversed-phase high-performance liquid chromatography. *Anal Biochem* 1992; 207:168–75
51. Garnero P, Gineyts E, Arbault P, et al. Different effects of bisphosphonate and estrogen therapy on free and peptide-bound bone cross-links excretion. *J Bone Miner Res* 1995;10:641–9
52. Eyre DR. Biochemical markers of bone metabolism. *Klin Lab* 1995;41:429–30
53. Seibel MJ, Duncan A, Robins SP. Urinary hydroxy-pyridinium crosslinks provide indices of cartilage and bone involvement in arthritic diseases. *J Rheumatol* 1989;16:964–70
54. Schneider DL, Barrett-Connor EL. Urinary N-telopeptide levels discriminate normal, osteopenic, and osteoporotic bone mineral density. *Arch Intern Med* 1997;157:1241–5
55. Chesnut CH III, Bell NH, Clark GS, et al. Hormone replacement therapy in post-menopausal women: urinary N-telopeptide of type I collagen monitors therapeutic effects and predicts response of bone mineral density. *Am J Med* 1997; 102:29–37
56. Last JA, Armstrong LG, Reiser KM. Biosynthesis of collagen crosslinks. *Int J Biochem* 1990;22: 559–64
57. Kuypers R, Tyler M, Kurth LB, et al. Identification of the loci of the collagen-associated Ehrlich chromogen in type I collagen confirms its role as a trivalent cross-link. *Biochem J* 1992;283: 129–36
58. Cloos PAC, Bonde M, Fledelius C, et al. Isomerized molecules in serum derived from bone resorption. In Papapoulos SE, et al., eds. *Osteoporosis 1996*. Amsterdam: Elsevier Science BV, 1996:227–31
59. Bonde M, Fledelius C, Qvist P, et al. Coated-tube radioimmunoassay for C-telopeptides of type I collagen to assess bone resorption. *Clin Chem* 1996;42:1639–44
60. Garnero P, Fledelius C, Bonde M, et al. Impaired isomerization of type I collagen C-telopeptide in Paget's disease: an index of bone quality. *J Bone Miner Res* 1996;11:M755
61. Overgaard K, Christiansen C. A new biochemical marker of bone resorption for follow-up on treatment with nasal salmon calcitonin. *Calcif Tissue Int* 1996;59:12–16
62. Christgau S, Alexandersen P, Schlemmer A, et al. Biological variation in the serum concentration of degradation products derived from the C-terminal telopeptide of type I collagen measured by a new version of the CrossLaps ELISA. *J Bone Miner Res* 1997;12:S577
63. Christiansen C, Riis BJ, Rødbro P. Screening procedure for women at risk of developing postmenopausal osteoporosis. *Osteoporosis Int* 1990;1: 35–40
64. Hansen MA, Overgaard K, Riis BJ, et al. Role of peak bone mass and bone loss in postmenopausal osteoporosis: 12 year study. *Br Med J* 1991; 303:961–4
65. Uebelhart D, Schlemmer A, Johansen JS, et al. Effect of menopause and estrogen treatment on the urinary excretion of pyridinium crosslinks. *J Clin Endocrinol Metab* 1991;72:367–73
66. Riis BJ, Hansen MA, Overgaard K, et al. Low bone mass and fast rate of bone loss at menopause: equal risk factors for future fracture: a 15-year follow-up study. *Bone* 1996;19:9–12
67. Garnero P, Hausherr E, Chapuy M-C, et al. Markers of bone resorption predict hip fracture in elderly women: the EPIDOS prospective study. *J Bone Miner Res* 1996;11:1531–8
68. Cummings SR, Black D, Ensrud K, et al. Urine markers of bone resorption predict hip bone loss and fractures in older women: the study of osteoporotic fractures. *J Bone Miner Res* 1996;11: 134

69. Van Daele PL, Seibel MJ, Burger H, et al. Case–control analysis of bone resorption markers, disability, and hip fracture risk: the Rotterdam study. *Br Med J* 1996;312:482–3

70. Ross PD, Wasnich RD, Knowlton WK. Skeletal alkaline phosphatase (TANDEM®-R Ostase®) measurements predict vertebral fractures: a prospective study. *J Bone Miner Res* 1997;12(Suppl 1):S150

16
Nutritional support for osteoporosis

A. Carey and B. Carey

'Let food be your medicine not medicine your food.'
Hippocrates

The incidence of osteoporosis is increasing despite the best attempts of the medical profession. More than 200 000 fractures now occur each year as a consequence of osteoporosis in England and Wales[1] and, in the 10 years from 1971, the incidence of fractured neck of femur in women doubled from 8 to 16 per 1000[2]. Other studies report similar incidences for fractures of both the hip and the wrist[3-5]. From the assessment of skeletons dating from 1729 to 1852, it is known that hip bone mineral density in women both before and after the menopause used to be significantly greater than it is in modern-day women[6].

WHY IS OSTEOPOROSIS INCREASING?

The number of patients suffering from osteoporosis is increasing as the number of elderly women and men in the society increases. A major risk factor for this in the female population is the number of years spent after the menopause while not receiving hormone replacement therapy. This does not explain why osteoporosis has also increased in premenopausal women and in men, in each age group, over the past 30 years. There are several possible explanations for this increasing incidence: decreased physical activity undertaken by Western populations; increased exposure to environmental pollution; and decreased nutritional content of the modern Western diet.

Exercise is now well recognized as essential for both the maintenance and development of bone[7]. Immobilization and weightlessness result in an accelerated bone loss. The benefits of exercise are not only for the young. A cohort of 12 women with a mean age of 84 years were entered into a 3-year exercise program and compared with age-matched controls. The exercise group increased their bone mineral density at the distal radius by an average of 2.3% compared to the control group who, on average, lost 3.3%[8]. An increasingly sedentary lifestyle in developed countries may partly explain the increasing incidence of osteoporosis. It was thought to be the reason for the difference in age-adjusted incidence of hip fractures between Sweden, 146 per 100 000 women, and South Africa, 7.5 per 100 000. The authors could not explain the difference on the basis of either hormonal status or dietary calcium intake[9].

Increased exposure to environmental toxic chemicals may also play a role in the development of osteoporosis. Aluminium, lead and cadmium have all been implicated in the recent increasing incidence of osteoporosis. Aluminium reduces the formation of new bone, increases its absorption[10] and increases urinary excretion of calcium[11]. Long-term use of antacids containing aluminium hydroxide is associated with osteomalacia and pseudofractures[12]. Aluminium is widely used in soft drinks cans, cookware and food additives. Levels of aluminium found in beverages from cans are six times higher than in the same drinks from bottles[13].

Lead toxicity causes diffuse osteoporosis and vertebral malformations[14]. The use of lead has been increasing dramatically over the past 50 years until recent environmental efforts to reduce it. American skeletons have been found to have 500 times higher concentrations of lead in their bones compared with those of Peruvian Indians living 1800 years ago[15].

Cadmium is an element commonly found in plastics, fertilizers and cigarette smoke which may also adversely affect bones causing osteomalacia, pathological fractures and increased urinary excretion of calcium[16,17]. All these environmental pollutants are dangerous at high levels and may lead to osteoporosis. The ability to safely metabolize them and minimize their toxic effects may be modified by an individual's nutritional state.

The modern Western diet no longer meets all nutritional needs even if it is perceived to be well balanced. Supplementation with a pint of milk a day for adolescent schoolgirls significantly increased bone mineral acquisition over 18 months, compared to a control group[18]. The mean intake of calcium in the group receiving supplementation was 1125 mg/day and their baseline calcium intake was 746 mg/day, which is not significantly different from the UK recommended intake of 800 mg/day for girls of this age. The authors concluded that the girls' baseline calcium intake and the UK reference range were inadequate for maximal bone mineral accrual in rapidly growing adolescents.

HOW MAY DIET CONTRIBUTE TO DEVELOPMENT OF OSTEOPOROSIS?

The past 20 years has seen growing concern about the quality of food. It is increasingly recognized that what we eat will have a dramatic effect on our health. The diets of many members of society are now seen to be inadequate, and poor nutritional status is leading to the development of many chronic diseases including cardiovascular disease and diabetes. A modern diet typically contains large amounts of refined sugar and flour, caffeine, alcohol, salt and processed foods. Each of these is associated with an increased risk of osteoporosis (Table 1).

Table 1 Foods to avoid

Refined flour	pasta
Refined sugar	sweets
Caffeine	coffee, tea, colas
Alcohol	
Sodium	table salt
Phosphorus	soft drinks
Processed foods	
Intensively farmed foods	

Refined flour

Refined flour makes up 30% of the calories in most Western diets. The practice of refining flour and other grains has become increasingly widespread over the past 100 years. During refinement, between 70 and 90% of the vitamin and mineral content is lost[19]. This is done on purpose to help storage and prevent the food being eaten by weevils. Refined flour together with refined sugar, which has absolutely no vitamin or mineral content, make up half the calories in most Western diets, so it is easy to see how nutritional deficiencies can develop.

Refined sugar

Osteoporosis can be induced in hamsters fed on a 56% sucrose diet[20]. A sugar load increases urinary excretion of calcium in humans, perhaps mediated by insulin inhibiting renal calcium absorption[21]. Individuals who develop renal stones have a greater urinary excretion of calcium in response to a glucose load[22] and are at increased risk of developing osteoporosis[23]. In 1973, Yudkin[24] identified that a large carbohydrate load caused a significant rise in fasting serum cortisol levels and suggested a further osteoporotic drive.

Caffeine

The evidence that caffeine has a direct osteoporotic effect is not strong, although caffeine has been shown to increase urinary calcium excretion in a dose-dependent fashion[25] and has been associated with increased risk of hip fracture[26].

Alcohol and smoking

Excessive alcohol consumption is well established as a risk factor for osteoporosis. Whether this is a primary effect of ethanol toxicity on the bone[27] or secondary to concurrent malnutrition is not established. Smoking has also long been identified as a risk factor. Smokers have elevated serum levels of cadmium which is known to have a direct toxic effect on bone.

Sodium and phosphorus

High sodium diets increase urinary calcium excretion and reducing the sodium intake reduces this loss[28]. For susceptible individuals with sodium-dependent hypercalcemia, a normal dietary intake of sodium increases the risk of both kidney stones and osteoporosis[29]. Animal studies have shown that excessive phosphorus intake also increases urinary calcium loss causing osteoporosis. In part, this may explain why high-protein diets do the same[30,31]. Of recent concern are the high-phosphorus drinks such as colas, which also contain large amounts of sugar and caffeine.

Food processing

Foods that are easily prepared, look enticing and have a prolonged shelf-life are now being made by the food technology industry. Development of these products may involve one, or a combination, of bleaching, irradiation, extraction with organic solvents, exposure to extremes of temperature or pH and the addition of other chemicals to preserve, texturize, color or otherwise modify the food. All these processes detract from the nutritional content of the food, while potentially adding to the 'toxic load' that the body has to metabolize.

Lysine, an essential amino acid which may have a role in bone metabolism, has been clearly shown to be denatured by the alkaline treatment used to make textured vegetable protein[32] and by heat, especially in the presence of sugars, as occurs during baking of pies and breads[33]. Lysine's role in bone metabolism is suggested by the rare genetic condition of lysinuric protein intolerance, in which individuals lose large amounts of lysine in their urine and develop osteoporosis in childhood[34].

Farming methods and food mineral content

Modern farming techniques are designed to increase the crop yield per unit area of land. The use of ammonia and inorganic fertilizers rather than manure, compost and crop rotation is leading to reduction in the soil mineral content of magnesium, manganese, zinc and copper[35]. There are many examples: in Florida, the soil has been found to be low in copper. Grazing animals often develop a deficiency that makes them susceptible to fractures which no longer occur when their diet is supplemented with copper[36].

These studies suggest that modern farming techniques are gradually depleting the soil of essential minerals, which results in food of lower nutritional value. Food is then refined and processed for convenience and storage, resulting in further reduction of the nutritional value. Finally, the modern diet that is high in simple carbohydrates, salt, caffeine and alcohol adds an osteoporotic drive that goes a long way towards explaining the increasing incidence of this disorder.

WHAT DIETARY MODIFICATIONS COULD BE MADE TO OPTIMIZE BONE DENSITY?

The formation of strong bones and maintenance of bone mass requires more than just adequate amounts of dietary calcium. Bone is a living structure with a wide range of nutritional needs. This was demonstrated by Albanese and colleagues[37] in 1981 when they showed that women receiving a micronutrient combination increased their bone mineral density three times more than those receiving only calcium. In another study, the addition of

Table 2 Foods to eat to prevent osteoporosis

Vitamin B6	wholegrains, fish, nuts, bananas, avocados
Folic acid	fresh vegetables, wheatgerm, brewer's yeast
Vitamin C	citrus fruits, green leafy vegetables, cauliflower, berries, potatoes
Vitamin D	fish and fish oils
Vitamin K	green vegetables
Boron	alfalfa, kelp, cabbage, leafy greens
Calcium	dark green leafy vegetables, broccoli, kelp, sesame seeds, almonds, mackerel (edible fish bones), dairy products
Copper	wholegrains, nuts, eggs, poultry, legumes, green leafy vegetables
Magnesium	dark green vegetables, apples, seeds, nuts, figs, lemons
Manganese	wholegrains, nuts, seeds, leafy vegetables, meat
Strontium	water but depends on geographical area
Zinc	oysters, fish, animal foods, pumpkin seeds, eggs

broad nutritional supplementation for a group of postmenopausal women receiving hormone replacement therapy resulted in an increase in the bone mineral density of 11% in 1 year, which was significantly greater than for those receiving hormone replacement therapy alone[38]. The vitamins and minerals which are known to be required for bone formation, and deficiencies of which may cause osteoporosis, are given in Table 2.

WHAT EVIDENCE IS THERE TO SUGGEST THAT NUTRITIONAL SUPPLEMENTS COULD BE OF VALUE IN TREATMENT OF OSTEOPOROSIS?

Table 3 lists minerals and vitamins to consider as nutritional supplements.

Minerals to consider

Boron

Boron exists in nature mainly as borax in combination with sodium and oxygen. It has been used medicinally in the Middle East by Arabian physicians for over 1000 years[39]. Boron is essential for normal plant growth and, when depleted, plants display a number of characteristic disorders such as top sickness in tobacco and brown heat in turnips. Boron is thought to play a role in hydroxylation reactions, such as those leading to production of the sex steroids and the

Table 3 Nutritional supplements for osteoporosis

	RDA	Suggestion
Mineral		
Boron	no value	1–2 mg
Calcium	800 mg	1000–1200 mg
Copper	2 mg	2 mg
Magnesium	350 mg	350–600 mg
Manganese	no value	15–20 mg
Strontium	—	0.5–3 mg
Zinc	15 mg	30 mg
Vitamin		
B6 (pyridoxine)	2.0 mg	5–25 mg
Folic acid	400 µg	1–5 mg
Vitamin C	30 mg	500 mg
Vitamin D	10 units	400 units
Vitamin K	300 µg	3–500 µg

RDA, recommended daily allowance

active metabolite 1,25-dihydroxyvitamin D. Animal studies indicate that boron deficiencies exacerbate the effects of vitamin D deficiency. In humans, the supplementation of a low-boron diet with 3 mg per day has been shown to increase serum 1,25-dihydroxyvitamin D levels[40]. In 12 postmenopausal women who were maintained on a low boron diet which was subsequently corrected, the urinary calcium excretion fell by 44% and serum concentrations of 17β-estradiol increased significantly[41].

There are no current recommendations for a daily allowance of boron. It has been suggested from animal studies that human requirements for boron should be in the order of 1–2 mg per day. Diets containing liberal amounts of vegetables, fruits and nuts will adequately achieve these levels. If it is suspected that the diet is suboptimal, then supplementation of 1–2 mg per day may be of benefit. Boron toxicity is not seen until there is long-term ingestion of more than 100 times this level. Indeed, there are parts of the world where diets typically contain 40 mg per day of boron and no side-effects are reported.

Calcium

Calcium is clearly an important component of bone and essential to its formation. The average calcium intake in women over 65 years is 480 mg per day[42] which is well below the recommended daily intake. Currently, many clinicians recommend supplementation with 1500 mg of calcium per day.

Women with osteoporosis have been shown to absorb less calcium than age-matched women with healthy bones[43]. However, supplementation with calcium and vitamin D for 2 years was found to correct the skeletal calcium levels in osteoporotic patients but did not improve bone mineral density[44]. Supplementation in combination with the other essential minerals and vitamins achieves better results. There is some concern that excessively high supplementation may lead to competition for absorption with other minerals such as zinc or magnesium and, consequently, to their depletion[45,46]. There are many forms of calcium available and no reason to recommend any particular one, except to note that the oxalate and carbonates are very poorly absorbed.

Copper

Animal studies have shown that copper deficiency reduces bone mineral content and bone strength[47,48]. In a dietary assessment, Holden and colleagues[49] found that 81% of men and women consumed less than two-thirds of the recommended daily allowance, suggesting that many of the population may have an inadequate copper intake.

Magnesium

The recommended daily allowance of this ubiquitous mineral is 350 mg per day. A typical diet contains approximately 250 mg per day, but recent work is now suggesting that an optimal intake should be in the order of 600 mg per day. Seventy per cent of the body magnesium is found in the teeth and bones. Many osteoporotic women have been found to be magnesium deficient, and the calcification that occurs in their bone matrices is not normal[50]. In a small controlled study of postmenopausal women where a combined supplementation program including 600 mg of magnesium was used in combination with hormone replacement therapy over a 9-month period, the group receiving the supplementation together with hormone replacement therapy increased their bone mineral density by 11% compared with 0.7% for the group receiving hormone replacement therapy alone[38].

Manganese

Manganese is predominately localized to bone and the endocrine glands. In the bone, it is required as a coenzyme in the production of mucopolysaccharides, upon which mineralization and calcification occur[51]. Animal studies have found that dietary deficiency of manganese can induce osteoporosis[52] and a group of osteoporotic women have been shown to have blood manganese levels which are only 25% those of age-matched controls[53]. A genetic predisposition may be important in those who develop osteoporosis from manganese deficiency. One such affected individual is Bill Walton, an American basketball player, who was found to be sustaining repeated fractures as a consequence of being osteoporotic. His calcium levels were normal but his serum manganese levels were very low.

Manganese is present in unrefined sugar cane and wheat germ but, during refinement, as much as 85% is lost. There is no recommended daily intake for this mineral. The average American diet contains 3–9 mg per day, which is considered to be at the lower end of acceptability.

Strontium

Strontium, like calcium, carries two positive charges and has been found to replace a small proportion of the calcium in hydroxyapatite crystals. Its function may be to add strength to the structure. Supplementation of strontium should be accompanied by vitamin D, to avoid blocking calcium absorption[54].

In 1955, a group of 32 osteoporotic patients were given supplements of strontium 1.7 g for between 3 months and 3 years. Radiological examination suggested an improvement in bone density in 78% of the subjects, while 84% reported a reduction in bone pain. However, the results are confounded because ten of the subjects also received estrogen and testosterone[55]. An animal study showed that adding 0.27% strontium to drinking water increased bone formation and decreased resorption[56].

Zinc

Although the recommended daily intake of zinc is 15 mg, nearly 70% of Americans obtain less than 10 mg from their diets[49]. In the elderly, the deficiency is closer to 90%[57]. The shortage in the modern diet is probably because of increased consumption of refined sugar and flour.

Zinc is used in a number of different enzymatic functions. It is required for cellular proliferation and protein synthesis. It has been shown to enhance the effects of vitamin D, promoting calcium absorption[58] and levels are low in individuals with osteoporosis[59]. There are a number of forms of zinc commonly available. The picolinate, citrate and chelated variations are well absorbed, the sulfate and oxide are not. Zinc interferes with copper metabolism, so overzealous replacement of zinc may create a deficiency of copper with disturbances of heart rhythm and cholesterol metabolism, unless copper is also supplemented.

Vitamins to consider

B6, pyridoxine

Animal studies have shown that a diet deficient in vitamin B6 causes osteoporosis[60], impaired cartilage formation[61] and prolonged fracture healing time[62]. The exact mechanism of action is not completely understood. Vitamin B6 is necessary for the conversion of the amino-acid metabolite homocysteine to cystathionine prior to its excretion[63]. Homocysteine increases after the menopause and interferes with collagen cross-linking in the bone matrix. In individuals with the recessive defect homocystinuria, vitamin B6 supplementation normalizes elevated homocysteine levels. Untreated, these individuals would develop severe atherosclerosis and osteoporosis in their early 20s, which is commonly fatal.

The modern Western diet does not provide the recommended daily allowance of vitamin B6. Deficiencies have been found in at least 30% of adolescent American girls[64] and, in the elderly, this figure increases to 86%[65]. A significant proportion of vitamin B6 is lost in the refining of grains, and further losses occur with cooking, canning and freezing of foods. There is increasing evidence to suggest that we now require more vitamin B6 than we did 50 years ago. This is because, during the past several decades, the environment has been flooded with chemicals which either prevent absorption of vitamin B6, potentiate its breakdown or inhibit its normal biochemical functions. Examples are found in cigarette smoke[66], metal manufacturing, food coloring, herbicides and plant growth regulators.

Folic acid

Folic acid was so named because it is found in high concentrations in foliage. The recommended daily allowance is 0.4 mg per day, and many diets do not achieve this[67]. Deficiencies occur when individuals consume a diet with a low vegetable content or when it is denatured by light, heat or many food processing techniques. Alcohol also interferes with folic acid absorption.

Folic acid, like vitamin B6, may be used in the metabolism of homocysteine. There are several pathways to ensure the elimination of this harmful metabolite. Although a woman's ability to metabolize homocysteine appears to be reduced after the menopause, it is possible to improve this with the addition of 5 mg of folic acid supplementation[68].

Vitamin C

Since the work of Linus Pauling in the early 1970s, this vitamin has received a great deal of attention. It has been attributed with a variety of functions including antioxidant, antibacterial and antiviral actions. Deficiency causes scurvy, a collagen disorder. Collagen makes up 90% of the bone matrix and, in animal studies, it is possible to induce osteoporosis with vitamin C deficiency[69]. The body cannot manufacture or store vitamin C and relies on what is eaten daily. As people get older, their ability to assimilate vitamin C (and probably many other vitamins and minerals) decreases. Biochemical deficiency has been detected in more than 20% of elderly subjects despite their ingesting twice the recommended daily allowance[70].

Vitamin D

The actions of vitamin D and its effects on bone metabolism are well known. The elderly are at risk of deficiency often because of a lack of fresh fish and dairy products, together with a lack of sunlight. Supplementation for the treatment of osteoporosis is well established.

Vitamin K

Outside of pediatrics and rare clotting disorders, vitamin K has received little attention. It is widely found in green vegetables, and measurements of prothrombin time suggest that vitamin K deficiency is uncommon. However, vitamin K appears to play an important role in bone metabolism. It is required to synthesize osteocalcin, a bone protein that forms the matrix structure upon which mineralization occurs[71]. In 1985 it became possible to measure serum levels of this vitamin. Hart and colleagues[72] identified suppressed levels of vitamin K in patients with hip fractures when compared to healthy age-matched controls. Other workers have shown that calcium excretion is reduced when healthy postmenopausal women with osteoporosis are given supplements of vitamin K[73]. These results suggest that, although postmenopausal women obtain sufficient vitamin K for functioning of the clotting mechanism, they may have inadequate levels to protect their bones. When considering a supplementation policy for osteoporosis, it would now seem appropriate to include this vitamin.

CONCLUSIONS

The incidence of osteoporosis is increasing. The financial and social consequences of this problem appear to be set to pose an enormous burden on health-care resources over the next 50 years. The debate regarding the exact causes of this epidemic will certainly continue. Refined convenience foods with low nutritional value, increased exposure to environmental toxins and limited use of hormone replacement therapy (outside the female members of the medical profession) compound the problem. Although traditional treatment may include estrogen replacement therapy, weight bearing exercise, calcium and vitamin D supplements and, in resistant cases, the use of bisphosphonates, there is no doubt that bone is a living structure and also needs to be supported in a complete nutritional fashion.

References

1. Kanis JA, Pitt FA. Epidemiology of osteoporosis. *Bone* 1992;13:S7–15

2. Wallace WA. The increasing incidence of fractures of the proximal femur: an orthopaedic epidemic. *Lancet* 1983;1:1413–14

3. Boyce WJ, Vessey MP. Rising incidence of fracture of the proximal femur. *Lancet* 1985;1:150–1
4. Johnell O, Nilsson B, Obrant K, *et al*. Age and sex patterns of hip fractures – changes in 30 years. *Acta Orthop Scand* 1984;55:290–2
5. Bengner U, Johnell O. Increasing incidence of forearm fracture. A comparison of epidemiologic patterns 25 years apart. *Acta Orthop Scand* 1985;56:158–60
6. Lees B, Molleson T, Arnett TR, *et al*. Differences in proximal femur bone density over two centuries. *Lancet* 1993;341:673–5
7. Pocock NA, Eisman JA, Yeates MG, *et al*. Physical fitness is a major determinant of femoral neck and lumbar spine bone mineral density. *J Clin Invest* 1986;78:618–21
8. Smith EL. Exercise for preventing osteoporosis: a review. *Physician Sportsmed* 1982;10:72–82
9. Chalmers J, Ho KC. Geographical variation in senile osteoporosis. The association with physical activity. *J Bone Joint Surg* 1970;52B:667–5
10. Kaehny WD. Newer understanding of aluminium metabolism. *Intermediate Metab* 1985;6:131–40
11. Spencer H, Kramer L, Norris C, *et al*. Antacid-induced calcium loss. *Arch Intern Med* 1983;143:657–9
12. Spencer H, Kramer L, Norris C, *et al*. Effect of small doses of aluminium-containing antacids on calcium and phosphorus metabolism. *Am J Clin Nutr* 1982;36:32–40
13. Gerrans C. Soft drinks tend to boost aluminium intake. *Med Tribune* 1992;23 July:17
14. Mongelli-Sciannameo N. Radiologic observations on skeletal apparatus of young person affected by chronic lead poisoning. In Campbell IR, Mergard EG, eds. *Biological Aspects of Lead: an Annotated Bibliography*, Abstr. 1355 (May). Washington DC: US Environmental Protection Agency, 1972:260
15. Settle DM, Patterson CC. Lead in Albacore: guide to lead pollution in Americans. *Science* 1980;207:1167–76
16. Anonymous. 'Ouch-ouch' disease: due to cadmium. *J Am Med Assoc* 1971;216:154
17. Scott R, Patterson PJ, Burns R, *et al*. Hypercalciuria related to cadmium exposure. *Urology* 1978;11:462–5
18. Cadogan J, Eastal R, Jones N, *et al*. Milk intake and bone mineral acquisition on adolescent girls: randomised, controlled interventional trial. *Br Med J* 1997;315:1255–60
19. Schroeder HA. Losses of vitamins and trace minerals resulting from processing and preservation of foods. *Am J Clin Nutr* 1971;24:562–73
20. Saffar JL, Sagroun B, de Tessieres C, *et al*. Osteoporotic effect of a high carbohydrate diet in golden hamsters. *Arch Oral Biol* 1981;26:393–7
21. Holl MG, Allen LH. Sucrose ingestion, insulin response and mineral metabolism in humans. *J Nutr* 1987;117:1229–33
22. Lemann J, Piering WF, Lennon EJ. Possible role of carbohydrate-induced calciuria in calcium oxalate kidney-stone formation. *N Engl J Med* 1969;280:232–7
23. Lawoyin S, Sismilich S, Browne R, *et al*. Bone mineral content in patients with calcium urolithiasis. *Metabolism* 1979;28:1250–4
24. Yudkin J. *Sweet and Dangerous*. New York: Bantam Books, 1973:112
25. Hollingbery PW, Bergman EA, Massey LK. Effect of dietary caffeine and aspirin on urinary calcium and hydroxyproline excretion in pre- and postmenopausal women. *Fed Proc* 1985;44:1149
26. Hernandez-Avila M, Colditz GA, Stampfer MJ, *et al*. Caffeine, moderate alcohol intake, and risk of fractures of the hip and forearm in middle-aged women. *Am J Clin Nutr* 1991;54:157–63
27. Dimond T, Stiel D, Lunzer M, *et al*. Ethanol reduces bone formation and may cause osteoporosis. *Am J Med* 1989;86:282–8
28. Goulding A. Osteoporosis: why consuming less sodium chloride helps to conserve bone. *NZ Med J* 1990;103:120–2
29. Silver J, Jubinger D, Friedlaender MM, *et al*. Sodium-dependent idiopathic hypercalciuria in renal stone formers. *Lancet* 1983;2:484–6
30. Draper H, Piche L, Gibson R. Effects of high protein intake from common foods on calcium metabolism in a cohort of postmenopausal women. *Nutr Res* 1991;11:273–81
31. Blank RP, Diehl HA, Ballard GT, *et al*. Calcium metabolism and osteoporotic ride absorption: a protein connection. *J Prosthet Dent* 1987;58:590–5
32. De Groot AP, Slump P. Effects of alkali treatment of proteins on amino acid composition and nutritive value. *J Nutr* 1969;98:45–56
33. Hurrell RF, Carpenter KJ. Mechanisms of heat damage proteins. *Br J Nutr* 1977;38:285–97
34. Carpenter TO, Levy HL, Holtrop ME, *et al*. Lysinuric protein intolerance presenting as childhood osteoporosis. *N Engl J Med* 1985;312:290–4
35. Hall RH. The agri-business view of soil and life. *J Holistic Med* 1981;3:157–66
36. Rose EF. The effects of soil and diet on disease. *Cancer Res* 1968;28:2390–2
37. Albanese AA. Effects of calcium and micronutrients on bone loss of pre- and postmenopausal women. Presented to the *American Medical Association*, Atlanta, GA, 24–26 January, 1981
38. Abraham GE, Grewal H. A total dietary program emphasising magnesium instead of calcium. Effect on the mineral density of calcaneous bone in postmenopausal women on hormone replacement therapy. *J Reprod Med* 1990;35:503–7

39. Pfeiffer CC, Jenney EH. The pharmacology of boric acid and boron compounds. *Bull Nat Formulary Comm* 1950;18:57–80
40. Nielsen FH. Effect of boron depletion and repletion on calcium and copper status indices in humans fed a magnesium-low diet. *FASEB J* 1989; 3:A760
41. Nielsen FH. Effect of dietary boron on mineral estrogen and testosterone metabolism in postmenopausal women. *Fed Am Soc Exp Biol* 1987;1:394–7
42. Heaney RP, Gallagher JC, Johnston CC, et al. Calcium nutrition and bone health in the elderly. *Am J Clin Nutr* 1982;36:986–1013
43. Spencer H. Absorption of calcium in osteoporosis. *Am J Med* 1964;37:223–34
44. Burnell JM, Baylink DJ, Chesnut CH 3d, et al. The role of skeletal calcium deficiency in postmenopausal osteoporosis. *Calcif Tissue Int* 1986;38: 187–92
45. Adham NF, Song MK. Effect of calcium and copper on zinc absorption in rats. *Nutr Metab* 1980;24:281–90
46. Smith KT, Luhrsen KR. Trace mineral interactions during elevated calcium consumption. *Fed Proc* 1986;45:374
47. Follis RH. Studies on copper metabolism. XVIII Skeletal changes associated with copper deficiency in swine. *Bull Johns Hopkins Hosp* 1955;97: 405–9
48. Wilson T, Katz JM, Gray DH. Inhibition of active bone resorption by copper. *Calcif Tissue Int* 1981; 33:35–9
49. Holden JM, Wolf WR, Merz W. Zinc and copper in self selected diets. *J Am Diet Assoc* 1979;75:23–8
50. Cohen L, Kitzes R. Infrared spectroscopy and magnesium content of bone mineral in osteoporotic woman. *Isr J Med Sci* 1981;17:1123–5
51. Leach RM, Muenster AM, Wein EM. Studies on the role of manganese in bone formation. II. Effect upon chondroitin sulfate synthesis in chick epiphyseal cartilage. *Arch Biochem Biophys* 1969;133:22–8
52. Strause L, Saltman P. Biochemical changes in rat skeleton following long term dietary manganese and copper deficiencies. *Fed Proc* 1985;44:752
53. Raloff J. Reasons for boning up on manganese. *Sci News* 1986;130:199
54. Rousselet F, El Solh N, Maurat JP, et al. Strontium and calcium metabolism. Interaction of strontium and vitamin D. *CR Soc Biol (Paris)* 1975;169:322–9
55. McCaslin FE, Janes JM. The effect of strontium lactate in the treatment of osteoporosis. *Proc Staff Meeting Mayo Clin* 1959;34:329–34
56. Marie PJ, Hott M. Short-term effects of fluoride and strontium on bone formation and resorption in the mouse. *Metabolism* 1986;35:547–51
57. Bogden JD, Oleske JM, Munves EM, et al. Zinc and immunocompetence in the elderly: baseline data on zinc nutriture and immunity in unsupplemented subjects. *Am J Clin Nutr* 1987;46: 101–9
58. Yamaguchi M, Sakashita T. Enhancement of vitamin D3 effect on bone metabolism in weanling rats orally administered zinc sulphate. *Acta Endocrinol* 1986;11:285–8
59. Atik OS. Zinc and senile osteoporosis. *J Am Geriatr Soc* 1983;31:790–1
60. Benke PJ, Fleshood HL, Pitot HC. Osteoporotic bone disease in the pyridoxine-deficient rat. *Biochem Med* 1972;6:526–35
61. Silberberg R, Levy BM. Skeletal growth in pyridoxine deficient mice. *Proc Soc Exp Biol Med* 1948;67:259–63
62. Dodds RA, Catterall A, Bitensky L, et al. Abnormalities in fracture healing induced by vitamin B6-deficiency in rats. *Bone* 1986;7:489–95
63. Seashore MR, Durant JL, Rosenberg LE. Studies on the mechanism of pyridoxine-responsive homocystinuria. *Pediatr Res* 1972;6:187–96
64. Kirksey A, Keaton K, Abernathy RP, et al. Vitamin B6 nutritional status of a group of female adolescents. *Am J Clin Nutr* 1978;31:946–54
65. Guilland JC, Bereksi-Reguig B, Lequeu B, et al. Evaluation of pyridoxine intake and pyridoxine status among aged institutionalised people. *Int J Vitam Nutr Res* 1984;54:185–93
66. Roepke JB, Kirksey A. Effect of smoking and vitamin B6 supplementation during pregnancy on maternal vitamin B6 status and infant birth weight. *Fed Proc* 1983;42:1066
67. Daniel WA, Graines EG, Bennett DL. Dietary intakes and plasma concentrations of folate in health adolescents. *Am J Clin Nutr* 1975;28: 363–70
68. Brattstrom LE, Hultberg BL, Hardebo JE. Folic acid responsive postmenopausal homocysteinemia. *Metabolism* 1985;34:1073–7
69. Wapnick AA, Lynch SR, Seftel HC, et al. The effect of siderosis and ascorbic acid depletion on bone metabolism with special reference to osteoporosis in the Bantu. *Br J Nutr* 1971;25: 367–76
70. Morgan AF, Gillum HL, Williams RI. Nutritional status of ageing. Serum ascorbic acid and intake. *J Nutr* 1955;55:431–48
71. Dodds RA, Catterall A, Bitensky L, et al. Effects on fracture healing of an antagonist of the vitamin K cycle. *Calcif Tissue Int* 1984;36:233

72. Hart JP, Shearer MJ, Klenerman L, *et al.* Electrochemical detection of depressed circulation vitamin K1 in osteoporosis. *J Clin Endocrinol Metab* 1985;60:1268–9

73. Knapen MH, Hamulyak JK, Vermeer C. The effect of vitamin K supplementation on circulating osteocalcin (bone GLA protein) and urinary calcium excretion. *Ann Intern Med* 1989;111:1001–5

17

Estrogens and neurotransmitters

A. R. Genazzani, C. Salvestroni, A. Spinetti, P. Monteleone and F. Petraglia

INTRODUCTION

In recent years, research findings from epidemiological and clinical studies have indicated that estrogen may be of critical importance not only for a woman's reproductive system, but also in many other biological functions. In particular, estrogen plays an important role in pain control, in thermoregulation, in mechanisms such as hunger and thirst, in psychophysical well-being and in cognitive functions.

During fetal life, estrogen influences central nervous system (CNS) development and sexual differentiation of tissues in specific brain areas, suggesting that some of the quantitative sex differences in specific cognitive functions that have been demonstrated in adult men and women may be due to different patterns of neuronal connectivity which develop prenatally because of different hormonal milieux between the sexes[1].

During a woman's fertile life, the interaction between gonadal steroids and neurotransmitters/neuropeptides modulates the ovulatory function by selectively acting at the hypothalamic level on the synthesis and release of gonadotropin-releasing hormone (GnRH)[2].

After the menopause, the rapid decline of gonadal steroids may account for some of the physical and psychological disturbances that, in turn, affect a woman's quality of life[3].

BRAIN AS A TARGET FOR ESTROGEN

Estrogens act on the CNS by both genomic and non-genomic mechanisms of action: genomic effects are permanent, and they are mediated by specific intracellular receptors, whereas non-genomic effects are due to a direct action on the neuronal membrane. This non-classical mechanism of action is characterized by rapid effect and short duration[1,4,5].

Estrogen receptors have been demonstrated in the cortex, limbic system, hippocampus, cerebellum, locus ceruleus, hypothalamus, preoptic area and amygdala[1,5]. In these brain areas, estrogens are able to modify the synthesis, release and metabolism of neurotransmitters such as norepinephrine, dopamine, acetylcholine, serotonin and melatonin. Neuropeptides directly influenced by estrogens include opioid peptides, corticotropin-releasing factor (CRF), neuropeptide Y (NPY) and galanin. Many of these neurotransmitters and neuropeptides, such as noradrenaline, dopamine, serotonin, β-endorphin and NPY, modulate the activity of hypothalamic centers for termoregulation, satiety/appetite and blood pressure, and participate in the limbic system in the regulation of mood tone and psychophysical well-being[1,6–8]. Consequently, by modulating these neurotransmitters, estrogens exert a global action on the whole female body, with relevant implications for well-being and quality of life[4,6]. Estrogens may also regulate the number of receptors for neurotransmitters and neuropeptides in the hypothalamus, thus increasing signal transduction at the postsynaptic level.

Estrogens influence the noradrenergic and dopaminergic activities in the brain. In particular, estrogens selectively increase norepinephrine activity and turnover in the brain, probably by both decreased norepinephrine reuptake and decreased monoamine oxidase (MAO), and catechol-o-methyl-transferase activity[9]. There is evidence that estrogen decreases D_2 receptors and probably also other dopaminergic receptors[10].

The hypothesis of specific neuroanatomical and neurophysiological effects of estrogens on brain function and structure may also explain how estrogens can influence cognitive functions. In fact, estrogens increase choline acetyltransferase, the rate-limiting enzyme for acetylcholine synthesis, thus enhancing cholinergic tone that has been demonstrated to be strictly linked to memory performance[11,12]. The hormonal influences on memory processes appear to involve actions on brain areas such as the hippocampus and the basal forebrain. Furthermore, experimental studies in female rats during the proestrus demonstrate that estrogens enhance synaptogenesis in the CA1 region of the hippocampus, an area of the brain known to be of critical importance for memory[13].

Although in human females sexual behavior is not tightly linked to the reproductive cycle, it is evident that endogenous estrogens greatly influence cognitive function in women. The facilitating action of estradiol on cognitive functions such as learning, short-term memory and attention seems to be directly related to genomic estrogenic effects, behaving as a growth factor at estrogen-responsive dendritic neurons, resulting in new synapse formation[14]. Estrogens may also have a direct action on the vasculature of the CNS, leading to smooth muscle relaxation and improved perfusion.

Estrogens can also modify the concentration and the availability of serotonin (5-HT), by stimulating the degradation of monoamine oxidase (MAO), the enzyme that catabolizes serotonin, and increasing the rate of free tryptophan to be metabolized to 5-HT, by displacing it from its binding sites on plasma albumin[6,15]. Sex differences in 5-HT levels have also been described in animal studies: higher levels have been demonstrated in the forebrain, rafe, frontal cortex and hypothalamus of female rats than in those of male rats. Moreover, estrogen administration positively affects serotoninergic tone in ovariectomized rats, by increasing postsynaptic responsivity and receptor activity[16,17].

Epidemiological studies indicate that women are more prone to develop anxiety disorders and depressive illness than men: sex differences derive from early experience, social and cultural factors and from the biological substrate, related to the hormonal milieu during sexual differentiation or during adulthood. The highest incidence of mood disorders in females occurs at times of rapidly fluctuating, mainly falling, estrogen levels during the postnatal, premenstrual and perimenopausal periods, confirming that estrogens play an excitatory role on the CNS through neurotransmitter receptor activation in estrogen-responsive neurons, leading to elevated mood, increased activity and antidepressant effects[4,5].

Experimental data on the effect of sex steroids on neuropeptides demonstrate that estrogens increase the synthesis and release of the endogenous opioid β-endorphin by the mediobasal hypothalamus through a direct action on opioid receptor activity[18,19]. In fact, cyclic changes in opiate μ-receptor density have been observed during the different phases of the estrous cycle in rats, and similar fluctuations of β-endorphin levels observed in the mediobasal hypothalamus of female rats are abolished by ovariectomy and then restored by estrogen administration[20].

Among opioid peptides, β-endorphin plays the most important role in the modulation of reproductive functions, by modulating the synthesis and secretion of hypothalamic GnRH and pituitary luteinizing hormone (LH) and follicle-stimulating hormone (FSH)[21]. In women, changes in plasma β-endorphin levels occur in relation to the most important reproductive events: puberty, pregnancy and the menopause[22]. During reproductive life, steroid hormones modulate the production and release of plasma β-endorphin: ovarian secretion of estradiol modulates plasma β-endorphin levels and, during the pre- and postovulatory phases of the menstrual cycle, the highest values of plasma β-endorphin levels have been demonstrated[23]. In pregnancy, there is a progressive increase in β-endorphin levels, with the highest concentrations occurring before delivery and during labor[24].

Experimental data derived from studies in female rats demonstrate that estrogen and progesterone exert a stimulatory effect on NPY synthesis in the arcuate nucleus and on peptide storage in the median eminence nerve terminals[25]. Studies based on intracerebroventricular injections of NPY in rats suggest that this neuropeptide can influence sexual behavior, food intake, the sleep–wakefulness cycle and also cardiovascular and neuroendocrine functions[26–30]. In ovariectomized rats, estrogen deficiency decreases NPY production and secretion. Recent findings also demonstrate several interactions between NPY and β-endorphin neurons at the hypothalamic level, suggesting that both estrogens and progestogens could indirectly exert modulatory effects on NPY, inducing β-endorphin release. Finally, estrogen was recently shown to upregulate NPY Y2 receptor levels, by inducing either an increased synthesis and membrane insertion of the receptor protein, or by decreasing receptor removal[25].

Galanin, a 29 amino-acid neuropeptide, has been demonstrated in the anterior pituitary gland in rats and in humans[31,32]. Galanin synthesis in rats is under the control of the sex steroids, particularly of the estrogens[31,33]. Galanin seems to inhibit the release of hypothalamic dopamine which, in basal conditions, inhibits prolactin release, thus stimulating lactotropes[34]. Moreover, galanin exerts an inhibitory effect on adrenocorticotropic hormone (ACTH) secretion by a direct inhibitory action on pituitary corticotropes[35].

NEUROENDOCRINE AND CLINICAL EFFECTS OF ESTROGEN DECLINE IN POSTMENOPAUSE

Experimental studies suggest that the decline of estrogen production by the ovary during perimenopause is associated with a reduction of the central content and activity of several neurotransmitters and neuropeptides, which is improved by estrogen administration. In women, clinical reports demonstrate that, even if the aging process itself may account for some psychophysical decline independent of any hormonal effect, the postmenopausal state represents an important risk factor not only for cardiovascular disease and osteoporosis, which are major causes of mortality and morbidity in women[7,8,36,37], but also for mood disorders, the so-called climacteric depression, and decreased cognitive functions such as short-term memory.

Most of the climacteric disturbances are related to neuroendocrine changes induced by estrogen withdrawal at specific sites of the CNS: vasomotor symptoms such as hot flushes and sweats, as well as changes in eating behavior or in blood pressure control, are consequences of estrogen deficiency in the hypothalamus, whereas mood changes, anxiety, depression, insomnia and headache/migraine seem to be related to estrogen-induced neuroendocrine changes in the limbic system.

Hot flushes are the most common and typical symptom, which is known to be related to a temporary derangement of the hypothalamic thermoregulatory set-point by sudden modifications of neurotransmitter/neuropeptide activity. Estrogen deficiency increases noradrenergic tone and decreases dopaminergic activity. Noradrenergic and dopaminergic systems modulate in turn both the GnRH and LH pulsatile release and the vasomotor/thermoregulatory system, as supported by the efficacy of clonidine, an α_2 receptor agonist, and veralipride, a dopamine antagonist, in the reduction of postmenopausal vasomotor symptoms[38,39]. Changes in the noradrenergic and dopaminergic systems could only in part explain the induction of hot flushes in postmenopausal women.

Experimental studies show that the castration of adult rats is associated, after 2 weeks, with reductions in the β-endorphin contents of the anterior pituitary and neurointermediate pituitary lobes as well as a reduction in plasma β-endorphin levels[18]. Similarly, surgical or spontaneous menopause in women is associated with a fall in circulating β-endorphin levels which are restored by hormone replacement therapy[40,41]. The reduction of the central β-endorphin neuron content seems to play an important role in the physiopathological mechanisms of postmenopausal hot flushes and sweats[42,43]. In fact, opioid peptides are involved in the neuroendocrine hypothalamic control of thermoregulatory centers, and hot flushes are accompanied by a sudden increase in plasma β-endorphin levels[43]. Several studies demonstrate that opioid peptides regulate GnRH synthesis and pulsatile release, which is mediated by aminergic activity and which affects thermoregulatory function[44]. The evidence of an inhibitory role for opioids on GnRH–LH secretion is given by the increment in frequency and amplitude of GnRH–LH release after administration of naloxone, an opioid receptor antagonist, in normal menstruating women[21]. The involvement of the central β-endorphin in the pathogenesis of vasomotor instability is confirmed by the observation that naloxone treatment inhibits postmenopausal hot flushes[45].

Finally, as opioidergic neurons are known to be involved in other brain functions, such as analgesia, mood and behavior control, menopause-induced changes of β-endorphin synthesis and secretion seem to be related to the pathogenesis of mood, behavior and nociceptive perception changes, typical of this age in a woman's life[44,46].

Other studies suggest that even norepinephrine and dopamine play significant roles in modulating mood, behavior, cognitive abilities and motor activity in postmenopausal women[4]. In fact, it has been found that dopaminergic tone decreases and noradrenergic tone increases in women following gonadectomy, with an increase in the norepinephrine/dopamine ratio[2].

Epidemiological findings suggest that postmenopausal women are more often affected by chronic degenerative diseases of the CNS, such as Parkinson's disease and Alzheimer's disease, than age-matched men. The physiopathological mechanism of these neurodegenerative diseases seems to be a prolonged period of estrogen deficiency. As mentioned above, estrogen levels greatly influence mood and cognitive function in women, so that, after the menopause, estrogen deficiency may be responsible for memory, sexuality and sleep disturbances, irritability, anxiety, depression and insomnia[1,4,5]. In particular, mood disorders seem to be related to the decreased serotoninergic synthesis and activity induced by estrogen withdrawal[4].

Furthermore, as estrogen increases levels of choline acetyltransferase, the enzyme involved in acetylocholine synthesis[47], and bearing in mind that a reduction in acetylcholine and of cholinergic tone occurs at the menopause, this could explain the decline in short-term memory[48]. Cholinergic mechanisms are critically involved in attentional processes and in learning and memory, cognitive domains that are also particularly affected by Alzheimer's disease[49–51]. It is suggested that postmenopausal deprivation may increase a woman's risk for developing Alzheimer's disease and, conversely, that estrogen replacement therapy may reduce the risk for Alzheimer's disease[52]. However, evidence for a cause-and-effect relationship remains inconclusive.

EFFECTS OF HORMONE REPLACEMENT THERAPY IN POSTMENOPAUSAL WOMEN

Estrogen therapy, primarily in combination with progestin as hormone replacement therapy (HRT), was introduced to alleviate perimenopausal symptoms such as hot flushes and vaginal dryness. However, clinical and epidemiological studies demonstrated that HRT exerts a positive effect not only on vasomotor instability, by reducing the number and intensity of hot flushes and sweats, but also improves psychological disturbances such as depressive symptoms, pain perception, affective and sexual behavior.

Experimental studies of HRT in animals show restoration of the noradrenergic tone, suggesting a feedback mechanism of sex steroids on catecholaminergic neurons[53]. Other studies of female castrated rats have demonstrated that estradiol exerts a reduction of noradrenaline release at the hypothalamic level[54]. Estrogens also directly modulate dopaminergic neuron activity, increasing dopaminergic release in the mediobasal hypothalamus[54].

Hormone replacement therapy is able to restore cholinergic tone in postmenopausal women, by increasing the activity of the choline acetyltransferase enzyme in several brain areas with increases of short-term memory and cognitive functions[55]. Clinical studies in postmenopausal women based on experimental studies of castrated rats have shown that HRT, and in particular estrogen, restores β-endorphin levels to normal premenopausal values[41], confirming the roles for central and peripheral concentrations of β-endorphin in the neuroendocrine modulation of vasomotor instability and psychological symptoms.

However, HRT is not effective in the reduction of vasomotor symptoms in about 25% of patients, in whom the use of other therapies should be evaluated, by using clonidine, an α_2 receptor agonist, and veralipride, a dopamine antagonist.

FUTURE PHARMACOLOGICAL APPROACH TO POSTMENOPAUSAL DISTURBANCES

The ideal postmenopausal HRT produces the beneficial effects of estrogens upon the skeletal tissue, cardiovascular system and brain without producing the adverse effects of estrogens upon reproductive tissues (uterus and breast). Such a selective estrogen profile might be achieved by exploiting a preferential tissue distribution or by synthesizing specific compounds that activate estrogen receptors only in desired tissues, while remaining inactive or acting as antagonists in reproductive tissues. In fact, certain compounds that were originally developed as estrogen antagonists for the prevention or treatment of breast cancer, for example tamoxifen, have been shown to produce estrogen agonist-like effects elsewhere in the body[56]. Further developments in the pharmacology and molecular biology of antiestrogens have led to the identification of a novel class of compounds referred to as 'selective estrogen receptor modulators' or SERMs[56]. The study of how these compounds interact with the estrogen receptor to create differing effects in various organs has led to the hypothesis that the estrogen receptor exists in the cell in multiple conformations that represent the inactive state, the active state and several intermediate states, and that ligands exert their biological activity by stabilizing a specific structure. These distinct conformations could result as a consequence of the ability of compounds to freeze the receptor in a specific conformation by blocking a processive interaction from the inactive to the active state[57].

Preclinical findings with raloxifene, another compound originally developed for the treatment of breast cancer, demonstrated that it represents an antagonist of the uterine estrogen receptor, in that it produces a nearly complete blockade of uterotrophic responses to estrogen because of the minimal agonist effect of raloxifene in this tissue[58]. Based on these findings, the search for an improved estrogen with a profile that obviates the need for inclusion of progestins during estrogen therapy is of critical importance, to determine whether a member of the SERM class will display an overall clinical profile approximating to an ideal estrogen for the prevention and treatment of postmenopausal disturbances in women.

References

1. Maggi A, Perez J. Role of female gonadal hormones in the CNS: clinical experimental aspects. *Life Sci* 1985;37:893–906
2. Speroff L, Glass RH, Kase NH. *Clinical Gynecological Endocrinology and Infertility*, 5th edn. Baltimore, MD: Williams and Wilkins, 1995
3. Lobo RA. *Treatment of Postmenopausal Women: Basic and Clinical Aspects.* New York: Raven Press, 1993
4. Sherwin BB. Hormones, mood and cognitive functioning in postmenopausal women. *Obstet Gynaecol* 1996;87:20–6
5. Smith SS. Hormones, mood and neurobiology – a summary. In Berg G, Hammar M, eds. *The Modern Management of the Menopause.* Carnforth, UK: Parthenon Publishing, 1993:204
6. Panay N, Sands RH, Studd JWW. Estrogen and behaviour. In Genazzani AR, Petraglia F, Purdy

RH, eds. *The Brain: Source and Target for Sex Steriod Hormones.* Carnforth, UK: Parthenon Publishing, 1996:257–76
7. Kannel WB, Hjortland MC, McNamara PM, *et al.* Menopause and the risk of cardiovascular disease: the Framingham study. *Ann Intern Med* 1976;85:447–52
8. Parrish HM, Carr LA, Hall PG. Time interval from castration in premenopausal women to development of excessive coronary atherosclerosis. *Am J Obstet Gynecol* 1967;99:155–62
9. Luine VN, Khylchevskaya R, McEwen BS. Effect of gonadal steroids on activities of monoamine oxidase and choline acetylase in rat brain. *Brain Res* 1975;86:293–306
10. McEwen BS. Non-genomic and genomic effects of steroids on neural activity. *Trends Pharmacol Sci* 1991;12:141–7
11. Luine VN. Estradiol increases choline acetyltransferase activity in specific basal forebrain nuclei and projection areas of female rats. *Exp Neurol* 1985;80:484–90
12. Bartus RT, Dean RL, Beer B, *et al.* The cholinergic hypothesis of geriatric memory dysfunction. *Science* 1981;217:208–17
13. Gould E, Wolley CS, Frankfurt M, *et al.* Gonadal steroids regulate dendritic spine density in hippocampal pyramidal cells in adulthood. *J Neurosci* 1990;10:1286–91
14. Garcia-Segura LM, Chowen JA, Parducz A, *et al.* Glial cells and estrogen-induced synaptogenesis and synaptic plasticity. In Genazzani AR, Petraglia F, Purdy RH, eds. *The Brain: Source and Target for Sex Steroid Hormones.* Carnforth, UK: Parthenon Publishing, 1996:191–200
15. Luine VN, McEwen BS. Effect of estradiol on turnover of type A monoamine oxidase in brain. *J Neurochem* 1977;28:1221–7
16. Di Paolo T, Daigle M, Picard V, *et al.* Effect of acute and chronic 17β estradiol treatment on serotonin and 5-hydroxiindole acetic acid content of discrete brain nuclei of ovariectomized rats. *Exp Brain Res* 1983;51:73–6
17. Johnson MD, Crowley WR. Acute effects of estradiol on circulating luteinizing hormone and prolactin concentrations and on serotonin turnover in individual brain nuclei. *Endocrinology* 1983;113:1935–41
18. Petraglia F, Penalva A, Locatelli V, *et al.* Effect of gonadectomy and gonadal steroid replacement on pituitary and plasma β-endorphin levels in the rat. *Endocrinology* 1982;111:1224–9
19. Genazzani AR, Petraglia F, Mercuri N. Effect of steroid hormones and antihormones on hypothalamic beta-endorphin concentrations in intact and castrated female rats. *J Endocrinol Invest* 1990;13:91–6
20. Petraglia F, Nappi RE, Ferrari AR, *et al.* Neuroendocrine aspects in reproductive medicine. In Rodríguez-Armas O, ed. *Fertility and Sterility: Progress in Research and Practice. Proceedings of XIV World Congress on Fertility and Sterility.* Carnforth, UK: Parthenon Publishing, 1994:277–86
21. Ferin M, Van Vugt D, Wardlaw S. The hypothalamic control of menstrual cycle and the role of endogenous opioid peptides. *Recent Prog Horm Res* 1984;40:441–85
22. Adler MW. Minireview: opioid peptides. *Life Sci* 1980;26:496–510
23. Yen SSC, Quigley ME, Reid RL, *et al.* Neuroendocrinology of opioid peptides and their role in the control of gonadotropin and prolactin secretion. *Am J Obstet Gynecol* 1985;152:485–93
24. Bridges RS, Ronsheim PM. Immunoreactive β-endorphin concentrations in brain and plasma during pregnancy in rats: possible modulation by progesterone and estradiol. *Neuroendocrinology* 1987;45:381–5
25. Parker SL, Carroll BL, Kalra SP, *et al.* Neuropeptide Y (NPY) Y2 receptors in hypothalamic neuroendocrine areas are up-regulated by estradiol and decreased by progesterone co-treatment in the ovariectomized rat. *Endocrinology* 1996;137:2896–900
26. Clark JT, Kalra PS, Kalra SP. Neuropeptide Y stimulates feeding but inhibits sexual behavior in rats. *Endocrinology* 1985;117:2435–42
27. Fuxe K, Agnati LF, Harfstrand A, *et al.* Central administration of neuropeptide Y induces hypotension bradypnea and EEG synchronization in the rat. *Acta Physiol Scand* 1983;118:189–92
28. Harfstrand A, Fuxe K, Agnati LF, *et al.* Studies on neuropeptide Y–catecholamine interactions in the hypothalamus and in the forebrain of the male rat. Relationship to neuroendocrine function. *Neurochem Int* 1986;8:355–76
29. McDonald JK, Lumpkin MD, Samson WK, *et al.* Neuropeptide Y affects secretion of luteinizing hormone and growth hormone in ovariectomized rats. *Proc Natl Acad Sci USA* 1985;82:561–4
30. Zini I, Merlo Pich E, Fuxe K, *et al.* Actions of centrally administered neuropeptide Y on EEG activity in different rat strains and in different phases of their circadian cycle. *Acta Physiol Scand* 1984;122:71–7
31. Kaplan LM, Gabriel SM, Koenig JI, *et al.* Galanin is an estrogen-inducible, secretory product of the rat anterior pituitary. *Proc Natl Acad Sci USA* 1988;85:7408–12
32. Hsu DW, Hooi CH, Hedley-Whyte ET, *et al.* Co-expression of galanin and adrenocorticotropic hormone in human pituitary and pituitary adenomas. *Am J Pathol* 1991;138:897–909

33. Vrontakis ME, Yamamoto T, Schroeder IC, *et al.* Estrogen induction of galanin synthesis in the rat anterior pituitary gland demonstrated by *in situ* hybridization and immunohistochemistry. *Neurosci Lett* 1989;100:59–64
34. Hsu DW, El-Azouzi M, Black PM, *et al.* Estrogen increases galanin immunoreactivity in hyperplastic prolactin-secreting cells in Fisher 344 rats. *Endocrinology* 1990;126:3159–67
35. Hooi SC, Maiter DM, Martin JB, *et al.* Galaninergic mechanisms are involved in the regulation of corticotropin and thyrotropin secretion in the rat. *Endocrinology* 1990;127:2281–8
36. Aitken JM, Hart DM, Anderson JB. Osteoporosis after oophorectomy for non-malignant disease in premenopausal women. *Brit Met J* 1973;2:325–8
37. Richeson LS, Wahner HW, Melton LJ III. Relative contributions of aging and estrogen deficiency to postmenopausal bone loss. *N Engl J Med* 1984;311:1273–5
38. Ginzburg J, Hardiman P. Adrenergic agonist for menopausal complaints. In Genazzani AR, Montemagno U, Nappi C, Petraglia F, eds. *The Brain and Female Reproductive Function.* Carnforth, UK: Parthenon Publishing, 1987:623–5
39. Melis G, Cagnacci A, Gambacciani M. Restoration of luteinizing hormone response to naloxone in postmenopausal women by chronic administration of the antidopaminergic drug veralipride. *J Clin Endocrinol Metab* 1988;66:964–9
40. Aleem FA, McIntosh T. Menopausal syndrome: plasma levels of β-endorphin in postmenopausal women using a specific radioimmunoassay. *Maturitas* 1985;13:76
41. Genazzani AR, Petraglia F, Facchinetti F, *et al.* Steriod replacement increases beta-endorphin and beta-lipotropin plasma levels in postmenopausal women. *Gynecol Obstet Invest* 1988;26:153–9
42. Meldrum DL, De Fazio J, Erlik Y, *et al.* Pituitary hormones during the menopausal hot flush. *Obstet Gynecol* 1984;64:752–6
43. Genazzani AR, Petraglia F, Facchinetti F, *et al.* Increase of proopiomelanocortin-related peptides during subjective menopausal flushes *Am J Obstet Gynecol* 1984;149:775–9
44. Yen SSC, Jaffe RB. *Reproductive Endocrinology.* Philadelphia: WB Saunders, 1991
45. Linghtman SL, Jacobs HS, Maguire AK, *et al.* Climacteric flushing: clinical and endocrine response to infusion of naloxone. *Br J Obstet Gynecol* 1981;88:919–24
46. O'Donohue TL, Dorse DM. The opiomelanotropinergic neuronal and endocrine system. *Peptides* 1982;3:383–95
47. Phillips S, Sherwin BB. Effects of estrogen on memory function in surgically menopausal women. *Psychoneuroendocrinology* 1992;17:485–95
48. Fillit H, Wenreb H, Cholst I, *et al.* Observation in a preliminary open trial of estradiol therapy for senile dementia – Alzheimer type. *Psychoneuroendocrinology* 1986;34:521–5
49. Coyle JT, Price DL, DeLong MR. Alzheimer's disease: a disorder of cortical cholinergic innervation. *Science* 1983;219:1184–90
50. Lawrence AD, Sahakian BJ. Alzheimer disease, attention, and the cholinergic system. *Alzheimer Dis Assoc Disord* 1995;9:43–9
51. Henderson VW, Buckwalter JG. Cognitive deficits in men and women with Alzheimer's disease. *Neurology* 1994;44:90–6
52. Fillit H. Estrogens in the pathogenesis and treatment of Alzheimer's disease in postmenopausal women. *Ann NY Acad Sci* 1994;743:233–8
53. Advis J, McConn S, Negro-Vilar A. Evidence that catecholaminergic and peptidergic (luteinizing hormone-releasing hormone) neurons in suprachiasmatic-medial preoptic, medial basal hypothalamus and median eminence are involved in estrogen negative feed back. *Endocrinology* 1980;107:892–902
54. Wise P, Rance N, Berraclough C. Effect of estradiol and progesterone on catecholamine turnover rates in discrete hypothalamic regions in ovariectomized rats. *Endocrinology* 1980;108:2186–93
55. Sar M. Estradiol is concentrated in tyrosine hydroxylase-containing neurons of the hypothalamus. *Science* 1989;223:938–40
56. Furr BJA, Jordan VC. The pharmacology and clinical uses of tamoxifen. *Pharmacol Ther* 1984;25:127–205
57. McDonnell DP, Clemm DL, Hermann T, *et al.* Analysis of estrogen receptor function *in vitro* reveals three distinct classes of antiestrogen. *Mol Endocrinol* 1995;9:659–69
58. Sato M, Glasebrook AL, Bryant HU. Raloxifene: a selective estrogen receptor modulator. *J Bone Miner Metab* 1995;12(Suppl 2):S9–20

18
Estrogens and cerebral blood flow

W. L. McCullough and K. F. Gangar

INTRODUCTION

Blood flow to virtually all organs studied is increased by postmenopausal estrogen use. This is likely to be an important element in the general cardiovascular protection afforded by estrogens[1]. Restriction to blood flow may occur because of vessel narrowing, tortuosity or increased vessel wall stiffness. Atherosclerosis is the usual cause of these changes. Primary prevention of cardiovascular disease is the most beneficial effect of postmenopausal estrogen because of the huge cost of these problems in terms of morbidity, mortality and health economics.

Estrogens reduce atherosclerosis formation by a variety of mechanisms. Simple reduction of serum low density lipoproteins and an increase in high density lipoproteins are two of these, but the contribution of these is likely to have been overestimated and probably only explain about 30% of the observed reduction in cardiovascular risk[2]. The remainder of the observed benefit may be explained and investigated by looking at the direct effects of estrogen on arteries. The effects of differing doses and routes of administration of estrogens and the influence of progestogens on cerebral blood flow may give some insight into the likely long-term effects of these combinations on cerebrovascular health. This relatively new area of research is expanding rapidly.

THE EPIDEMIOLOGICAL DATA

Estrogen and mortality from cerebrovascular disease

Stampfer and colleagues[3] found no significant difference in the incidence of ischemic or hemorrhagic stroke between users and non-users of estrogen in the Nurses' Health Study. The Framingham Study[4] detected an increased risk of stroke in postmenopausal women ever exposed to estrogen. A large Danish study[5] showed no difference in stroke mortality between postmenopausal women who did or did not use estrogens. These three studies included mainly middle-aged women but the authors of the Californian Leisure World cohort study reported the findings for a group whose median age was 73 years[6]. The relative risk of mortality from stroke in estrogen users in this retirement community was 0.53 (95% confidence interval (CI), 0.31–0.91). In a highly selected cohort of long-term estrogen users in the United Kingdom, the observed/expected ratio of deaths from stroke was 0.54 (95% CI, 0.24–0.84) compared to the UK female population[7].

It could be argued that ischemic cerebrovascular disease occurs in older women. Studies which include younger cohorts would be likely to detect a high proportion of hemorrhagic strokes which are not clearly related to atherosclerosis. Support for this hypothesis comes from a Scandinavian population-based cohort which, by virtue of its size, permitted age stratification of the data[8]. There was no advantage for estrogen users in the groups up to 59 years. In the over 60s, however, there was a significant reduction in the incidence of stroke amongst those who had used estrogen. The results of very large long-term prospective trials (The Women's Health Initiative and the MRC/MRCGP trial) examining all aspects of risk–benefit for HRT will provide more insight into the impact of estrogen, with and without progestogen, on cerebrovascular mortality.

Estrogens and Alzheimer's disease

Estrogen deficiency is likely to be one of several factors modifying the neuronal injury and loss leading to Alzheimer's disease. The effects of estrogen are not only to increase cerebral blood flow but also to promote growth and survival of cholinergic neurons (especially those found in the amygdalo-hippocampal region, responsible for memory and cognitive ability), to stimulate secretase metabolism of the amyloid beta precursor protein (the histological hallmark of Alzheimer's disease[9]) and to suppress apolipoprotein E (accelerates the deposition of β amyloid[10]).

A possible role for estrogen in preventing or delaying Alzheimer's disease was suggested by Fillit and colleagues[11] in an open study. In their prospective nested case–control study, Paganini-Hill and Henderson[12] reported reduced Alzheimer's disease-related mortality with estrogen use at any time previously (relative risk, 0.69; 95% CI, 0.46–1.03). A postal questionnaire was used to collect data on estrogen use and follow-up was undertaken by examination of health records and death certificates.

In a prospective community-based study reported by Tang and colleagues[13], normal elderly women, free of dementia, were asked to record estrogen use in the past. They were followed for 1–5 years and diagnosis of Alzheimer's disease was based on an internationally agreed standard with blinding of the physicians to estrogen use. The data analysed by survival analysis plot suggested that women are most protected from Alzheimer's disease if estrogen has been taken for more than 1 year. The authors suggest that estrogen delays the onset of Alzheimer's disease rather than preventing it.

A full understanding of the role of estrogens and progestogens in reducing the impact of stroke and dementia on health economies is becoming increasingly important in an otherwise healthy aging population.

THE PHYSIOLOGY OF CEREBRAL BLOOD FLOW

The internal carotid arteries supply roughly two-thirds of the cerebrum; the vertebro-basilar arteries supply the remainder of the cerebrum and the cerebellum and midbrain[14]. In disease, anastomoses maintain blood flow through the anterior and posterior communicating arteries, forming a ring of arteries, the circle of Willis. Cerebral blood flow in the average human brain is 750 ml of blood per minute (50 ml per minute per 100 g of brain tissue)[15]. The most important influence on cerebral blood flow is the partial pressure of carbon dioxide in the circulating blood. A change of 1 mmHg results in alteration of the total cerebral blood flow by 5%.

Methods of measuring cerebral blood flow

The classic method described in 1945 used inhalation of a low-concentration nitrous oxide[16]. Fick's principle was used to estimate the dilution. The method was highly invasive, requiring cannnulation of the femoral artery and jugular vein. Modern methods of measurement of cerebral blood flow have reproduced the findings and chronic cannulation is no longer necessary in studies of the effect of estrogen on cerebral blood flow!

Blood flow is the product of the cross-sectional area and blood flow velocity. The complexities of normal laminar flow, vessel wall distensibility and varying blood viscosity make real-time flow estimates from non-invasive measurements of vessel diameter and Doppler shift subject to error. Nevertheless, the internal carotid artery pulsatility index has been accepted as a surrogate measure of cerebral blood flow[14].

Pulsatility index

Obstetricians and gynecologists have become familiar with analysis of umbilical and uterine flow velocity waveforms. When pulsed wave Doppler ultrasound is applied to any artery, a characteristic, or signature, flow velocity waveform is produced.

The pulsatility index is derived from the flow velocity waveform and is calculated as the difference between end-systolic flow and end-diastolic flow divided by the mean of the two. Physiologically, the contributing elements are arterial compliance, or distensibility, and peripheral resistance, or 'run off', distal to the point of sampling (Figure 1). Gangar and Vyas[17] carefully controlled for blood pressure and the various sensory inputs to the cranium which can alter significantly the total cerebral blood flow and affect the regional distribution of blood.

Using this methodology, they showed that transdermal estrogen at physiological doses, when given to postmenopausal women, led to a significant reduction in the pulsatility index (Figure 2). A lower pulsatility index is associated with increased run-off and improved vessel wall compliance and therefore greater flow. The reduction of the pulsatility index after administration of estrogens to postmenopausal women was again demonstrated by Penotti and colleagues[18] and Vyas and Jackson[19], adding temporal control data and placebo-controlled groups, respectively. Such results are not confined to postmenopausal women. Shamma and colleagues[20] used measurements of cerebral blood flow velocity and pulsatility index and found these correlated with estradiol levels during controlled ovarian hyperstimulation in premenopausal women. Belfort and colleagues[21] reported fluctuations in blood flow through the central retinal artery according to *all* the phases of a woman's reproductive life.

Single-photon emission computed tomography (SPECT scan)

Ohkura and colleagues[22] reported the use of a SPECT scan to investigate the effect of postmenopausal estrogens on cerebral blood flow. The mean cerebral blood flow in ten postmenopausal women increased from 44 ml/100 g per min to 47.2 ml/100 g per min ($p < 0.02$) after 3 weeks of treatment with 0.625 mg of conjugated equine estrogens. The mean percentage change

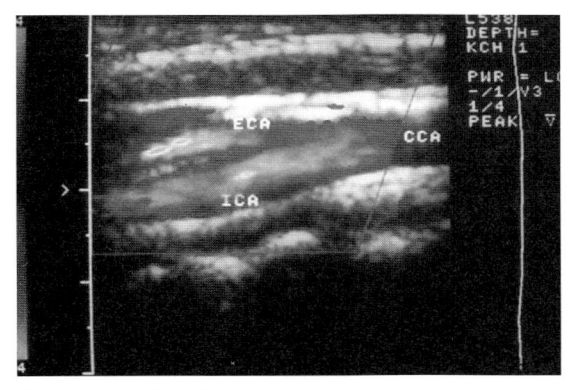

Figure 1 Color flow Doppler image of the bifurcation of the common carotid artery. The sampling point for internal carotid artery pulsatility index was chosen as 1 cm from the bifurcation

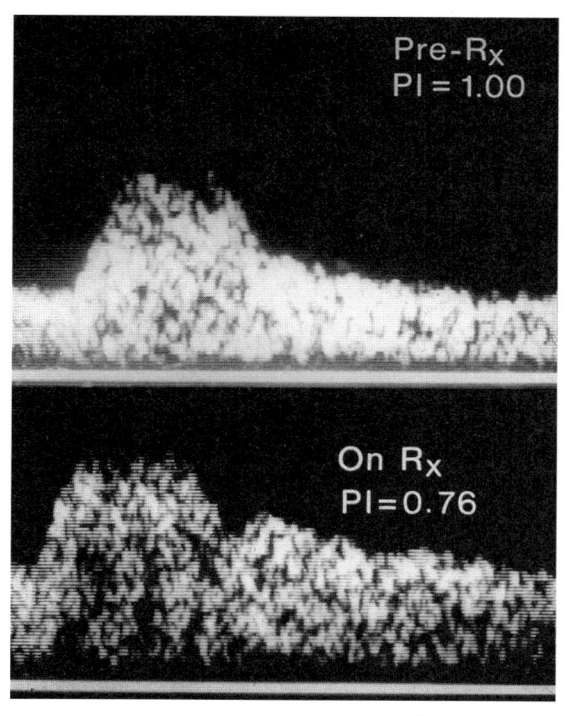

Figure 2 Internal carotid artery Doppler waveforms before (upper) and after treatment (lower) with estrogen patches. Reduction in pulsatility index is illustrated

in cerebral blood flow was 7.4% (standard error ± 2.2%). This is an important result, as SPECT scanning is the current definitive method of measuring cerebral blood flow.

VASCULAR MORPHOLOGY STUDIES

Apart from reducing vessel wall distensibility, atherosclerosis may form subintimal plaques. These plaques are the site of platelet aggregation and clot formation. Clot may either propagate to completely block the artery or embolize to block a more distal branch of the arterial tree, both with dire neurological consequences.

Duplex ultrasound gives information about the extent of atherosclerosis in an artery and has been used to study the effects of estrogen on the carotid artery. By this method, two observations can be made on the individual artery. The intimal–medial thickness is measured (Figures 3 and 4) and plaque formation can be quantified (Figure 5).

The Cardiovascular Health Study, a population-based study of risk factors for coronary heart disease and stroke in the elderly, investigated these parameters in 2955 women of 65 years or older. Current or prior use of estrogen was associated with reduced intimal–medial thickness and carotid stenosis grade[23]. Further data from the Cardiovascular Health Study collaboration compared estrogen only and estrogen with progestogen users and showed that both groups were associated with decreased measures of subclinical carotid atherosclerosis. Furthermore, there was no significant difference between the two groups of users of hormone replacement therapy[24]. In this observational analysis, there was no evidence of a negative effect of progestogen use.

The Asymptomatic Carotid Atherosclerosis Progression Study (ACAPS) investigators found

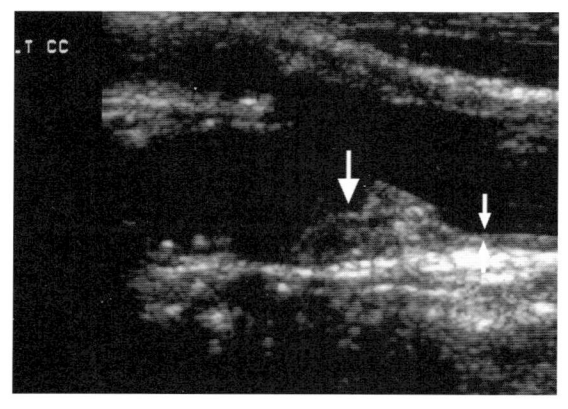

Figure 4 An example of an abnormal carotid artery showing increased intimal–medial thickness (between thin arrows) and plaque formation with ulceration (thick arrow). Reproduced with permission from Dr K. Dewbury, Consultant Radiologist, Southampton General Hospital

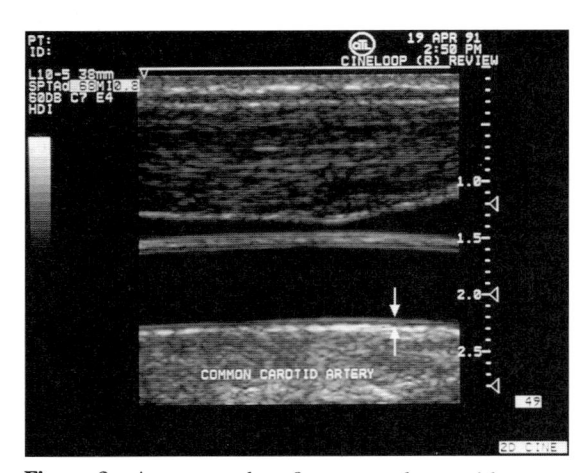

Figure 3 An example of a normal carotid artery demonstrating a normal intimal–medial thickness (between white arrows). Reproduced with permission from Dr K. Dewbury, Consultant Radiologist, Southampton General Hospital

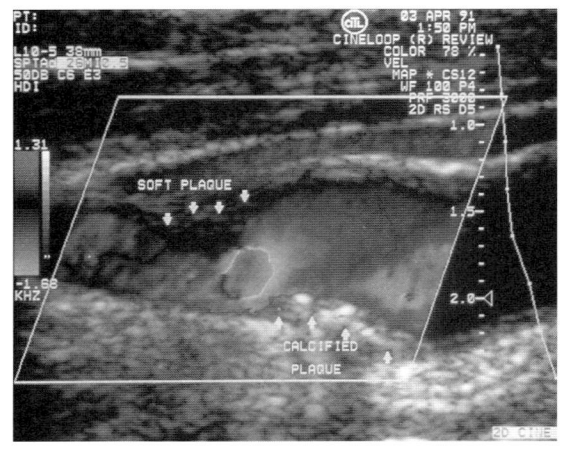

Figure 5 Color flow Doppler image of common carotid artery showing plaques

a significant difference in intimal–medial thickness between oestrogen users and non-users in the placebo group of a 3-year study intended to investigate the effect of lovastatin, a lipid lowering agent[25]. Akkad and colleagues[26] studied intimal thickness and plaque length and thickness in 17 postmenopausal women with known carotid disease. Reduction in plaque thickness (–18%, $p = 0.004$) was significant after only 6 months of treatment with unopposed estrogen.

These interesting studies suggest that Duplex ultrasound is another useful non-invasive method of assessing the effect of various regimens of hormone replacement therapy on carotid atherosclerosis.

PROGESTOGENS AND CEREBRAL BLOOD FLOW

The influence of progestogens alone on cerebral blood flow and surrogate measures has not been studied. The observational data presented above from the Cardiovascular Health Study suggest no diminution of the positive influence of estrogen when progestogen is added[24]. These patients are obviously not randomized, there are no controls and the parameters studied have not been directly linked to clinical end-points. The same is true of data from a small study by Gangar and colleagues[27] which investigated the pulsatility index of the internal carotid in postmenopausal women before and 4 months after using continuous combined hormone replacement therapy. The results showed a significant reduction in pulsatility index and therefore improved vascular function. The magnitude of the change was similar to that seen in earlier studies using transdermal[17] and oral estrogens alone[19]. Penotti and colleagues[18] similarly observed no modification of the positive influence of transdermal estrogen on internal carotid and middle cerebral artery pulsatility indices when cyclical medroxyprogesterone acetate was added. Further studies, using randomized controls, will be needed to validate these findings.

CONCLUSION

Cerebrovascular disease is a high-ranking cause of mortality in all developed countries. The most devastating effect of this disease is that it ranks number one as a cause of chronic disability. Any therapeutic option which might reduce or prevent this must be urgently and rigorously investigated.

Well-designed, prospective, randomized double-blind placebo-controlled trials of hormone replacement therapy in primary and secondary prevention of carotid atherosclerosis are needed to clarify the situation. The role of cerebral blood flow measures and surrogate measures need to be validated by long-term studies with hard clinical end-points. These vascular function tests might usefully be combined with measures of vascular morphology in future investigations. SPECT scanning requires injection with radioactive technetium and the main limitation of the technique is the cost and availability of such scanning facilities. In contrast, most hospitals have access to the equipment and expertise necessary to perform pulsatility index, intimal–medial thickness and plaque measurements with a high degree of reproducibility.

References

1. Collins P, Beale CM. *The Cardioprotective Role of HRT: a Clinical Update.* Carnforth, UK: Parthenon Publishing, 1996
2. Bush T. Submission to the American Food and Drug Administration, 1993
3. Stampfer MJ, Colditz GA, Willett WC, *et al.* Postmenopausal estrogen therapy and cardiovascular disease. *N Engl J Med* 1991;325:756–62
4. Wilson PWF, Garrison RJ, Castelli WP. Postmenopausal estrogen use, cigarette smoking and cardiovascular morbidity in women over 50; the Framingham Study. *N Engl J Med* 1985;313:1038–43
5. Boysen G, Nyboe J, Appleyard M, *et al.* Stroke incidence and risk factors for stroke in Copenhagen, Denmark. *Stroke* 1988;19:1345–53.

6. Paganini-Hill A, Ross RK, Henderson BE. Postmenopausal oestrogen treatment and stroke: a prospective study. *Br Med J* 1988;297:519–22
7. Hunt K, Vessey M, McPherson K. Mortality in a cohort of long-term users of hormone replacement therapy: an updated analysis. *Br J Obstet Gynaecol* 1990;97:1080–6
8. Falkeborn M, Persson I, Terent A, *et al.* Hormone replacement therapy and the risk of stroke. *Arch Intern Med* 1993;153:1201–9
9. Jaffe AB, Toran-Allerand CD, Greengard P, *et al.* Estrogen regulates metabolism of Alzheimer's amyloid beta precursor protein. *J Biol Chem* 1994;269:13065–8
10. Paganini-Hill A. Oestrogen replacement therapy and Alzheimer's disease. *Br J Obstet Gynaecol* 1996;103:80–6
11. Fillit H, Weinreb H, Cholst I, *et al.* Observations in a preliminary open trial of estradiol therapy for senile dementia – Alzheimer's type. *Psychoneuroendocrinology* 1986;11:337–45
12. Paganini-Hill A, Henderson VW. Estrogen deficiency and risk of Alzheimer's disease in women. *Am J Epidemiol* 1994;140:256–61
13. Tang M-X, Jacobs D, Stern Y, *et al.* Effect of oestrogen during menopause on risk and age at onset of Alzheimer's disease. *Lancet* 1996;348:429–32
14. Walton J, ed. *Brain's Diseases of the Nervous System*, 10th edn. Oxford: Oxford University Press, 1993
15. Parent A, ed. *Carpenter's Human Neuroanatomy*, 9th edn. Philadelphia: Williams and Wilkins, 1995
16. Kety SS, Schmidt CF. The determination of cerebral blood flow in man by the use of nitrous oxide in low concentrations. *Am J Physiol* 1945;143:53
17. Gangar KF, Vyas S, Whitehead MI, *et al.* Pulsatility index in the internal carotid artery in relation to transdermal oestradiol and time since menopause. *Lancet* 1991;338:839–42
18. Penotti M, Nencioni T, Gabrelli L, *et al.* Blood flow variations in internal carotid and middle cerebral arteries induced by postmenopausal hormone replacement therapy. *Am J Obstet Gynecol* 1993;169: 1226–32
19. Vyas S, Jackson P. A randomised controlled study of the influence of oral oestrogens on internal carotid pulsatility index. Presented at the *FIGO XV World Congress Conference*, Copenhagen, August, 1997
20. Shamma FN, Fayad P, Brass L, *et al.* Middle cerebral artery blood velocity during controlled ovarian hyperstimulation. *Fertil Steril* 1992;57:1022–5
21. Belfort MA, Saade GR, Snabes M, *et al.* Hormonal status affects reactivity of the cerebral vasculature. *Am J Obstet Gynecol* 1995;172:1273–8
22. Ohkura T, Iwasaki N, Yaoi Y. The effect of low-dose estrogen treatment on brain blood flow. Presented at the *VIII International Menopause Congress*, Sydney, 1996
23. Manolio TA, Furberg CD, Shemnanski L, *et al.* Associations of postmenopausal estrogen use with cardiovascular disease and its risk factors in older women. The CHS Collaborative Research Group. *Circulation* 1993;88:2163–71
24. Jonas HA, Kronmal RA, Psaty BM, *et al.* Current estrogen–progestin and estrogen replacement therapy in elderly women: association with carotid atherosclerosis. CHS Collaborative Research Group. Cardiovascular Health Study. *Am J Epidemiol* 1996;6: 314–23
25. Espeland MA, Applegate W, Furberg CD, *et al.* Estrogen replacement therapy and progression of intimal–medial thickness in the carotid arteries of postmenopausal women. ACAPS Investigators. Asymptomatic Carotid Atherosclerosis Progression Study. *Am J Epidemiol* 1996;142:1011–19
26. Akkad A, Hartshorne T, Bell PR, *et al.* Carotid plaque regression on oestrogen replacement: a pilot study. *Eur J Endovasc Surg* 1996;11:347–8
27. Gangar KF, McCullough WL. Continuous combined hormone replacement therapy and cardiovascular protection. *Eur Menopause* 1996;3:147–50

19
Estrogens and prevention of Alzheimer's disease

V. W. Henderson

INTRODUCTION

Menopause management has come to entail much more than the amelioration of hot flushes or atrophic vaginitis associated with the loss of ovarian estrogen production. The primary prevention of other disorders linked to postmenopausal estrogen deficiency, such as cardiovascular disease and osteoporosis, must also concern the older woman's physician. One of the most feared consequences of aging is the marked loss of mental abilities characteristic of dementia. Dementia is most commonly caused by Alzheimer's disease, a progressive neurodegenerative disorder whose prevalence among the elderly doubles about every 4.5 years[1]. Women are affected more often than men, in part because there are more elderly women than men, but women also appear to be at greater risk for Alzheimer's disease even after adjusting for age[2–4].

Alzheimer's symptoms begin insidiously and progress slowly over a number of years[5] (Table 1). The first clinical manifestation is almost always memory loss, in particular the inability to learn and recall new information. Eventually, patients manifest other difficulties affecting speech, visuospatial skills, calculation and abstract reasoning. Depression, apathy, agitation or delusions are occasionally prominent, but focal neurological deficits are not part of the initial clinical picture. As validated by

Table 1 Diagnostic criteria for Alzheimer's disease. Derived from reference 5

'Probable' Alzheimer's disease
Dementia; i.e. cognitive deterioration severe enough to interfere with usual daily activities, not attributable solely to disturbance of consciousness, and affecting both
   memory (ability to learn and recall new information)
   at least one other area of cognition
Cognitive defects began insidiously after age 39 years and gradually worsened over a period of at least 6 months
Based on thorough medical evaluation – one that includes neurological assessment, mental status testing and appropriate laboratory tests – no other illness that could account for patient's dementia

'Possible' Alzheimer's disease
Criteria for 'probable' Alzheimer's disease, except for
   atypical variations in onset, presentation or clinical course
   presence of second illness sufficient to produce dementia but which is not viewed as primary cause of dementia
   single, gradually progressive severe cognitive deficit in absence of another identifiable cause

'Definite' Alzheimer's disease
Dementia
Histopathological verification of Alzheimer's pathology by brain biopsy or by autopsy examination of brain

neuropathological criteria, a carefully considered clinical diagnosis of Alzheimer's disease[5] will be correct at least 80–90% of the time.

The pathological hallmark of Alzheimer's disease is the accumulation of neurofibrillary tangles within vulnerable neurons of the brain and neuritic plaques in the brain parenchyma between neuronal bodies. Neurofibrillary tangles are composed largely of paired helical filaments derived from an excessively phosphorylated form of tau, a microtubule-associated protein. Neuritic plaques typically include a central core of β-amyloid surrounded by distended neuronal processes (neurites) that contain paired helical filaments. The β-amyloid protein can also be deposited in the cerebral vasculature. Within the plaque, the presence of microglia, reactive astrocytes, cytokines and acute phase reactants suggests a concomitant inflammatory process[6].

ALZHEIMER'S DISEASE RISK FACTORS

Point mutations in genes on chromosomes 14, 1 and 21, inherited as autosomal dominant disorders, are largely responsible for uncommon early-onset forms of Alzheimer's disease that present during the fourth, fifth and sixth decades of life[7]. These genetic defects are rarely associated with dementia that begins after age 60 years, but the risk of late-onset Alzheimer's disease is strongly influenced by normal variations (polymorphisms) of apolipoprotein E, a lipid-transport protein encoded on chromosome 19 and involved in neuronal repair[8]. Of the three common apolipoprotein E alleles (ε2, ε3 and ε4), the ε4 allele is associated with increased risk[9], especially in women[10].

The presence of an ε4 allele is neither sufficient nor necessary for the development of Alzheimer's disease[11], and it is likely that a number of non-genetic factors cause or modify the risk of Alzheimer's disease through interactions in a multifactorial model that includes various environmental and genetic contributions. Evidence reviewed below suggests that estrogen deprivation after the menopause is one of the exogenous factors that increases a woman's Alzheimer's risk. Apart from age, female sex and genetic predisposition, other likely risk factors include a preceding history of head injury or depression and low educational attainment[12].

ESTROGEN, THE BRAIN AND ALZHEIMER'S DISEASE

Estrogen effects on the brain

As with other steroid hormones, many estrogen effects on the brain are mediated through nuclear receptors and the transcriptional regulation of specific gene products[13]; other estrogen actions, however, do not require genomic interactions[14]. Two estrogen receptors (alpha and beta) have been identified, whose distributions differ in different brain regions[15]. It is believed that estrogen and other gonadal steroids influence dynamic processes by which neurites are extended, synaptic connections are formed and neuronal circuits are modelled[16–20]. Estrogen interactions with growth and neurotrophic factors appear especially important in this regard[21–23].

Estrogen levels decline markedly after the menopause[24]. In addition to estrogen actions on neuronal plasticity, the loss of estrogen affects the development or manifestations of Alzheimer's disease in other ways. Estrogen influences a number of neurotransmitter actions, including those of acetylcholine. Neurons in the basal forebrain region, which supply cholinergic input to large regions of the hippocampus and neocortex, possess estrogen receptors[25], and these cells are severely impacted by pathological alterations of Alzheimer's disease[26]. In ovariectomized female rats, estradiol increases cholinergic markers in the basal forebrain and its projection target areas[27,28]. Therapeutic strategies that increase brain levels of acetylcholine improve cognitive skills of Alzheimer's patients, and demented women receiving estrogens may be more apt to benefit from cholinergic treatment than patients not receiving hormone replacement[29].

Experimental brain lesions that interrupt cholinergic pathways elevate apolipoprotein E levels in denervated regions[30], but despite cholinergic deficits, Alzheimer's patients actually have reduced levels of apolipoprotein E in the brain[31]. Non-neuronal elements within the central nervous system respond to estrogen with increased expression of apolipoprotein E[32].

Antioxidant[33] and anti-inflammatory[34,35] properties of estrogen may be important in Alzheimer's disease. Free radicals are implicated in several neurodegenerative disorders of aging, including Alzheimer's disease. Neurotoxic effects of the β-amyloid protein are potentiated by free radicals[36], and antioxidant therapy (e.g. with alpha-tocopherol[37]) may retard the progression of Alzheimer's symptoms. Inflammatory processes are implicated in certain aspects of neuritic plaque formation[6]. There is suggestive evidence that anti-inflammatory drugs might lower the risk of Alzheimer's disease[38], and anti-inflammatory agents have been used for Alzheimer's symptoms[39].

Dementia caused by Alzheimer's pathology may be potentiated by the co-occurrence of ischemic cerebrovascular disease[40], but it is controversial whether hormone replacement lowers the older woman's risk of stroke[41]. Notably, however, the postmenopausal use of estrogen reduces atherosclerotic narrowing of the carotid arteries[42] and augments cerebral blood flow[43,44].

Estrogen effects on cognition and mood in healthy women

Cognitive skills may be influenced by sex steroids. Some behavioral consequences of estrogen exposure in the developing brain are thought to be permanent, but estrogen is also believed to influence behavior transiently. A study of cross-gender hormone therapy in transsexual men and women implies that estrogen and testosterone exert reciprocal effects on cognition, with estrogen associated with enhanced verbal fluency and testosterone with better visuospatial abilities[45].

Large case–control and cohort studies have been inconsistent in suggesting important cognitive effects of postmenopausal hormone replacement[46–48]. However, several smaller observational studies of healthy women during different phases of the menstrual cycle[49–51] and of postmenopausal women receiving hormone replacement therapy[52–54] imply that estrogen can benefit a number of skills, including fine motor abilities, verbal fluency and creativity. Interventional studies point to particularly noticeable estrogen effects on verbal memory[55,56]. The magnitude of such putative estrogen effects, although modest, may nonetheless be clinically relevant.

In addition to effects on cognition, estrogen can enhance mood and subjective well-being in the perimenopausal and postmenopausal period[57–61]. The manner by which estrogen affects mood is uncertain but may involve augmentation of brain levels of noradrenaline or serotonin[62–64], monoaminergic neurotransmitters whose deficiency is implicated in depression. Although mood can influence cognitive performance, the effect of estrogen on cognition appears to be independent of mood[54,55].

Estrogen effects on cognition in women with Alzheimer's disease

Henderson and colleagues[65] observed that Alzheimer's patients receiving estrogens perform better on a global measure of cognitive ability than women with Alzheimer's disease who do not receive estrogen. In separate analyses involving women matched for age, education and duration of dementia symptoms, differences favoring the estrogen group were apparent on several neuropsychological measures[66]. The greatest difference occurred on a naming (semantic memory) task[66], the same type of task that is more severely impacted for women than men with Alzheimer's disease[67]. Cognitive differences in this study could not be attributed to mood[66].

Several investigators have used estrogen to treat women with Alzheimer's disease (reviewed by Henderson[68]). Most studies have been small, uncontrolled and of short duration. Only one peer-review double-blind study has been published to date. Honjo and co-workers[69] treated 14 Alzheimer's patients with either oral conjugated estrogens (1.25 mg/day) or a placebo. After 3 weeks, women in the estrogen arm improved significantly over baseline levels with regard to three outcome measures, while those in the placebo arm did not change significantly. Between-group differences at 3 weeks were significant for one of these three measures.

Preliminary results of a second double-blind study have been presented by Asthana and associates[70]. Ten women received transdermal estradiol (50 mg/day) or a placebo patch for 8 weeks. Significant group differences for two measures of verbal memory favored subjects in the active treatment arm, but other psychometric measures did not differ significantly between groups. Finally, Birge[71] has announced an interim analysis of a 9-month double-blind trial of oral conjugated estrogens (0.625 mg/day cycled with medroxyprogesterone) or placebo. Five of 10 estrogen-treated women improved on a clinician interview-based impression of change. Ten Alzheimer's women in the placebo group remained the same with regard to this measure or declined over the course of the trial.

ESTROGEN REPLACEMENT THERAPY AND ALZHEIMER'S DISEASE RISK

Epidemiological evidence of reduced risk

Compared to elderly women without dementia, women with Alzheimer's disease are significantly less likely to use hormone replacement[65]. It is possible, however, that prescribing practices may have confounded findings in this and similar studies. Estrogen might be considered a discretionary medication, and some physicians could be reluctant to continue hormone therapy after their patients develop dementia. Conversely, the perception that estrogen may palliate Alzheimer's disease symptoms could induce some physicians to begin hormone therapy only after dementia has become apparent.

Strong support for a protective role of estrogen replacement comes from recent epidemiological investigations where information on estrogen use was obtained prospectively, before some study participants became demented (Table 2). The largest such study is from the Leisure World retirement community cohort in southern California[72]. Participants in this nested case–control study provided information on hormone replacement when the cohort was established by postal survey in the early 1980s. Among cohort members who subsequently died, diagnoses suggestive of Alzheimer's disease were listed on death certificates of 248 women. Thirty-eight per cent of these women had used some form of estrogen, compared to 49% of matched controls whose death certificates did not indicate Alzheimer's disease. The estrogen 'ever-users' were shown to have about a one-third reduction in their risk of

Table 2 Epidemiological studies of estrogen replacement therapy and Alzheimer's disease in which information on estrogen use was collected before onset of dementia

Study location/study authors	Number of Alzheimer's disease cases	Number of non-demented controls	Source of information on estrogen use	Risk estimate	95% confidence interval
Seattle, Washington Brenner et al., 1994[76]	107	120	pharmacy records	1.1	0.6–1.8
Leisure World, California* Paganini-Hill and Henderson, 1996[72]	248	1198	self	0.65	0.49–0.88
New York City Tang et al., 1996[73]	167	957	self	0.5	0.25–0.9
Baltimore, Maryland Kawas et al., 1997[74]	34	438	self	0.46	0.21–1.00
Rochester, Minnesota Waring et al., 1997[75]†	222	222	medical records	0.4	0.2–0.8

*1994 analysis from Leisure World[77] considered 138 cases and 550 controls: relative risk estimate was 0.69; †preliminary report

Alzheimer's disease when compared to women who had never used estrogen (Table 2). Similar risk reductions were found in analyses from Leisure World that considered only oral estrogen replacement therapy (odds ratio (OR) = 0.70, 95% confidence interval (CI) = 0.50–0.98)[72]. Although Alzheimer's disease is almost certainly under-reported on death certificate records, any resulting bias would reduce the likelihood of detecting any effect of hormone replacement rather than falsely suggest benefit in the absence of an effect.

In an ethnically diverse community-based cohort study from the northern Manhattan area of New York City[73], 13% of older women reported having used oral estrogens. Over a follow-up period of 1–5 years, ever-users of oral estrogen faced a 50% lower risk of Alzheimer's disease (Table 2). Among women with newly diagnosed Alzheimer's disease, the age at onset was earlier in the never-user group. In this study, possession of the ε4 allele of apolipoprotein E did not modify the protective effect of estrogen[73]. However, in a European population-based study of early-onset Alzheimer's disease, preliminary analyses suggested that the protective effect of estrogen was limited to women with the ε4 allele (OR = 0.14, 95% CI = 0.02–0.87)[78].

In the Baltimore Longitudinal Study of Aging, follow-up of 472 eligible women detected 34 new cases of definite, probable or possible Alzheimer's disease. Approximately 45% of women had used oral or transdermal estrogen preparations. Ever-users in this cohort had a risk of Alzheimer's disease of about one-half that of women who had never used these forms of estrogen[74] (Table 2).

Preliminary analyses from Rochester, Minnesota, also suggest that estrogen use helps prevent Alzheimer's disease. This population-based case–control study considered all forms of estrogen used for at least 6 months after the menopause but before the onset of dementia (or before the corresponding year in the matched control group)[75]. The frequency of estrogen use was lower among Alzheimer's disease cases (5%) than non-demented controls (12%), and the risk reduction among estrogen users was greater than one-half (Table 2).

Different conclusions were reached in a case–control study of members of a Seattle health maintenance organization. Computerized pharmacy records of 107 women diagnosed with definite or probable Alzheimer's disease were compared with records of control subjects without dementia[76]. About 50% of subjects in each group had used some form of estrogen, with 23% of cases and 28% of controls having used an oral preparation. As in the Leisure World study, the risk of an Alzheimer's diagnosis was reduced by about 30% among women who had previously used oral estrogens, but in the Seattle study, the magnitude of reduction was not statistically significant (OR = 0.7, 95% CI = 0.4–1.5). Moreover, primary analyses based on all estrogen preparations showed no protective effect of hormone replacement (Table 2).

Strength of exposure

The hypothesis that estrogen replacement protects against Alzheimer's disease would be bolstered by demonstration that women with greater estrogen exposures are at lower risk than those exposed to lower amounts. Epidemiological evidence lends partial support to this contention. In the Leisure World cohort, there were significant trends for lower risk to be associated with both larger doses of the most commonly prescribed oral estrogen preparation and with longer durations of estrogen use[72]. In the highest dose category (≥ 1.25 mg/day) conjugated estrogens), the relative risk estimate was 0.54 (95% CI = 0.32–0.92), and in the longest duration category (≥ 15 years of estrogen therapy), the estimate was 0.44 (95% CI = 0.26–0.75). Similarly, the Rochester, Minnesota analysis indicated decreasing risk with increasing duration of estrogen use and with increasing total cumulative dose[75]. Information on dosage was not obtained in the New York City study, but there was a significant effect for duration of estrogen use on disease risk. Women who had used estrogen for more than a year (average 14 years) had a relative risk estimate of only 0.13 (95% CI = 0.02–0.92)[73]. However, no significant effect of treatment duration was evident in the smaller Baltimore cohort[74], and the number of estrogen prescriptions did not have a significant impact on Alzheimer's risk in the Seattle study[76].

ALZHEIMER'S PREVENTION: CLINICAL IMPLICATIONS

There are compelling reasons why a postmenopausal woman and her physician may opt for estrogen replacement after the menopause[79,80]. Well-established beneficial effects on cardiovascular disease and overall mortality[81–83] appear to outweigh cancer risks and other known hazards, and there is additional strong evidence favoring estrogen use for the prevention of osteoporosis[84,85]. As reviewed above, there is a robust biological rationale for the relevance of estrogens to Alzheimer's disease. Estrogen appears to influence cognition in healthy women and possibly improves cognitive skills in women with Alzheimer's disease.

Epidemiological studies of estrogen and Alzheimer's disease generally suggest that estrogen replacement therapy may reduce Alzheimer's risk by about one-third to one-half (Table 2). However, evidence regarding Alzheimer's disease prevention is observational rather than experimental. Moreover, the number of studies is relatively small, and results are not uniformly consistent. For these reasons, firm conclusions on Alzheimer's prevention are not yet possible.

Although basic laboratory work indicates that neurotrophic and other estrogen actions vary among different estrogen compounds, no convincing human data address possible differences with regard to Alzheimer's protection. Most of the epidemiological studies on estrogen and Alzheimer's disease risk have been conducted in the United States, where conjugated estrogens are the most commonly prescribed estrogen preparation. Prescribing patterns differ in Europe. However, findings from the Italian longitudinal study on aging, which are based on current estrogen use, also imply a protective effect of estrogen[86]. Based on limited information, both opposed and unopposed estrogens appear to protect against Alzheimer's disease. Epidemiological data on dosage necessarily reflect patterns of clinical practice, but treatment over a longer period of time may afford better protection[72,73,75], and within the range of estrogen dosages examined, greater doses may also enhance protection[72]. Future studies also must consider the possibility that estrogen replacement therapy might benefit some women more than others, with subgroups of women defined, for example, by apolipoprotein E genotype, the presence of cerebrovascular disease or by other risk factors.

ACKNOWLEDGEMENTS

This research is supported in part by grants from the National Institutes of Health (AG05142), the Alzheimer's Association, and Wyeth-Ayerst Laboratories; the Bowles Clinic for Alzheimer's and Related Disorders; and gifts from Mrs E. Lent and Mr and Mrs R. Miller. Among colleagues at the University of Southern California, the author particularly acknowledges contributions of Drs A. Paganini-Hill, G. Buckwalter and L. Schneider for work cited in this review.

References

1. Jorm AF, Korten AE, Henderson AS. The prevalence of dementia: a quantitative integration of the literature. *Acta Psychiatr Scand* 1987;76:465–79
2. Mölsä PK, Marttila RJ, Rinne UK. Epidemiology of dementia in a Finnish population. *Acta Neurol Scand* 1982;65:541–52
3. Rorsman B, Hagnell O, Lanke J. Prevalence and incidence of senile and multi-infarct dementia in the Lundby study: a comparison between the time periods 1947–1957 and 1957–1972. *Neuropsychobiology* 1986;15:122–9
4. Katzman R, Aronson M, Fuld P, *et al*. Development of dementing illnesses in an 80-year-old volunteer cohort. *Ann Neurol* 1989;25:317–24
5. McKhann G, Drachman D, Folstein MF, *et al*. Clinical diagnosis of Alzheimer's disease: report of the NINCDS–ADRDA Work Group under the

auspices of Department of Health and Human Services Task Force on Alzheimer's Disease. *Neurology* 1984;34:939–44
6. McGeer PL, McGeer EG. The inflammatory response system of brain: implications for therapy of Alzheimer and other neurodegenerative diseases. *Brain Res Rev* 1995;21:195–218
7. Pericak-Vance MA, Haines JL. Genetic susceptibility to Alzheimer disease. *Trends Genet* 1995;11:504–8
8. Poirier J. Apolipoprotein E in animal models of CNS injury and in Alzheimer's disease. *Trends Neurosci* 1994;17:525–30
9. Strittmatter WJ, Saunders AM, Schmechel D, et al. Apolipoprotein E: high-avidity binding to β-amyloid and increased frequency of type 4 allele in late-onset familial Alzheimer disease. *Proc Natl Acad Sci USA* 1993;90:1977–81
10. Farrer LA, Cupples LA, van Duijn CM, et al. Apolipoprotein E genotype in patients with Alzheimer's disease: implications for the risk of dementia among relatives. *Ann Neurol* 1995;38:797–808
11. Kukull WA, Schellenberg GD, Bowen JD, et al. Apolipoprotein E in Alzheimer's disease risk and case detection: a case–control study. *J Clin Epidemiol* 1996;49:1143–8
12. Graves AB, Kukull WA. The epidemiology of dementia. In Morris JC, ed. *Handbook of Dementing Illnesses.* New York: Marcel Dekker, 1994:23–69
13. Katzenellenbogen JA, O'Malley BW, Katzenellenbogen BS. Tripartite steroid hormone receptor pharmacology: interaction with multiple effector sites as a basis for the cell- and promotor-specific action of these hormones. *Mol Endocrinol* 1996;10:119–31
14. Wong M, Thompson TL, Moss RL. Nongenomic actions of estrogens in the brain: physiological significance and cellular mechanisms. *Crit Rev Neurobiol* 1996;10:189–203
15. Shughrue PJ, Komm B, Merchenthaler, I. The distribution of estrogen receptor-β mRNA in the rat hypothalamus. *Steroids* 1996;61:678–81
16. Chung SK, Pfaff DW, Cohen RS. Estrogen-induced alterations in synaptic morphology in the midbrain central gray. *Exp Brain Res* 1988;69:522–30
17. Toran-Allerand CD. Organotypic culture of the developing cerebral cortex and hypothalamus: relevance to sexual differentiation. *Psychoneuroendocrinology* 1991;16:7–24
18. Brinton RD. 17β-estradiol induction of filopodial growth in cultured hippocampal neurons within minutes of exposure. *Mol Cell Neurosci* 1993;4:36–46
19. Woolley CS, McEwen BS. Roles of estradiol and progesterone in regulation of hippocampal dendritic spine density during the estrous cycle in the rat. *J Comp Neurol* 1993;336:293–306
20. Keefe D, Garcia-Segura M, Naftolin, F. New insights into estrogen action on the brain. *Neurobiol Aging* 1994;15:495–7
21. Miranda RC, Sohrabji F, Toran-Allerand CD. Presumptive estrogen target neurons express mRNA for both the neurotrophins and neurotrophin receptors: a basis for potential developmental interactions of estrogen with neurotrophins. *Mol Cell Neurosci* 1993;4:510–25
22. Sohrabji F, Miranda RC, Toran-Allerand CD. Estrogen differentially regulates estrogen and nerve growth factor receptor mRNAs in adult sensory neurons. *J Neurosci* 1994;14:459–71
23. Shughrue PJ, Dorsa DM. Estrogen modulates the growth-associated protein GAP-43 (neuromodulin) mRNA in the rat preoptic area and basal hypothalamus. *Neuroendocrinology* 1993;57:439–47
24. Burger HG. The endocrinology of the menopause. *Maturitas* 1996;23:129–36
25. Toran-Allerand CD, Miranda RC, Bentham WD, et al. Estrogen receptors colocalize with low-affinity nerve growth factor receptors in cholinergic neurons of the basal forebrain. *Proc Natl Acad Sci USA* 1992;89:4668–72
26. Coyle JT, Price DL, DeLong MR. Alzheimer's disease: a disorder of cortical cholinergic innervation. *Science* 1983;219:1184–90
27. Luine V. Estradiol increases choline acetyltransferase activity in specific basal forebrain nuclei and projection areas of female rats. *Exp Neurol* 1985;89:484–90
28. Gibbs RB, Pfaff DW. Effects of estrogen and fimbria/fornix transection on p75^{NGFR} and ChAT expression in the medial septum and diagonal band of Broca. *Exp Neurol* 1992;116:23–39
29. Schneider LS, Farlow MR, Henderson VW, et al. Effects of estrogen replacement therapy on response to tacrine in patients with Alzheimer's disease. *Neurology* 1996;46:1580–4
30. Poirier J, Hess M, May PC, et al. Astrocytic apolipoprotein E mRNA and GFAP mRNA in hippocampus after entorhinal cortex lesioning. *Mol Brain Res* 1991;11:97–106
31. Bertrand P, Poirier J, Oda T, et al. Association of apolipoprotein E genotype with brain levels of apolipoprotein E and apolipoprotein J (clusterin) in Alzheimer disease. *Mol Brain Res* 1995;33:174–8
32. Stone DJ, Rozovsky I, Morgan TE, et al. Astrocytes and microglia respond to estrogen with increased apoE mRNA *in vivo* and *in vitro*. *Exp Neurol* 1997;143:313–18
33. Sack MN, Rader DJ, Cannon ROI. Oestrogen and inhibition of oxidation of low-density

lipoproteins in postmenopausal women. *Lancet* 1994;343:269–70
34. Ershler WB. Interleukin-6: a cytokine for gerontologists. *J Am Geriatr Soc* 1993;41:176–81
35. Hashimoto S, Katou M, Dong Y, *et al.* Effects of hormone replacement therapy on serum amyloid P component in postmenopausal women. *Maturitas* 1997;26:113–19
36. Sagara Y, Dargusch R, Klier FG, *et al.* Increased antioxidant enzyme activity in amyloid β protein-resistant cells. *J Neurosci* 1996;16:497–505
37. Sano M, Ernesto C, Thomas RG, *et al.* A controlled trial of selegiline, alpha-tocopherol, or both as treatment for Alzheimer's disease. *N Engl J Med* 1997;336:1216–22
38. Rich JB, Rasmussen DX, Folstein MF, *et al.* Nonsteroidal anti-inflammatory drugs in Alzheimer's disease. *Neurology* 1995;45:51–5
39. Rogers J, Kirby LC, Hempelman SR, *et al.* Clinical trial of indomethacin in Alzheimer's disease. *Neurology* 1993;43:1609–11
40. Snowdon DA, Greiner LH, Mortimer JA, *et al.* Brain infarction and the clinical expression of Alzheimer disease. *J Am Med Assoc* 1997;277:813–17
41. Paganini-Hill A. Estrogen replacement therapy and stroke. *Prog Cardiovasc Dis* 1995;38:223–42
42. Espeland MA, Applegate W, Furberg CD, *et al.* Estrogen replacement therapy and progression of intimal–medial thickness in the carotid arteries of postmenopausal women. *Am J Epidemiol* 1995;142:1011–19
43. Belfort MA, Saade GR, Snabes M, *et al.* Hormonal status affects the reactivity of the cerebral vasculature. *Am J Obstet Gynecol* 1995;172:1273–8
44. Ohkura T, Teshima Y, Isse K, *et al.* Estrogen increases cerebral and cerebellar blood flows in postmenopausal women. *Menopause* 1995;2:13–18
45. Van Goozen SHM, Cohen-Kettenis PT, Gooren LJG, *et al.* Gender differences in behaviour activating effects of cross-sex hormones. *Psychoneuroendocrinology* 1995;20:343–63
46. Barrett-Connor E, Kritz-Silverstein D. Estrogen replacement therapy and cognitive function in older women. *J Am Med Assoc* 1993;269:2637–41
47. Schmidt R, Fazekas F, Reinhart B, *et al.* Estrogen replacement therapy in older women: a neuropsychological and brain MRI study. *J Am Geriat Soc* 1996;44:1307–13
48. Szklo M, Cerhan J, Diez-Roux AV, *et al.* Estrogen replacement therapy and cognitive functioning in the Atherosclerosis Risk in Communities (ARIC) study. *Am J Epidemiol* 1996;144:1048–57
49. Hampson E. Variations in sex-related cognitive abilities across the menstrual cycle. *Brain Cognit* 1990;14:26–43
50. Phillips SM, Sherwin BB. Variations in memory function and sex steroid hormones across the menstrual cycle. *Psychoneuroendocrinology* 1992;17:497–506
51. Krug R, Stamm U, Pietrowsky R, *et al.* Effects of menstrual cycle on creativity. *Psychoneuroendocrinology* 1994;19:21–31
52. Kampen DL, Sherwin BB. Estrogen use and verbal memory in healthy postmenopausal women. *Obstet Gynecol* 1994;83:979–83
53. Robinson D, Friedman L, Marcus R, *et al.* Estrogen replacement therapy and memory in older women. *J Am Geriatr Soc* 1994;42:919–22
54. Kimura D. Estrogen replacement therapy may protect against intellectual decline in postmenopausal women. *Horm Behav* 1995;29:312–21
55. Phillips SM, Sherwin BB. Effects of estrogen on memory function in surgically menopausal women. *Psychoneuroendocrinology* 1992;17:485–95
56. Sherwin BB, Tulandi T. 'Add-back' estrogen reverses cognitive deficits induced by a gonadotropin-releasing hormone agonist in women with leiomyomata uteri. *J Clin Endocrinol Metab* 1996;81:2545–9
57. Schneider MA, Brotherton PL, Hailes J. The effect of exogenous oestrogens on depression in menopausal women. *Med J Aust* 1977;2:162–3
58. Sherwin BB. Affective changes with estrogen and androgen replacement therapy in surgically menopausal women. *J Affect Disord* 1988;14:177–87
59. Ditkoff EC, Crary WG, Cristo M, *et al.* Estrogen improves psychological function in asymptomatic postmenopausal women. *Obstet Gynecol* 1991;78:991–5
60. Best NR, Rees MP, Barlow DH, *et al.* Effect of estradiol implant on noradrenergic function and mood in menopausal subjects. *Psychoneuroendocrinology* 1992;17:87–93
61. Gerdes LC, Sonnendecker EWW, Polakow ES. Psychological changes effected by estrogen–progestogen and clonidine treatment in climacteric women. *Am J Obstet Gynecol* 1982;142:98–104
62. Greengrass PM, Tonge SR. The accumulation of noradrenaline and 5-hydroxytryptamine in three regions of mouse brain after tetrabenazine and iproniazid: effects of ethinyloestradiol and progesterone. *Psychopharmacologia* 1974;39:187–91
63. Ball P, Knuppen R, Haupt M, *et al.* Interactions between estrogens and catechol amines. III. Studies on the methylation of catechol estrogens, catechol amines and other catechols by the catechol-O-methyltransferases of human liver. *J Clin Endocrinol Metab* 1972;34:736–46
64. Cohen IR, Wise PM. Effects of estradiol on the diurnal rhythm of serotonin activity in

microdissected brain areas of ovariectomized rats. *Endocrinology* 1988;122:2619–25
65. Henderson VW, Paganini-Hill A, Emanuel CK, *et al.* Estrogen replacement therapy in older women: comparisons between Alzheimer's disease cases and nondemented control subjects. *Arch Neurol* 1994;51:896–900
66. Henderson VW, Watt L, Buckwalter JG. Cognitive skills associated with estrogen replacement in women with Alzheimer's disease. *Psychoneuroendocrinology* 1996;21:421–30
67. Henderson VW, Buckwalter JG. Cognitive deficits of men and women with Alzheimer's disease. *Neurology* 1994;44:90–6
68. Henderson VW. Estrogen replacement therapy for the prevention and treatment of Alzheimer's disease. *CNS Drugs* 1997;8:343–51
69. Honjo H, Ogino Y, Tanaka K, *et al.* An effect of conjugated estrogen to cognitive impairment in women with senile dementia – Alzheimer's type: a placebo-controlled double blind study. *J Jpn Menopause Soc* 1993;1:167–71
70. Asthana S, Craft S, Baker LD, *et al.* Transdermal estrogen improves memory in women with Alzheimer's disease (abstr.). *Soc Neurosci Abstr* 1996;22:200
71. Birge SJ. The role of estrogen in the treatment of Alzheimer's disease. *Neurology* 1997;48 (Suppl 7):S36–41
72. Paganini-Hill A, Henderson VW. Estrogen replacement therapy and risk of Alzheimer's disease. *Arch Intern Med* 1996;156:2213–17
73. Tang MX, Jacobs D, Stern Y, *et al.* Effect of oestrogen during menopause on risk and age at onset of Alzheimer's disease. *Lancet* 1996;348:429–32
74. Kawas C, Resnick S, Morrison A, *et al.* A prospective study of estrogen replacement therapy and the risk of developing Alzheimer's disease: the Baltimore Longitudinal Study of Aging. *Neurology* 1997;48:1517–21
75. Waring SC, Rocca WA, Petersen RC, *et al.* Postmenopausal estrogen replacement therapy and Alzheimer's disease: a population-based study in Rochester, Minnesota (abstr.). *Neurology* 1997;48 (Suppl.2):A79
76. Brenner DE, Kukull WA, Stergachis A, *et al.* Postmenopausal estrogen replacement therapy and the risk of Alzheimer's disease: a population-based case–control study. *Am J Epidemiol* 1994;140:262–7
77. Paganini-Hill A, Henderson VW. Estrogen deficiency and risk of Alzheimer's disease in women. *Am J Epidemiol* 1994;140:256–61
78. Van Duijn C, Meijer H, Witteman JCM, *et al.* Estrogen, apolipoprotein E and the risk of Alzheimer's disease (abstr.). *Neurobiol Aging* 1996;16(Suppl.):S79–80
79. American College of Physicians. Guidelines for counseling postmenopausal women about preventive hormone therapy. *Ann Intern Med* 1992;117:1038–41
80. Lobo RA. Benefits and risks of estrogen replacement therapy. *Am J Obstet Gynecol* 1995;173:982–90
81. Ettinger B, Friedman GD, Bush T, *et al.* Reduced mortality associated with long-term postmenopausal estrogen therapy. *Obstet Gynecol* 1996;87:6–12
82. Folsom AR, Mink PJ, Sellers TA, *et al.* Hormonal replacement therapy and morbidity and mortality in a prospective study of postmenopausal women. *Am J Public Health* 1995;85:1128–32
83. Stampfer MJ, Colditz GA. Estrogen replacement and coronary heart disease: a quantitative assessment of the epidemiologic evidence. *Prevent Med* 1991;20:47–63
84. Barzel US. Estrogens in the prevention and treatment of postmenopausal osteoporosis: a review. *Am J Med* 1988;85:847–50
85. Belchetz PE. Hormonal treatment of postmenopausal women. *N Engl J Med* 1994;330:1062–71
86. Baldereschi M, DiCarol A, Maggi S, *et al.* Estrogen replacement therapy and the risk of dementia in the Italian longitudinal study on aging (abstr.). *Eur J Neurol* 1996;3(Suppl.5):85–6

20
Hormone replacement therapy and breast cancer mortality

L. Bergkvist

INTRODUCTION

Estrogen and combined estrogen–progestogen treatments are widely used to relieve climacteric symptoms, and are very effective in doing so. These drugs also have positive effects on the skeleton, reducing the incidence of hip fractures and other osteoporotic fractures by almost 50%[1–3], and the incidence of cardiovascular disease by approximately 50%[4–6]. There is also a positive effect on Alzheimer's disease, especially on cognitive functions[7]. There are, however, some adverse effects that have made many physicians reluctant to prescribe the drugs, and patients afraid to use them. Since the mid-1970s it has been known that unopposed estrogen use can increase the risk of endometrial cancer[8,9]. Addition of progestogens seems to diminish this risk and to bring the incidence back to baseline level[10]. The other main possible negative effect of estrogen treatment is a proposed effect on breast cancer incidence. Theoretically, there are several factors indicating that the incidence of breast cancer might be affected by estrogen. Estrogens are needed for a proper development of the breast, and breast cancer is 100 times more common in females than in males. Several endocrine factors related to menarche, menopause and childbearing have implications on breast cancer risk. Over 50 studies have been published on the relationship between exogenous estrogen treatment and breast cancer risk[11]. The results are reassuring, concerning ever-use of estrogen or estrogen–progestogen combinations: there is no overall increased risk for a woman that has ever used estrogens[12–20]. However, long-term treatment seems to increase the risk slightly, maybe in the order of 30–50% after 10–20 years of treatment[12,14,21]. The increased risk does not seem to be lowered by the addition of progestogens[14,17,22,23]. There is a possibility, however, that the increased risk is confined to current users only[17], a situation parallel to that seen for oral contraceptive pills[24]. The tumors developing after estrogen treatment have been found to be clinically less advanced, with more ductal carcinoma *in situ* (DCIS), fewer lymph-node metastases and higher grade than tumors arising in women without estrogens[21,25], and the prognosis has been shown to be better, at least among women over 50 years with ongoing treatment at the time of diagnosis[26]. It is unclear whether this merely reflects a better medical surveillance with earlier detection among treated women, or if the treatment itself has any impact on the type or aggressiveness of the cancer that develops after exogenous hormone use. A more stable estimate of the long-term effects of estrogen treatment would be to study breast cancer mortality among users of estrogen. A problem involved in this type of study is finding a proper baseline risk for comparison, and there have been but few attempts to date in the literature to address this question.

The purpose of this paper is to summarize the results of these studies and to discuss the difficulties involved in the interpretation.

PREVIOUS RESULTS

The results of previous studies on breast cancer mortality in relation to estrogen treatment are summarized in Table 1.

In 1987, Kathryn Hunt and her colleagues first published data on mortality in breast cancer among women receiving hormone replacement therapy[27]. The study group consisted of 4544 women recruited while on hormone treatment, from several menopause clinics in Britain. All women had at least 1 year of treatment prior to recruitment. They were followed prospectively and data were obtained from a National Health Service register, from treating doctors and hospitals and from the patients themselves through mailed questionnaires. Despite an increased incidence of breast cancer among estrogen users (relative risk, RR 1.59), they reported a significantly lowered breast cancer mortality (RR 0.55; 95% confidence interval, CI 0.28–0.96). In a later follow-up of the cohort[28], with an additional 4 years of follow-up, they found that the overall mortality from breast cancer was still below that of the background population, but the 95% confidence interval now included unity (RR 0.76; 95% CI 0.45–1.06). Analyzing mortality within different time periods from start of treatment showed a trend of increasing mortality with increasing latency, RR being 0.38 with latency 0–4 years, RR 0.74 after 5–9 years and RR 0.97 after more than 10 years of latency. The trend, however, was not statistically significant.

In 1993, Yuen and co-workers[29], and later in 1996, Persson and associates[23] reported mortality data from a Swedish cohort, consisting of 23 000 estrogen-treated women. These women were recruited through collection of estrogen-containing prescription forms from the pharmacies in the Uppsala Health Care Region in Sweden. Complete follow-up was ascertained through linkage of the national registration numbers of the cohort women to the Swedish Cancer Registry and the Causes of Death Registry. In the mortality analysis, treatment was characterized only from the prescription forms. Observed mortality rates from breast cancer within the cohort were compared with those of the background population. In the first follow-up, adjustments were made to account for the fact that background mortality rates were based on all women dying from breast cancer irrespective of whether they had their first cancer diagnosed recently or 20 years ago, whereas the cohort mortality was based only on incident cancers. Despite these adjustments, which increased the mortality rate ratios compared to unadjusted, the standard mortality ratio (SMR) was lower than unity at 0.81 (CI 0.64–1.02). In the second follow-up, no such corrections were performed. The overall breast cancer mortality was significantly lowered (SMR 0.5; CI 0.4–0.6). For women on combined estrogen–progestogen treatment, a trend of increasing mortality rates with time was found. The SMR was 0.2 with less than 5 years of follow-up, 0.6 after 5–9 years of follow-up and 1.0 after more than 10 years.

The third study which has reported on breast cancer mortality is the Nurses' Health Study from the USA. The cohort consists of a total of 121 700 nurses from 30 to 55 years old at recruitment, which started in 1976. In their latest published follow-up from 1995, Colditz and colleagues[17] report on 69 500 postmenopausal women, of whom 1935 developed breast cancer and 359 died from the disease. The relative risk of death was 1.14 among current users of estrogen, 0.80 among past users, 0.99 among current users with less than 5 years of use and 1.45

Table 197 Summary of mortality estimates in relation to postmenopausal estrogen treatment

Authors	Relative risk	95% confidence interval
Hunt et al.[27]	0.55	0.28–0.96
Hunt et al.[28]	0.76	0.45–1.06
Yuen et al.[29]	0.81*	0.64–1.02
Persson et al.[23]	0.5	0.4–0.6
Colditz et al.[17]	1.14**	0.85–1.51
Ettinger et al.[30]	1.89	0.43–8.36
Willis et al.[31]	0.84	0.75–0.94

*Adjusted for healthy drug-user effect; **current users

(CI 1.01–2.09) among current users with more than 5 years of use.

Ettinger and co-workers[30], in 1996, published data from a case–control study of 232 postmenopausal women who had used hormone replacement therapy for at least 5 years, compared with 222 postmenopausal age-matched non-users. They found a non-significant increase in death rates from breast cancer among users, compared to non-users (RR 1.89; CI 0.43–8.36).

Finally, Willis and associates[31] published data in 1996 from a large prospective US study, the Cancer Prevention Study II. After 9 years of follow-up in a cohort of 422 000 postmenopausal women, 1469 breast cancer deaths were observed. Ever-use of estrogen replacement therapy (ERT) was associated with a significantly decreased risk of fatal breast cancer (RR 0.84; CI 0.75–0.94). There was a trend of decreasing risk with younger age at first use of ERT. Women with a natural menopause before age 40 had the lowest risk (RR 0.59).

DISCUSSION

The interpretation of these data is not straightforward. Seemingly, there is no increased mortality from breast cancer among estrogen users, and the results are even compatible with a reduced mortality. However, there are a number of methodological considerations to be made before such a conclusion can be reached.

There is an obvious possibility of selection bias among estrogen-treated women. Traditionally, breast cancer is considered to be a contraindication to treatment with exogenous hormones. A cohort of estrogen-treated women, therefore, will be made up of persons free of the disease at the onset of treatment. Mortality rates among estrogen-treated women, thus, are based only on newly diagnosed incident cases and, when compared with background mortality rates, which are composed of deaths both from incident cases and cases diagnosed many years ago, they are falsely low. The Swedish study[29] made an attempt to adjust for this in the first analysis and the adjusted rates were higher than the unadjusted, but still showed a non-significant decreased mortality from breast cancer among estrogen-treated women. The previous study, using external rates[27,28], did not adjust for such bias, and the figures, therefore, may underestimate the true mortality rate.

There is also a possibility of detection bias among estrogen-treated women, owing to better medical surveillance and higher participation in mammographic screening programs and, perhaps, also a difference in health awareness and behavior among women actively seeking medical help for climacteric symptoms. This leads to earlier diagnosis of breast cancer and lead time bias, but also a shift towards more favorable stages and less spread of the disease at diagnosis. This certainly affects survival estimates, but may also affect mortality rates provided the disease is detected in a curable stage. Detection bias may possibly operate in all studies.

Two of the cohort studies have provided data from two different periods of follow-up and have consistently shown that the mortality rates are very low during the first years of follow-up and then increase to reach unity[23,27–29]. This fits with the bias resulting from selection of women without breast cancer in the cohorts as well as detection bias. Within the first years of follow-up, there is a deficiency of deaths compared with the background rate, simply because there are no old cases of breast cancer and the incident cases are detected early. In addition, as these cases have a long expected survival or may even potentially be cured, they do not contribute in the same way as more advanced cases from the background population to the mortality rates. It will be very interesting to see what happens at the next follow-up of these two cohorts. There is some cause for concern that the increased incidence rates noted in both these studies will also have an effect on the mortality, but it could be that the cancers developing during estrogen therapy actually are less aggressive, and that the mortality will stay low, despite higher incidence.

The Nurses' Health Study shows that the increased incidence and mortality are confined only to current users of hormones[17]. The other studies have not analyzed their data in a way that makes it possible to determine the effect of recency of use. If the effect of estrogen wears off after cessation of treatment, which seems plausible, studies with aggregated data from a mixture of current and past users might show falsely low estimates.

If cancers developing after estrogen treatment are less aggressive, the survival of such patients will be long, and any rise in mortality rates owing to the increased incidence will not be expected until maybe 15–20 years after diagnosis. The follow-up time for all studies, thus, might be too short to detect such an increased mortality rate.

There are indications from the Nurses' Health Study that older women are the ones most profoundly affected, their relative risks for breast cancer being higher than those of younger women. Also, there are many indications in the literature that the risk of developing breast cancer increases with longer duration of estrogen therapy. Taking these two factors into consideration, one could expect that the long term-treatments which are necessary for protection against osteoporosis and cardiovascular disease may lead to a moderate increase in breast cancer incidence and later on, perhaps, also breast cancer mortality. On the other hand, the study of Willis and colleagues[31] demonstrates a significantly decreased mortality from breast cancer among women who first used ERT at less than 40 years of age, but no clear trend with duration of use. There are, however, some limitations of this study concerning duration of treatment. No information on use was obtained after the start of the study in 1982, and follow-up was continued to 1991. It should also be kept in mind that current studies are of the effects on the breast among women taking hormones for menopausal symptoms, as the indication of protection against osteoporosis and cardiovascular disease is rather new and, in some countries, not yet an accepted indication. It is not known for sure that the effects on breast cancer incidence and mortality will be similar among nonsymptomatic women. Their risk profiles, including the susceptibility of the breast parenchyma, might be quite different, as the symptoms of menopause are related to the levels of circulating hormones, or at least changes in them.

CONCLUSION

In conclusion, there is to date no indication of an increase in breast cancer mortality among women using hormone replacements for the treatment of climacteric symptoms, and there is even a possibility of a lowered breast cancer mortality. It is, however, for reasons discussed above, quite obvious that the results from the studies of breast cancer mortality among menopausal women treated with sex hormones must be interpreted with great care. Further studies with long-term follow-up and careful design must be awaited, before it can be completely ruled out that the increase in breast cancer incidence, shown in many studies especially among women with ongoing long-term estrogen treatment, will eventually be followed by an increased mortality from breast cancer. Ongoing randomized trials, such as the Women's Health Initiatives in the United States, also seem to be promising with regard to the possibility of giving an unbiased answer.

References

1. Weiss NS, Ure CL, Ballarch JH, *et al.* Decreased risk of fractures of the hip and lower forearm with postmenopausal use of estrogen. *N Engl J Med* 1980;303:1195–8
2. Kiel DP, Felson DT, Anderson JJ, *et al.* Hip fracture and the use of estrogens in postmenopausal women. *N Engl J Med* 1987;317:1169–74
3. Naessén T, Persson I, Adami HO, *et al.* Hormone replacement therapy and the risk of first hip fracture. A prospective population based cohort study. *Ann Intern Med* 1990;113:95–103
4. Stampfer MJ, Colditz GA. Estrogen replacement therapy and coronary heart disease: a quantitative assessment of the epidemiologic evidence. *Prev Med* 1991;20:47–63
5. Stampfer MJ, Colditz GA, Willett WC, *et al.* Postmenopausal estrogen therapy and cardiovascular disease: ten year follow-up from the

Nurses' Health Study. *N Engl J Med* 1991;325: 756–62

6. Falkeborn M, Persson I, Adami HO, *et al.* The risk of acute myocardial infarction after estrogen and estrogen–progestin replacement. *Br J Obstet Gynaecol* 1992;99:821–8

7. Paganini-Hill A, Hendersson VW. Estrogen deficiency and risk of Alzheimer's disease in women. *Am J Epidemiol* 1994;140:256–61

8. Herrington LJ, Weiss NS. Postmenopausal unopposed estrogens. Characteristics of use in relation to the risk of endometrial carcinoma. *Ann Epidemiol* 1993;3:308–18

9. Grady D, Gebretsadik T, Kerlikowske K, *et al.* Hormone replacement therapy and endometrial cancer risk: a meta analysis. *Obstet Gynecol* 1995;85:304–13

10. Persson I, Adami HO, Bergkvist L, *et al.* Risk of endometrial cancer after treatment with oestrogens alone or in conjunction with progestogens: results of a prospective study. *Br Med J* 1989; 298:147–51

11. Bergkvist L, Persson I. Hormone replacement therapy and breast cancer. A review of current knowledge. *Drug Safety* 1996;15:360–70

12. Steinberg KK, Thacker SB, Smith J, *et al.* A meta-analysis of the effect of estrogen replacement therapy on the risk of breast cancer. *J Am Med Assoc* 1991;265:1985–90

13. Dupont WD, Page DL. Menopausal estrogen replacement therapy and breast cancer. *Arch Intern Med* 1991;151:67–71

14. Bergkvist L, Adami HO, Persson I, *et al.* The risk of breast cancer after estrogen and estrogen–progestin replacement. *N Engl J Med* 1989;321: 293–7

15. Schairer C, Byren C, Keyl PM, *et al.* Menopausal estrogen and estrogen–progestin replacement therapy and the risk of breast cancer (United States). *Cancer Causes Control* 1994;5:491–500

16. Stanford JL, Weiss NS, Voigt LF, *et al.* Combined estrogen and progestin hormone replacement in relation to risk of breast cancer in middle-aged women. *J Am Med Assoc* 1995;274:137–42

17. Colditz GA, Hankinsson SE, Hunter DJ, *et al.* The use of estrogens and progestins and the risk of breast cancer in postmenopausal women. *N Engl J Med* 1995;332:1589–93

18. Newcomb PA, Longnecker MP, Storer BE, *et al.* Long-term hormone replacement therapy and risk of breast cancer in postmenopausal women. *Am J Epidemiol* 1995;142:788–95

19. Schuurman AG, van den Brandt PA, Goldbohm RA. Exogenous hormone use and the risk of postmenopausal breast cancer: results from The Netherlands cohort study. *Cancer Causes Control* 1995;6:416–24

20. La Vecchia C, Negri E, Franchesi S, *et al.* Hormone replacement treatment and breast cancer risk: a cooperative Italian study. *Br J Cancer* 1995; 72:244–8

21. Brinton LA, Hoover R, Fraumeni JF. Menopausal oestrogens and breast cancer risk: an expanded case–control study. *Br J Cancer* 1986; 54:825–32

22. Ewertz M. Influence of non-contraceptive exogenous and endogenous sex hormones on breast cancer risk in Denmark. *Int J Cancer* 1988;42: 832–8

23. Persson I, Yuen J, Bergkvist L, *et al.* Cancer incidence and mortality in women receiving estrogen and estrogen–progestin replacement therapy. Long-term follow-up of a Swedish cohort. *Int J Cancer* 1996;67:327–32

24. Collaborative group on hormonal factors in breast cancer. Breast cancer and hormonal contraceptives: collaborative reanalysis of individual data on 53 297 women with breast cancer and 100 239 women without breast cancer from 54 epidemiological studies. *Lancet* 1996;347: 1713–27

25. Bonnier P, Romain S, Giacalone PL, *et al.* Clinical and biological prognostic factors in breast cancer diagnosed during postmenopausal hormone replacement therapy. *Obstet Gynecol* 1995;85: 11–17

26. Bergkvist L, Adami H-O, Persson I, *et al.* Prognosis after breast cancer diagnosis in women exposed to estrogen and estrogen–progestin replacement therapy. *Am J Epidemiol* 1989;130: 221–8

27. Hunt K, Vessey M, McPherson K, *et al.* Long-term surveillance of mortality and cancer incidence in women receiving hormone replacement therapy. *Br J Obstet Gynaecol* 1987;94: 620–35

28. Hunt K, Vessey M, McPherson K. Mortality in a cohort of long-term users of hormone replacement therapy: an updated analysis. *Br J Obstet Gynaecol* 1990;97:1080–6

29. Yuen J, Persson I, Bergkvist L, *et al.* Hormone replacement therapy and breast cancer mortality in Swedish women: results after adjustment for 'healthy drug-users' effect. *Cancer Causes Control* 1993;4:369–74

30. Ettinger B, Friedman GD, Bush T, *et al.* Reduced mortality associated with long-term postmenopausal estrogen therapy. *Obstet Gynecol* 1996;87: 6–12

31. Willis DB, Calle EE, Miracle-McMahill L, *et al.* Estrogen replacement therapy and risk of fatal breast cancer in a prospective cohort of post-menopausal women in the United States. *Cancer Causes Control* 1996;7:449–57

21
Estrogens after breast cancer

S. L. Nand, J. A. Eden and B. G. Wren

INTRODUCTION

Breast cancer is the most common cause of deaths from cancer in females in Australia and in most developed countries. The management of breast cancer has changed considerably over the past few decades, and it has become a highly treatable disease. Overall, almost 80% of women with primary breast cancer are alive 5 years after treatment. For women with small invasive cancers (less than 10 mm), the 10-year survival rate is approximately 90%[1].

According to the Australian Bureau of Statistics, breast cancer was responsible for 3.9% of the deaths of Australian women aged over 55 years in 1993. In the same year, ischemic heart disease accounted for 31% of the deaths while 14% died of stroke[2].

Breast cancer mortality for women aged 25–44 years has remained remarkably stable since 1909[3]. However, for women over the age of 50, breast cancer mortality rose dramatically in the first half of the 20th century and has remained stable since around 1950.

This rise in breast cancer mortality for older women occurred when the contraceptive pill and hormone replacement therapy (HRT) were not being used. The reasons for this rise in breast cancer mortality are most likely related to women having fewer pregnancies and delaying childbirth to a later age. Premature deaths from infectious diseases are now rare owing to public health measures and immunization programs. Safer childbirth has seen maternal mortality rates plummet since the beginning of the 20th century. It is not surprising, therefore, that in the western world most women will spend one-third of their life in the postmenopausal state. Women are now able to live long enough to suffer from the diseases associated with aging, such as heart disease, stroke, osteoporosis and cancer.

Many women who are treated for breast cancer will subsequently undergo the menopause, either as a result of cancer treatment or as a natural process. As adjuvant chemotherapy is increasingly being used for premenopausal women with both node-negative and node-positive breast cancers, chemotherapy-induced premature menopause will also be seen with increasing frequency. For young women made prematurely menopausal, the risk of premature coronary artery disease and osteoporosis is higher than those who reach menopause at the expected age[4].

Estrogen replacement therapy improves quality of life by relieving menopausal symptoms and decreases the risk of cardiovascular disease and osteoporosis[5,6]. However, there has been considerable controversy regarding the use of estrogens after breast cancer. Most surgeons advise against HRT after breast cancer. However, in the past, the potent estrogen stilbestrol has been used to treat advanced breast cancer with similar results to those of other endocrine treatments such as bilateral oophorectomy or Tamoxifen[7].

Because of the inconclusive data regarding risk, the known deleterious consequences of menopause and the improved survival of women treated for breast cancer, physicians have now begun to question whether the common advice against HRT in breast cancer survivors is appropriate.

Risk factors for breast cancer

The two major risk factors for breast cancer are female gender and age. Other risk factors include positive family history of breast cancer, reproductive history (trend to smaller families and later childbearing), obesity, western lifestyle and diet, and moderate alcohol (ethanol) intake[8].

SEX HORMONES AND THEIR EFFECT ON BREAST TISSUES

Breast cell internal signaling system

The internal signaling systems of all cells are extremely complex and involve a series of accelerators and inhibitors which maintain a fine balance between mitosis, apoptosis (programmed cell death) and/or specialized differentiation of the cell. These signaling systems are composed of a series of proteins and enzymes which assemble and activate or inhibit cell progress, depending on their relative concentrations in the cell.

Cell cycle activity is traditionally divided into four phases known as G_1, S, G_2 and M phases. Gap1 (G_1) phase involves recruitment and stimulation of cells to begin synthesis of DNA (S phase). Following duplication of DNA, there is a further resting phase (G_2) before the cell begins mitotic cell division (M phase). The rate of cell division is controlled by the speed with which the cell passes through the G_1 phase. Within the G_1 phase, there is a critical 'restriction point' (R point) through which every cell must pass[9,10]. The R point is now known to be retinoblastoma protein (pRb) which must be phosphorylated before the cell will progress. The production of cyclins and cyclin-dependent kinases which assemble to induce phosphorylation of pRb is under the influence of estrogen. Conversely, progesterone/progestogens increase the production of those specific protein inhibitors which block the assembly of these enzyme activators.

In the normal breast alveolar or ductal cell, the assembly and activation of the cyclin/cyclin-dependent kinase (CDK) enzymatic complex results in phosphorylation of retinoblastoma protein (pRb). This hyperphosphorylation of pRb results in an increase in mitogenesis as the cell is driven from the G_1 phase into S, G_2 and M phase activity. Estrogen increases production of cyclin D_4 which is responsible for early phosphorylation of pRb.

The protein inhibitors p16, p18, p21, p27, p53 and p57 all interfere or block the assembly and activation of cyclins and CDK[10–15]. Progestogens appear to increase the production of some of these protein inhibitors and thus reduce mitogenesis. Some of these same protein inhibitors are thought to be responsible for differentiation of immature alveolar cells into mature secretory cells.

Progestogens have a biphasic action on the breast cell[16]. Initially, progestogens increase production of cyclin E which accelerates phosphorylation of pRb in the later portion of G_1 phase activity, but progestogens also increase production of p16, p21 and p27 which also inhibit assembly and activation of cyclin D_4 and CDK_2 in the early part of the G_1 phase[9,16–18]. Thus, progestogens initially induce a surge of mitogenesis but, when given continually for more than 10 days, they produce inhibition of mitosis. In fact, when a woman is found to have metastases following treatment for breast cancer, progestogens in high dosage are often prescribed to slow down the rate of growth and, hopefully, to provide a remission.

Estrogen

Estrogen has been implicated in the pathogenesis of breast cancer by most researchers. Two theories have been proposed in recent years to explain the possible link between estrogens and breast cancer. Henderson and colleagues[19] suggested that it is a woman's total lifetime

Table 1 Studies on effect of pregnancy after breast-cancer diagnosis on prognosis

Study	Year	No. of patients	Result of survival
Holleb and Farrow[21]	1962	52	no adverse effect
Rissanen[22]	1968	33	no adverse effect
Cooper and Butterfield[23]	1970	40	no adverse effect
Harvey et al.[24]	1981	41	no adverse effect
Ariel and Kempner[25]	1989	47	no adverse effect
Sutton et al.[26]	1990	50	possible benefit
Von Schoultz et al.[27]	1995	50	possible benefit

exposure to estrogen that determines breast cancer risk. A woman who has an early menarche and late menopause and takes HRT for over 10 years, therefore, will have an increased risk of developing breast cancer. Key and Pike[20] have postulated that estrogen increases the risk of breast cancer but that adding a progesterone or a progestogen makes it even worse, and the two hormones have a synergistic adverse effect on the breast.

These two theories fail to explain the protective effect of an early first pregnancy. Both estrogen and progesterone are markedly elevated in pregnancy, and so a woman who has her first child early and then goes on to have several subsequent babies should have the highest risk of breast cancer of all. However, the converse is true[8]. Obviously, the impact of sex hormones on normal breast and breast cancer risk are far more complex. Studies[21–27] have shown that pregnancies after the diagnosis of breast cancer do not have an adverse effect on survival (Table 1).

The overall experience with oral contraceptives over the past few decades has shown no definitive evidence that exogenous estrogen and progestin increase the risk of breast cancer. This exposure has not been shown to have a protective effect, either. However, a lack of obvious detrimental effect is a substantial argument against linking breast cancer to exogenous sex hormone treatment.

Table 2 summarizes some of the reasons why estrogens are implicated in the development of breast cancer. There are many unknown aspects of the impact of estrogen on the breast. It is still not clear what impact endogenous ovarian estrogen has on breast tissue levels of estradiol[28,29]. Breast tissues, particularly breast fat and stromal tissue, are capable of local synthesis of estrogen[29–31]. It has also been shown that the majority of breast cancers are surrounded by fat with a higher aromatase activity than fat taken from different quadrants in the same breast[30]. Bulbrook and colleagues[28] were unable to demonstrate a relationship between serum (total free), urinary or salivary estrogens and breast cancer risk. The breast can metabolize estradiol into inert estrogens such as estrone sulfate or into the ubiquitous catecholestrogens[32]. Hence, the importance of the role of local breast estrogen in promoting or initiating breast cancer may be quite significant.

Table 2 Reasons why estrogens are implicated in development of breast cancer

Breast cancer is more common among women than men
Estrogen stimulates growth of some breast cancer cell lines in culture
Estrogen stimulates proliferation of breast ductal tissue
Breast cancer risk relates to reproductive markers such as age at menarche, first pregnancy and menopause
Premature menopause reduces risk of breast cancer development
Bilateral oophorectomy is effective palliative therapy for advanced breast cancer
Serum levels of estradiol predict breast cancer risk
Cessation of hormone replacement therapy (HRT) may induce regression of breast cancer

Davidson and Lippman[33] have reviewed the potential role of estrogens in the regulation of cancer cell growth. Estrogens stimulate and induce several intracellular proteins and enzymes in breast cancer cell lines. In cell culture studies, estrogen has been shown to interact in a complex fashion with a number of growth factors that can promote malignant cell growth, enhance invasiveness and accelerate the development of metastases. It is clear that the impact of sex steroids on the breast is very complicated and appears to be modulated by several factors.

Progesterone and progestogens

Breast cancer cells have few differences compared with the parent cell from which they originate, with the main difference being either overexpression of those factors that induce uncontrolled mitogenesis, or loss of some of those inhibitors that induce quiescence, apoptosis or specialized cell function.

It is the action of various hormones on the processes in the G_1 phase of breast cell function that allows hormones to be used to reduce breast cancer mitogenesis. Estrogen leads to an increase in production of cyclins and CDKs, thus increasing the rate of phosphorylation of pRb and mitogenesis. Antiestrogens such as Tamoxifen block the action of estrogen in the early part of the G_1 phase and, thus, act as a canceristatic agent[34].

Some clinical studies have suggested that progestogens increase mitogenesis[35-37] while others have suggested a suppression of mitosis during the luteal phase[38]. Most of these results have been based on circumstantial evidence obtained following post-mortem examination of young women who had died suddenly, or were obtained at routine biopsy on young women during a particular phase of their menstrual cycle. The problems in determining exactly when ovulation and progesterone production occurred in these young women are obvious and, therefore, these research results are often viewed with caution. One recent study, however, in which a high-dose progesterone gel was rubbed into the breast tissue of women for 10–13 days prior to elective breast biopsy, demonstrated that progesterone inhibits mitogenesis. Chang and colleagues[39] demonstrated a 60–80% reduction in indicators of mitogenesis when compared with results from women using a placebo gel or an estrogen gel.

There are at least three studies, one a prospective study in premenopausal women and two others in postmenopausal women, taking combined estrogen and progestogen, which suggest that continuous progestogen reduces the risk of developing breast cancer by up to 50%. Plu-Bureau and co-workers[40] gave norethisterone 10 mg daily to 599 women for up to 10 years. There was a 50% reduction in the incidence of breast cancer when compared with results from a similar group of women receiving a non-hormonal therapy regimen. Ewertz[41] also showed a 40% reduction in developing breast cancer in women who were given continuous combined estrogen and progestogen hormonal therapy. Eden and colleagues[42] also treated women who had known breast cancer with either continuous progestogen or combined continuous estrogen and progestogen therapy, and recorded a much lower rate of new or recurrent cancer.

Other studies have demonstrated that women with breast cancer and evidence of metastases have a considerable reduction in rate of progression of their secondary tumors when high-dose progestogens are used[43-45].

HORMONE REPLACEMENT THERAPY AND BREAST CANCER RISK

The studies to date on the risk of breast cancer in women on HRT are imperfect in that no large, prospective, double-blind, randomized trials have been conducted. Studies under way such as the Women's Health Initiative study, the Wisdom Trial and the HABIT study from Scandinavia should provide a better risk profile.

There have been many cohort and case–control studies of women using HRT and these have yielded inconsistent results. Several meta-analyses[46-51] have been published to attempt to clarify the situation (Table 3). There is a possibility of a slightly increased risk of breast cancer associated with long duration (5 or more years) of postmenopausal estrogen use. However, the epidemiological data on this relationship are not consistent or uniform. Overall, they suggest

Table 3 Meta-analyses on risk of breast cancer with hormone replacement therapy (HRT) use

Reference	No. of studies	Ever use, RR (95% CI)	Duration of use, RR (95% CI)
Armstrong[46]	–	1.01 (0.95–1.08)	no effect
Dupont and Page[47]	28	1.07 (1.01–1.05)	no conclusion
Steinberg et al.[48]	16	1.0	> 15 years, 1.3 (1.2–1.6)
Grady et al.[49]	10	1.0	≥ 10 years, 1.25 (1.04–1.51)
Sillero-Arenas et al.[50]	37	1.06 (1.0–1.12), current users 1.63	≥ 8 years, 1.2
Colditz et al.[51]	31	1.4 (1.2–1.63) (current users)	> 10 years, 1.23 (1.08–1.4)

RR, relative risk; CI, confidence interval

that the risk of developing breast cancer is not increased with short-term use of HRT.

Users of HRT see their physicians more frequently than non-users and have more frequent mammography, so studies to date probably overestimate the risk. Most studies include all HRT users and do not define the type of regimen that they are using. It is likely that the type of estrogen used and the type and regimen of progestogen used will affect breast cancer risk. A study from Uppsala, Sweden[52,53], concluded that estrogen use was associated with a slight increase in breast cancer (relative risk 1.1). They also found a relationship with duration of use, with a relative risk of 1.7 after 9 years. This increased risk was associated with the use of estradiol (56% of women) at a dose approximately equivalent to 1.25 mg conjugated estrogens. No increase in risk was noted with the use of conjugated estrogens 0.625 mg (22% of women) or other types of estrogen.

The Cancer and Sex Hormone (CASH) Study[54] of the Centers for Disease Control and Prevention (CDC) has not detected an overall increase in breast cancer with postmenopausal estrogen use and found no relation with a duration of use of up to 20 years or longer.

The Nurses' Health Study[55,56] was established in 1976 when 121 700 female registered nurses aged between 30 and 55 years of age completed a mailed questionnaire. Every 2 years, a follow-up questionnaire was mailed to these women, which asked them to update information on various risk factors including hormone usage. During the period 1976–92, 1935 cases of breast cancer were identified among more than 69 000 postmenopausal women. The analysis showed that women who had previously used estrogen (ever or for 10 or more years) were not at increased risk of breast cancer. However, the relative risks for current users were 1.46 (95% confidence interval (CI) 1.22–1.74) for 5–9 years of use and 1.46 (95% CI 1.20–1.76) for 10 or more years of use. This study has greater credibility than most because of its large numbers and 16 years of follow-up. However, as estrogen users are more likely to be examined frequently, detection bias is still a concern. Current users had a 14% higher prevalence of mammography compared with never users. The risk of dying from breast cancer was 0.80 (95% CI 0.60–1.07) for past users, 0.99 (CI 0.66–1.48) for current users with less than 5 years of use and 1.45 (CI 1.01–2.09) with 5 or more years of use.

As long-term current estrogen replacement therapy (ERT) users reduce their risk of death from cardiovascular disease and fractures, then more cases of breast cancer should be seen owing to disease substitution. There is some early evidence to suggest that long-term HRT users taking a sequential therapy may have a higher risk of breast cancer than those taking continuous combined treatment[41]. Interestingly, estrogen–testosterone preparations seem to be associated with the highest risk of developing breast cancer[48].

It has been reported that, although the use of HRT may possibly be associated with a small increased risk of developing breast cancer, there is an overall reduction in mortality from the disease. This may be due to surveillance bias, but also raises the possibility that the use of HRT may induce a more favorable type of breast cancer. A number of studies have shown that HRT users who develop breast cancer are more likely to have breast-only disease, and have significantly smaller tumors than their non-HRT using controls[53,57–60]. Several studies have attempted to investigate the impact of HRT usage on the grade and type of tumor. There appears to be no clear relationship between the use of HRT and estrogen receptor status[60]. There is some evidence that HRT users who develop breast cancer do have tumors with histologically better indices[60].

ESTROGEN REPLACEMENT THERAPY AND SURVIVAL OF BREAST CANCER PATIENTS

One of the concerns about prescribing ERT to women with a history of breast cancer is fear that dormant cancer cells may become activated. However, there is very little evidence to support this concern. If this were the case, then women diagnosed with breast cancer after the menopause should have a better prognosis than those with premenopausal breast cancer. This is not the case and, in fact, there is worsening in the prognosis for women diagnosed with breast cancer after the menopause[61].

Users of ERT have been shown to have a better prognosis when diagnosed with breast cancer when compared with women with no record of exposure to it[53,58,59,62,63]. Bergkvist and colleagues[53] compared the survival among women with breast cancer in a cohort exposed to ERT before diagnosis with women of the background population diagnosed with breast cancer at the same time. Women with a history of ERT exposure had significantly better observed and relative survival rates when compared with those who had no history of ERT exposure.

Gambrell[63] found a mortality rate of 22% among those diagnosed with breast cancer while using hormones, and 46% among those not using hormones ($p < 0.002$). Fifty-seven per cent of hormone users were node-negative and 42% of non-users were node-negative. Within this node-negative group, the mortality rate was 8% for hormone users and 25% for non-users ($p < 0.05$). Hunt and co-workers[58] reported a relative risk of mortality of 0.55 for ERT users compared with national rates. Henderson and associates[59] observed a 19% reduction in mortality from breast cancer among ERT users when compared with non-users who developed breast cancer.

Willis and colleagues[64] reported 1469 breast cancer deaths in a cohort of 422 373 postmenopausal women after 9 years of follow-up. After adjusting for 11 other potential risk factors, they showed that ever-use of ERT was associated with a significantly decreased risk of fatal breast cancer (relative risk, (RR) = 0.84, 95% CI = 0.75–0.94). No increase in fatal breast cancer risk was observed with estrogen use status (baseline/former), age at first use, duration of use or years since last use. Their findings suggest that ever-use of ERT is associated with a 16% decreased risk of fatal breast cancer.

These findings may be explained by various confounding variables. Women taken ERT are known to have breast examinations and mammograms more regularly and, hence, may be diagnosed at an earlier stage than non-users. Estrogen replacement therapy may promote the development of estrogen-dependent tumors that regress on withdrawal of estrogen. Nevertheless, the literature clearly suggests that the use of ERT prior to diagnosis may have a beneficial effect on survival.

USE OF HORMONE REPLACEMENT THERAPY AFTER BREAST CANCER

Estrogen replacement therapy has been shown to be beneficial for women with menopausal symptoms and risk of long-term problems such as cardiovascular disease and osteoporosis. For women who have had breast cancer and are suffering from severe menopausal symptoms, should ERT be an option in their management? Vassilopoulou-Sellin and Zolinski[65] surveyed 224 women with breast cancer, asking a series of questions regarding menopause, including symptoms related to estrogen deficiency, concerns about osteoporosis and heart disease, and attitudes and perceptions regarding ERT. Seventy-seven per cent of women were postmenopausal at the time of completion of the survey. Of these women, 8% had taken ERT at some point subsequent to their cancer

Table 4 Studies on use of hormone replacement therapy (HRT) in women with breast cancer

Reference	No. of patients and stage of disease	Type and duration of HRT	Outcome
Stoll and Parbhoo[67]	50	0.625 mg CEE, 0.15 mg norgestrol for 3–6 months	no relapses
Wile et al.[68,69]	25, all stages	unknown, mean duration of use 35 months	three recurrences, one of whom died from progressive disease
Di Saia[70]	77, all stages	CEE and in 83% combined with a progestin, mean duration of use 27 months	three alive with metastases, three deaths, two progressive disease
Powles et al.[71]	35, all stages	CEE + 75 µg levonorgestrel, mean duration 14.6 months	no deaths, two progressive disease
Bluming et al.[72]	70, early stage disease	not stated	two progressive disease
Eden et al.[42]	90	continuous combined HRT, usually CEE and 50 mg MPA	7% relapse in users compared with 17% in controls

CEE, conjugated equine estrogen; MPA, medroxyprogesterone acetate

diagnosis. Approximately 78% were afraid that ERT might precipitate a cancer recurrence but were also concerned about the risk of osteoporosis (70%) and heart disease (72%). Of these women, 44% indicated that they would consider taking ERT under medical supervision.

Canney and Hatton[66] surveyed 108 patients successfully treated for breast cancer to ascertain the prevalence of menopausal symptoms using the Greene Climacteric Scale. During the first year after treatment, 70% of women suffered menopausal symptoms and, overall, 60% of women surveyed were affected. Adjuvant treatment with Tamoxifen was the largest contributing factor for the development of these symptoms.

Clinical trials[42,67–72] of breast cancer survivors who have been prescribed HRT have not shown an increased risk of tumor recurrence or death from progressive disease (Table 4). In the largest series to date, Eden and colleagues[42] have reported on 90 women treated with continuous combined estrogen/progestogen therapy using a moderate dose of progestogen (usually medroxyprogesterone acetate (MPA) 50 mg daily). The 90 HRT users were compared with 180 matched controls. Interestingly, the risk of recurrence was significantly lower among the hormone users compared with the controls. It is likely that these results are biased towards a favorable result. In a recently updated reanalysis of the data (unpublished) using a larger series of 167 women who had used continuous combined therapy, no effect of using HRT on tumor occurrence or overall survival was demonstrated. A Cox proportional hazard model was used to ascertain any difference between the group using HRT and the controls.

Stoll and Parbhoo[67] gave 0.625 mg of conjugated equine estrogen and 0.15 mg of noregestrel per day for severe hot flushes and sweats and followed the subjects for 2 years. No relapses occurred. In a case–control study of ERT use in 25 breast cancer survivors, Wile and co-workers[68] matched each patient with two non-ERT controls for stage, age and duration of observation. The average duration of observation of patients receiving ERT was 2 years. There was one cancer-related death in the treated group and two in the control group. In a subsequent report, when mean observation period was 35 months, it was revealed that the type of ERT varied[69]. By this stage, three women receiving ERT had relapsed.

Despite these encouraging results, it is clear that caution is still necessary. Until a randomized prospective trial is undertaken to examine the effect of HRT on tumor recurrence rate and overall survival in patients with a history of breast cancer, this uncertainty will continue.

Dhodapkar and associates documented results from four women who were treated with HRT after a diagnosis of breast cancer[73]. Each had a recurrence of their disease and, when the HRT was stopped, tumor regression followed. Interestingly, Stoll and Parbhoo gave HRT to 65 postmenopausal women with advanced breast cancer and, in 22% of them, the disease regressed after 6 months of treatment[67].

Vassilopoulou-Sellin and Theriault[74] are currently conducting a prospective clinical trial of ERT in breast cancer survivors. Eligibility criteria include stage I or stage II breast cancer with no evidence of disease for at least 2 years since therapy if estrogen-receptor negative disease, or for at least 10 years if estrogen-receptor status is unknown. This groundbreaking trial should be an important step in the study of ERT in breast cancer survivors. Prospective trials are also under way in the United Kingdom, Sweden and Australia.

MANAGEMENT OF MENOPAUSE IN WOMEN WITH PERSONAL HISTORY OF BREAST CANCER

Relief of menopausal symptoms

Progestogens alone have been shown to be effective treatment for hot flushes, but often in higher doses than are normally used as part of HRT. Depot-Provera[75], oral medroxyprogesterone acetate (MPA) in a dose of at least 20 mg a day, and norethisterone 5–10 mg daily[76,77] have all been shown to significantly reduce menopausal flushes when compared with a placebo. Around 15% of women will have some progestogen side-effects but the majority will not, and this therapy will be effective in about 60% of cases. Progestogens have a long history of use in the management of breast cancer, and most oncologists will permit their patients to receive this therapy as an alternative to estrogen replacement. However, there have been no prospective randomized trials demonstrating the safety of such an approach. Sometimes, formal stress reduction, avoiding aggravating factors such as hot drinks, spicy food and overheating the body, can also be very useful[78,79]. Vaginal dryness may be managed with vaginal moisturizers and poorly absorbed topical estrogens[78,79].

However, in a relatively significant number of women, menopausal symptoms will be so severe and persistent that they will only respond to estrogen replacement.

Long-term aspects

It is well known that menopausal women are at increased risk of cardiovascular disease and osteoporotic fractures, and that long-term HRT will reduce the risk of these two common diseases[80,81].

Osteoporosis can now be reduced with a number of non-estrogen therapies including bisphosphonates, calcitonin or perhaps progestogen alone[80]. Weight-bearing exercise and a calcium supplement may also be useful. Lifestyle changes such as a diet low in animal fat and high in fiber, an exercise regimen, the control of hyperlipidemia and hypertension and the avoidance of cigarette smoking should all reduce the risk of cardiovascular disease. There is also increasing evidence that Tamoxifen usage reduces the risk of cardiovascular disease as well as preserving bone mass[82–84]. However, it is interesting to note that nearly one-half of the women with breast cancer surveyed by Vassilopoulou-Sellin and Zolinski[65] were willing to consider hormone replacement if appropriately supervised.

CONCLUSION

The use of hormone replacement therapy (HRT) after breast cancer remains a controversial issue. Small case–control and cohort studies performed to date suggest that it may be safe to use HRT for short periods after breast cancer. However, it is apparent that there is an urgent need for a randomized controlled prospective study to examine the impact of progestogen used to treat menopausal symptoms, and the impact of combined continuous hormone replacement therapy after breast cancer.

References

1. Tabar L, Duffy SW, Burhenne LW. New Swedish breast cancer detection results for women aged 40–49. *Cancer* 1993;72:1437–48
2. Australian Bureau of Statistics. *Causes of Death, Australia 1993.* Catalogue no. 3303.0. Canberra: Australian Bureau of Statistics
3. Eden JA. The use of hormone replacement therapy in women previously treated for breast cancer. *Contemp Rev Obstet Gynaecol* 1995;7:20–4
4. Barret-Connor E, Bush TL. Estrogen and coronary artery disease in women. *J Am Med Assoc* 1991;265:1861–7
5. Hammond CB, Maxon WS. Current status of estrogen therapy for menopause. *Fertil Steril* 1982;37:5–25
6. Stampfer MJ, Colditz GA. Oestrogen replacement therapy and coronary artery disease: a quantitative assessment of epidemiologic evidence. *Prev Med* 1991;20:47–63
7. Rose C, Mouridsen HT. Endocrine management of advanced breast cancer. *Horm Res* 1989;32 (Suppl 1):189–97
8. Gail MH, Benichou J. Assessing the risk of breast cancer in individuals. *Cancer Prev* 1992;1:1–15
9. Musgrove EA, Hui R, Sweeney KJE, et al. Cyclins and breast cancer. *J Mammary Gland Biol Neoplasia* 1996;1:153–62
10. Norton L, Rosen PP, Rosen M. Refining the origins of breast cancer. *Nat Med* 1995;1:1250–1
11. Watts CKW, Brady A, Sarcevic I, et al. Anti oestrogen inhibition of cell cycle progression in breast cancer cells is associated with inhibition of cyclin-dependent kinase activity and decreased retinoblastoma protein phosphorylation. *Mol Endocrinol* 1995;9:1804–13
12. Weinberg RA. The retinoblastoma protein and cell cycle control. *Cell* 1995;81:323–30
13. Sherr CJ, Roberts JM. Inhibitors of mammalian G_1 cyclin-dependent kinases. *Genes Dev* 1995;9:1149–63
14. Hunter T, Pine J. Cyclins and cancer II: cyclin D and CDK inhibitors come of age. *Cell* 1994;79:573–82
15. Sherr CJ. G_1 phase progression: cycling on cue. *Cell* 1994;79:551–5
16. Musgrove EA, Hamilton JA, Lee CSL, et al. Growth factor, steroid, and steroid antagonist regulation of cyclin gene expression associated with changes in T-47D human breast cancer cell cycle progression. *Mol Cell Biol* 1993;13:3577–87
17. Musgrove EA, Lee CSL, Cornish AL, et al. Anti progestin inhibition of cell cycle progression in T-47D breast cancer cell is accompanied by induction of the cyclin-dependent kinase inhibitor p21. *Mol Endocrinol* 1997;11:1–13
18. Sutherland RL, Watts CKW, Musgrove EA. Cell cycle control by steroid hormones in breast cancer: implications for endocrine resistance. *Endocr Relat Cancer* 1995;2:87–96
19. Henderson BE, Ross R, Berstein L. Oestrogens as a cause of human cancer. *Cancer Res* 1988;48:246–53
20. Key TJ, Pike MC. The role of oestrogens and progestogens in the epidemiology and prevention of breast cancer. *Eur J Cancer* 1988;24:29–43
21. Holleb AL, Farrow JH. The relation of carcinoma of the breast and pregnancy in 283 patients. *Surg Gynecol Obstet* 1962;115:65–71
22. Rissanen PM. Pregnancy following treatment of mammary carcinoma. *Acta Radiol Ther* 1968;8:415–22
23. Cooper DR, Butterfield J. Pregnancy subsequent to mastectomy for cancer of the breast. *Ann Surg* 1970;171:429–33
24. Harvey JC, Rosen PP, Ashikari R, et al. The effect of pregnancy on the prognosis of carcinoma of the breast following mastectomy. *Surg Gynecol Obstet* 1981;153:723–5
25. Ariel IM, Kempner R. The prognosis of patients who become pregnant after mastectomy for breast cancer. *Int Surg* 1989;74:185–7
26. Sutton R, Buzdar AU, Hortobagyi GN. Pregnancy and offspring after adjuvant chemotherapy in breast cancer patients. *Cancer* 1990;65:847–50
27. Von Schoultz E, Johannson H, Wilking N, et al. Influence of prior and subsequent pregnancy on breast cancer prognosis. *J Clin Oncol* 1995;13:430–4
28. Bulbrook RD, Leake RE, George WD. Oestrogens in initiation and promotion of breast cancer. In Beck JS, ed. *Oestrogen and the Human Breast.* Edinburgh: Royal Society of Edinburgh, 1989:67–76
29. Blankenstein MA, Szymczak J, Daroszewski J, et al. Oestrogens in plasma and fatty tissue from breast cancer patients and women undergoing surgery for non-oncological reasons. *Gynecol Endocrinol* 1992;6:13–17
30. Bulun SE, Price TM, Aitken J, et al. A link between breast cancer and local oestrogen biosynthesis suggested by quantification of breast at opposed tissue aromatase cytochrome P450 transcripts using competitive polymerase chain reaction after reverse transcription. *J Clin Endocrinol Metab* 1992;77:1622–8

31. Miller WR, Mullen P. Factors influencing aromatase activity in the breast. *J Steroid Biochem Mol Biol* 1993;44:597–604
32. Fishman J, Schneider J, Herschchopf RJ, *et al.* Increased oestrogen 16α-hydroxylase activity in women with breast and endometrial cancer. *J Steroid Biochem* 1984;20:1077–81
33. Davidson NE, Lippman ME. The role of oestrogens in growth regulation of breast cancer. *Crit Rev Oncol* 1989;1:89–111
34. Wilcken M, Sarcevic B, Musgrove EA, *et al.* Differential effects of retinoids and anti oestrogens on cell cycle progression and cell cycle regulatory genes in human breast cancer cells. *Cell Growth Differentiation* 1996;7:65–74
35. Musgrove EA, Lee CSL, Sutherland RL. Progestins both stimulate and inhibit breast cancer cell cycle progression while increasing expression of transforming growth factor α, epidermal growth factor receptor, c-*fos* and c-*myc* genes. *Mol Cell Biol* 1991;11:5032–43
36. Ferguson DJP, Anderson TJ. Morphological evaluation of cell turnover in relation to the menstrual cycle in the resting human breast. *Br J Cancer* 1981;44:177–81
37. Longacre TA, Bartow SA. A correlative morphological study of human breast and endometrium in the menstrual cycle. *Am J Surg Pathol* 1986;10:382–93
38. Vogel PM, Georgiade NG, Fetter BF, *et al.* The correlation of histologic changes in the human breast with the menstrual cycle. *Am J Pathol* 1981;104:23–4
39. Chang K-T, Fournier S, Lee TTY, *et al.* Influences of percutaneous administration of estradiol and progesterone on human breast epithelial cell cycle *in vivo. Fertil Steril* 1995;63:785–91
40. Plu-Bureau G, Sitruk-Ware R, Thalabard JC, *et al.* Progestogen use and decreased risk of breast cancer in a cohort of pre-menopausal women with benign breast disease. *Br J Cancer* 1994;70:270–7
41. Ewertz M. Influence of non-contraceptive exogenous and endogenous sex hormones on breast cancer risk in Denmark. *Int J Cancer* 1988;42:832–8
42. Eden JA, Bush T, Nand S, *et al.* A case–control study of combined continuous estrogen–progestin replacement therapy among women with a personal history of breast cancer. *Menopause* 1995;2:67–72
43. Robustelli della Cuna G, Pavesi L, Preti P, *et al.* High doses of medroxyprogesterone acetate in breast cancer: controlled studies. *Adv Clin Oncol* 1988;1:45–56
44. Robustelli della Cuna G, Bernardo-Strada MR. High dose medroxyprogesterone acetate combined with chemotherapy for metastatic breast cancer. *Endocr Relat Tumours* 1980;53–63
45. Blassey HC, Bartsch HH, Kanne D, *et al.* The pharmacokinetics of high-dose medroxyprogesterone acetate in the therapy of advanced breast cancer. *Cancer Chemother Pharmacol* 1982;8:77–81
46. Armstrong BK. Oestrogen therapy after the menopause – boon or bane? *Med J Aust* 1988;148:213–14
47. Dupont WD, Page DL. Menopausal oestrogen replacement therapy and breast cancer. *Arch Intern Med* 1991;151:67–72
48. Steinberg KK, Thacker SB, Smith SJ, *et al.* A meta-analysis of the effect of oestrogen replacement therapy on the risk of breast cancer. *J Am Med Assoc* 1991;265:1985–90
49. Grady D, Rubin SM, Petitti DB, *et al.* Hormone therapy to prevent disease and prolong life in postmenopausal women. *Ann Intern Med* 1992;117:1016–37
50. Sillero-Arenas M, Delgado-Rodriguez M, Rodriguez-Canteras R, *et al.* Menopausal hormone replacement therapy and breast cancer; a meta-analysis. *Obstet Gynecol* 1992;79:286–94
51. Colditz GA, Egan KM, Stampfer MJ. Hormone replacement therapy and risk of breast cancer: results from epidemiologic studies. *Am J Obstet Gynecol* 1993;168:1473–80
52. Bergkvist L, Adami HO, Perrson I, *et al.* The risk of breast cancer after estrogen and estrogen–progestin replacement. *N Engl J Med* 1989;321:393–7
53. Bergkvist L, Adami HO, Perrson I, *et al.* Prognosis after breast cancer diagnosis in women exposed to oestrogen and oestrogen/progestogen replacement therapy. *Am J Epidemiol* 1989;130:221–8
54. Wingo PA, Layde PM, Lee NC, *et al.* The risk of breast cancer in postmenopausal women who have used estrogen replacement therapy. *J Am Med Assoc* 1987;257:209–15
55. Colditz GA, Stampfer MJ, Willett WC, *et al.* Type of postmenopausal hormone use and risk of breast cancer: 12-year follow-up from the Nurses' Health Study. *Cancer Causes Control* 1992;3:433–9
56. Colditz GA, Hankinson SE, Hunter DJ *et al.* Use of estrogens and progestins and the risk of breast cancer in postmenopausal women. *N Eng J Med* 1995;332:1589–93
57. Colditz GA, Stampfer MJ, Willett WC, *et al.* Prospective study of oestrogen replacement therapy and risk of breast cancer in postmenopausal women. *J Am Med Assoc* 1990;264:2648–53
58. Hunt K, Vessey M, McPherson K, *et al.* Long term surveillance of mortality and cancer incidence in women receiving hormone replacement therapy. *Br J Obstet Gynaecol* 1987;94:620–35

59. Henderson BE, Paganini-Hill A, Ross RK. Decreased mortality in users of oestrogen replacement therapy. *Arch Intern Med* 1991;151:75–8
60. Harding C, Knox FW, Faragher EB, *et al.* Hormone replacement therapy and tumour grade in breast cancer: prospective study in screening unit. *Br Med J* 1996;312:1646–7
61. Adami HO, Malker B, Holmberg L., *et al.* The relation between survival and age at diagnosis in breast cancer. *N Engl J Med* 1986;315:559–63
62. Criqui MH, Suarez L, Barret-Connor E, *et al.* Postmenopausal estrogen use and mortality. *Am J Epidemiol* 1988;128:606–14
63. Gambrell DR. Proposal to decrease the risk and improve the prognosis of breast cancer. *Am J Obstet Gynecol* 1984;150:119–28
64. Willis DB, Calle EE, Miracle-McMahill HL, *et al.* Estrogen replacement therapy and risk of fatal breast cancer in a prospective cohort of post menopausal women in the United States. *Cancer Causes Control* 1996;7:449–57
65. Vassilopoulou-Sellin R, Zolinski C. Estrogen replacement therapy in women with breast cancer: a survey of patients' attitudes. *Am J Med Sci* 1992;304:145–9
66. Canney PA, Hatton MQF. The prevalence of menopausal symptoms in patients treated for breast cancer. *Clin Oncol* 1994;6:297–9
67. Stoll BA, Parbhoo F. Treatment of menopausal symptoms in breast cancer patients. *Lancet* 1988;1:278–9
68. Wile AG, Opfell RW, Margileth DA, *et al.* Hormone replacement therapy does not affect breast cancer outcome. *Proc Am Soc Clin Oncol* 1991;10:58
69. Wile AG, Opfell RW, Margileth DA. Hormone replacement therapy in previously treated breast cancer patients. *Am J Surg* 1993;165:372–5
70. Di Saia PJ. Hormone replacement therapy in patients with breast cancer. *Cancer Suppl* 1993;71:1490–1500
71. Powles TJ, Hickish T, Casey S, *et al.* Hormone replacement therapy after breast cancer. *Lancet* 1993;341:60–1
72. Bluming AZ, Wile AG, Schain W, *et al.* Hormone replacement therapy in women with previous treated primary breast cancer. In *Proceedings of the Annual Meeting of the American Society of Clinical Oncology*, 1994;13, abstr. 137
73. Dhodapkar MV, Ingle JN, Ahmann DL. Oestrogen replacement therapy withdrawal and regression of metastatic breast cancer. *Cancer* 1995;75:43–6
74. Vassilopoulou-Sellin R, Theriault RL. Randomized prospective trial of estrogen-replacement therapy in women with a history of breast cancer. *J Natl Cancer Inst Monograph* 1994;16:153–9
75. Lobo RA, McCormick W, Singer F, *et al.* Depot medroxyprogesterone acetate compared with conjugated oestrogens for the treatment of postmenopausal women. *Obstet Gynecol* 1994;3:1–5
76. Schiff I, Tulchinsky D, Cramer D, *et al.* Oral medroxyprogesterone in the treatment of postmenopausal symptoms. *J Am Med Assoc* 1980;244:1443–5
77. Paterson MEL. A randomised double-blind cross-over trial into the effect of norethisterone on climacteric symptoms and biochemical profiles. *Br J Obstet Gynaecol* 1992;89:464–72
78. Eden JA. Oestrogen and the breast-myths about oestrogen and breast cancer. *Med J Aust* 1992;157:175–7
79. Eden JA. Oestrogen and the breast – the management of the menopausal women with breast cancer. *Med J Aust* 1992;157:247–50
80. Law MR, Wald NJ, Meade TW. Strategies for prevention of osteoporosis and hip fracture. *Br Med J* 1991;303:453–9
81. Stampfer MJ, Colditz GA, Willett WC, *et al.* Postmenopausal oestrogen and cardiovascular disease. *N Engl J Med* 1991;325:756–62
82. Love RR, Mazess RB, Barden HS, *et al.* Effects of Tamoxifen on bone density in postmenopausal women with breast cancer. *N Engl J Med* 1992;326:852–6
83. Fornandert Rutqvist LE, Sjoberg HE, Blomquist L, *et al.* Long term adjuvant Tamoxifen in early breast cancer: effect on bone mineral in postmenopausal women. *J Clin Oncol* 1990;8:1019–24
84. McDonald CC, Stewart HJ. Fatal myocardial infarction in the Scottish adjuvant Tamoxifen trial. *Br Med J* 1991;303:435–7

22

The cardioprotective effects of estrogens

F. Grodstein and M. J. Stampfer

Cardiovascular diseases remain the leading cause of death in women in industrialized countries. Several lines of evidence strongly support the role of estrogen in reducing women's risk of heart disease. Rates of coronary heart disease (CHD) are relatively low among premenopausal women, but rise sharply with age. Furthermore, the ratio of rates between men and women grows narrower with increasing age. Also, young women with bilateral oophorectomy are at increased risk of CHD, unless they are treated with estrogen[1]. Consistent evidence from over 40 epidemiological studies demonstrates that postmenopausal women who use estrogen therapy after the menopause have significantly lower rates of heart disease than women who do not take estrogen[2]. In support of the epidemiological data, large clinical trials have reported substantial improvement in the lipid profile[3] and enhanced blood flow[4] among women taking estrogen.

Whether estrogen use can lead to regression of atherosclerotic lesions, and if coronary events are reduced in women with established coronary artery disease have not been well studied. This chapter briefly reviews the studies of estrogen therapy and primary prevention of heart disease, and then specifically discusses the results of those investigations which examine estrogen use after diagnosis of CHD. Also summarized is the biological support for an effect of estrogen on heart disease in healthy women and those with established disease.

EPIDEMIOLOGICAL DATA ON ESTROGEN AND CORONARY HEART DISEASE

Estrogen and primary prevention of coronary heart disease

Several epidemiological approaches have been used to study the association between estrogen and the risk of CHD. Case–control studies compare estrogen use in women with CHD and those without CHD; cross-sectional studies of women undergoing angiography compare the extent of coronary disease in estrogen users and non-users; and cohort studies compare rates of CHD among women taking estrogen with those not taking estrogen.

The hospital-based case–control studies have provided the least convincing evidence of a protection against heart disease in estrogen users; a meta-analysis summarizing these studies (Figure 1) yielded a pooled relative risk of 1.33 (95% confidence interval, CI 0.93–1.91)[2]. Of all the study designs, however, the hospital-based case–control studies carry the greatest likelihood of bias, primarily because of problems in the selection of hospitalized controls.

In contrast, population- or community-based case–control studies do not have this problem in the control selection process because all subjects are chosen from the general population. As expected, these studies show consistent, protective associations between estrogen and CHD, with a summary relative risk of 0.80 (95% CI 0.68–0.97)[2] (Figure 1).

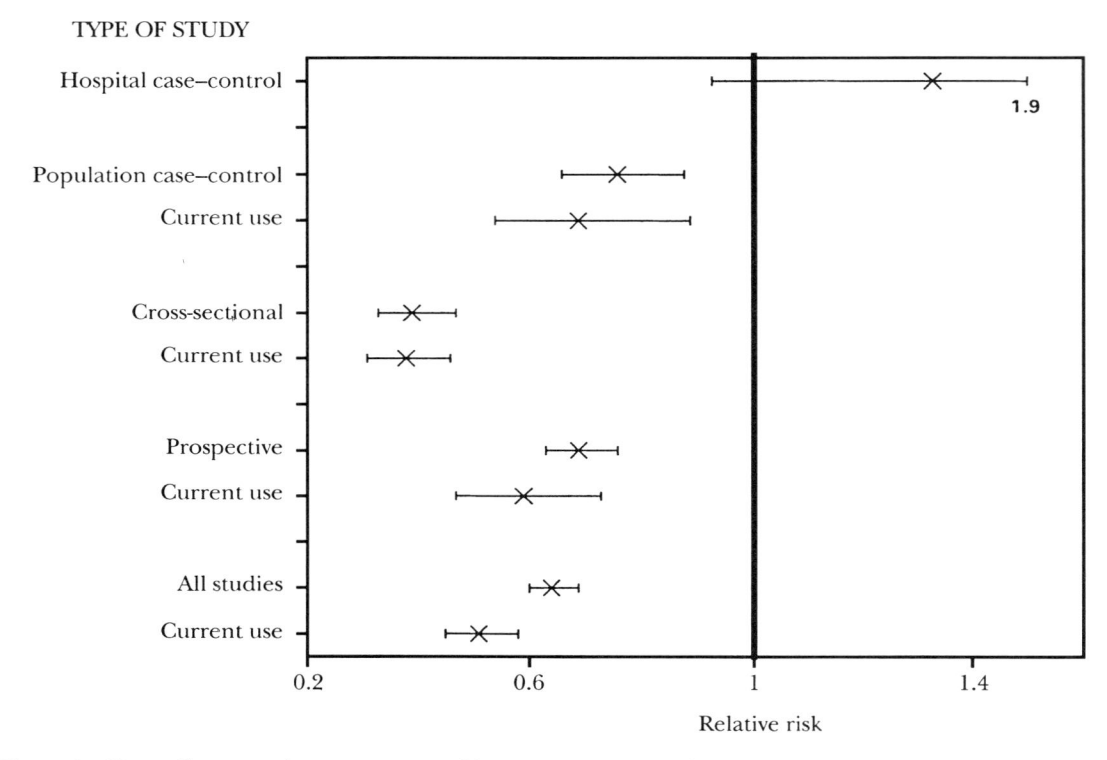

Figure 1 Heart disease and postmenopausal hormones: meta-analysis of ever- and current use compared to never use. From reference 2

In the cross-sectional angiography studies, the risk estimates for the effect of estrogen on heart disease are among the lowest reported. In these studies, the degree of coronary artery occlusion was assessed among users and non-users of postmenopausal estrogens in women undergoing coronary arteriography. The summary relative risk from the angiographic studies (Figure 1), comparing women with occlusion to those without, was 0.40 (95% CI 0.33–0.48).[2]

The prospective study is methodologically the best of the observational study designs, primarily because all women are healthy when recruited into the study; thus, reporting of estrogen use is unbiased, and there is no issue of control selection. Virtually all of the prospective studies have observed a protective effect of estrogens on coronary heart disease; the meta-analysis for the cohort studies (Figure 1), comparing ever- and never-users, yielded a pooled relative risk of 0.71 (95% CI 0.65–0.77)[2].

The meta-analysis of all of the epidemiological studies assessing ever- versus never-use (Figure 1), with relative risks ranging from 0.17 to 4.2, resulted in a summary relative risk of 0.65 (95% CI 0.61–0.69)[2]. However, evidence from many of these studies indicates that current estrogen users enjoy greater protection against heart disease than past users. Thus, combining investigations of current, past and ever-use in a summary estimate such as this is misleading because the results will be directly affected by the proportions of past and current use in the studies included. Summary estimates based on analyses of current use, where such data were provided, were recalculated; as expected, the estimates were lower than those derived by combining studies of any estrogen use (Figure 1)[2]. For the population-based case–control studies, the pooled relative risk for current estrogen use was 0.69 (95% CI 0.50–0.95), for the cross-sectional studies, it was 0.39 (95% CI 0.31–0.48), and for the internally controlled prospective studies, the summary estimate was 0.60 (95% CI 0.50–0.72). The pooled relative risk for current estrogen use, combining all three study designs, was 0.53 (95% CI 0.47–0.60).

Epidemiological studies of cardiovascular disease and estrogen in women with coronary disease

There are a growing number of studies on secondary prevention of heart disease and estrogen use (Table 1), although the differing methodologies preclude a coherent meta-analysis of the results. Three studies followed estrogen users and non-users for recurrent cardiovascular events after angioplasty or coronary artery surgery. O'Keefe and colleagues examined 337 women after angioplasty, of whom 137 were taking estrogen and 200 did not use estrogen[5]. After 7 years, there were fewer recurrent cardiovascular events in the estrogen group (12%) than in the control women (35%); after adjustment for differences in risk factors, the authors observed a marked and highly significant decrease in the risk of cardiovascular death or non-fatal myocardial infarction (MI) (relative risk, RR 0.38; 95% CI 0.19–0.89). Using a similar design, Kim and associates followed 293 women after coronary angioplasty, and compared the outcome among 100 subjects who used hormones both before angioplasty and during follow-up to the 193 women who had never used hormones[6]. The results were nearly identical to those of O'Keefe; survival or freedom from infarction at 7 years was 89% for women taking hormones and 66% for non-users. In a study of 1091 women after coronary artery bypass surgery, Sullivan and co-workers[7] reported that estrogen users had improved survival at 5 and 10 years (98.8% vs. 80.7% and 69.3% vs. 46.3%, respectively). After adjusting for confounding factors such as age and the number of diseased vessels, estrogen use remained strongly inversely correlated with survival (RR 0.34; $p = 0.001$).

Four other studies have assessed the risk of recurrent disease among women with a prior diagnosis of cardiovascular disease (CVD), comparing hormone users and non-users. In the

Table 1 Epidemiological studies of postmenopausal hormone use in women with coronary artery disease

Study	Design	n	Estrogen users	Estrogen non-users
Henderson et al.[8]; Leisure World Cohort	prospective: subjects with prior angina/MI		mortality 28/1000	mortality 42/1000
Bush et al.[9]; Lipid Research Clinics	prospective: subjects with prevalent CVD	236	CVD death rate 13.8/10 000	CVD death rate 66.3/10 000
Kim et al.[6]	survival analysis after PTCA	293	5-year survival 98%, 7-year survival 95%	5-year survival 90%, 7-year survival 78%
Sullivan et al.[7]	survival analysis after CABG	1091	5-year survival 99%, 10-year survival 69%; RR 0.34, ($p = 0.001$)	5-year survival 81%, 10-year survival 46%
Sullivan et al.[10]	survival analysis after angiography	2268	5-year survival with severe CAD 97%, 10-year survival 97%	5-year survival with severe CAD 81%, 10-year survival 60%
O'Keefe et al.[5]	prospective: after angioplasty	337	RR 0.38 (95% CI 0.19–0.89) for CVD death or MI	—
Newton et al.[11]; Group Health Cooperative	prospective: subjects with prior MI	726	RR 0.64 (95% CI 0.32–1.30) for current use and death/MI	—

MI, myocardial infarction; CVD, cardiovascular disease; PTCA, percutaneous transluminal coronary angioplasty; CABG, coronary artery bypass graft; RR, relative risk; CAD, coronary artery disease; CI, confidence interval

Leisure World Study[8], a prospective study, hormone users with a history of angina or MI at baseline had approximately a 35% decreased risk of mortality compared to those not taking hormones. Similarly, in the Lipid Research Clinics cohort[9], among women with prevalent CVD, those taking hormones ($n = 74$) had an 80% lower cardiovascular death rate than non-users ($n = 162$) (death rates were 13.8/10 000 and 66.3/10 000, respectively; RR 0.21; approximate 95% CI 0.03–1.6). Sullivan and colleagues[10] followed 2268 women presenting for angiography: 446 with no detectable coronary artery disease, 644 with mild-to-moderate disease and 1178 with severe disease. Among those with no disease, the 5-year survival among estrogen users was the same as that for non-users (98%). However, among those with mild to moderate disease, estrogen users had better 5-year survival (98% vs. 91%). The difference was even more marked for those with severe disease (97% vs. 81%). Thus, the most substantial benefit was for women with the worst disease at baseline. Finally, Newton and associates[11] conducted a prospective study of 726 women who survived a first MI; current estrogen therapy after MI was associated with a significantly lower rate of reinfarction and death (RR 0.64; 95% CI 0.32–1.30), although there was little relation to past use (RR 0.90; 95% CI 0.62–1.31).

Evaluation of strength of epidemiological data

Virtually all of the evidence for both primary and secondary prevention derives from observational studies. In observational studies, the participants and their physicians decide whether to use estrogen therapy. Often, the health status of the patient has an important influence on this decision and, thus, could influence the results of studies. Women who use estrogen see a physician more regularly than those who do not, and this increased medical care may decrease their risk of CHD. Furthermore, women who choose to use estrogen may also choose to lead generally healthier lifestyles than those who do not take such medication.

Thus, some have argued that estrogen use is merely a marker, rather than a cause, of good health. In the Nurses' Health Study of primary prevention of coronary disease[12], it was shown that increased medical care among estrogen users could not be responsible for the benefit observed. In a substudy, only women who reported regular visits to their physician (50% of the cohort) were included in the analysis, and the results were similar to those found in all subjects: the relative risk for major CHD (CHD death or non-fatal MI) was 0.52 (95% CI 0.37–0.74) for current hormone use.

Several studies have compared the CHD risk factor profile of estrogen users and non-users. In general population studies, estrogen users tend to have a more favorable cardiac risk profile than non-users, even apart from hormone use. In a cohort of postmenopausal women, Barrett-Connor[13] observed that those taking estrogens reported better healthcare behavior, including more screening tests such as blood cholesterol measurement and mammograms. Among 9704 women in a study of osteoporotic fractures[14], users tended to be better educated and less obese, and drank alcohol and participated in sports more often than non-users. Similarly, in a prospective study of randomly selected premenopausal women in Pennsylvania, Matthews and colleagues[15] observed a better cardiovascular risk factor profile prior to hormone use among the women who subsequently took hormones at menopause than among women who did not.

However, variations in health status between hormone users and non-users largely reflect sociological heterogeneity, and are not generally biological phenomena. One would expect hormone users in the general population to be of higher socioeconomic status than non-users; they can afford medical care. Yet, such socioeconomic variation may not be present in a study which consists entirely of registered nurses or women living in a specific retirement community. Thus, in both the Nurses' Health Study[12] and the Leisure World Study[8], few important differences in risk factor status have been found in estrogen users compared to non-users. The results from these and other studies have been adjusted for a large number of risk factors; these adjustments often have only a modest effect on the benefits seen among estrogen users, indicating a similar overall risk factor status for hormone users and non-users. In the Leisure World Study[8], the age-adjusted relative risk of all-cause mortality was 0.80 (95% CI 0.70–0.87) for estrogen users compared to non-users; after further adjustment for high blood pressure, history of angina, MI or stroke, alcohol use, smoking, body mass index and age at menopause, the relative risk was virtually the same (RR 0.79, 95% CI 0.71–0.88). In the study of secondary prevention among women from the Group Health Cooperative of Puget Sound[11], the age-adjusted relative risk of reinfarction was 0.64 and of death was 0.50 with current estrogen use; adjustment for multiple risk factors had little impact on these results (RR 0.72 for reinfarction and 0.53 for death). An analysis restricted solely to women in the Nurses' Health Study[12] who were free from major CHD risk factors (obesity, cigarette smoking, diabetes, hypertension and high cholesterol) still revealed approximately a 50% decrease in the risk of heart disease for current estrogen users. Similarly, in the secondary prevention study from the Group Health Cooperative[11], results from an analysis of women without risk factors were similar to those for the entire cohort. In summary, to explain the benefit as a result of confounding by health status, one would have to presume unknown risk factors which are extremely strong predictors of CHD and very closely associated with estrogen use.

BIOLOGICAL MECHANISMS FOR ESTROGEN'S PROTECTIVE EFFECT

Lipid profile

In experimental studies among postmenopausal women, estrogen reduces low-density lipoprotein (LDL) and raises high-density lipoprotein (HDL). In summarizing estrogen's influence on lipids, Bush and Miller reviewed a substantial body of experimental work and estimated that, on average, 0.625 mg/day of estrogen led to a 10% increase in HDL and a 4% decrease in LDL[16]. In other studies, this regimen increased HDL by an average of 16% and reduced LDL by an average of 15%[17]. The Postmenopausal Estrogen/Progestin Interventions (PEPI) Trial is the largest trial to provide information on estrogen and cholesterol levels[3]. In 175 women aged 45–64 years, randomized for 3 years to estrogen, LDL decreased by 14.5 mg/dl and HDL increased by 5.6 mg/dl compared to a LDL decrease of 4.1 and a HDL decrease of 1.2 for the 175 women on placebo. A 1-mg/dl increase in HDL is associated with approximately a 3% decrease in risk of coronary disease, and a 1-mg/dl decrease in LDL is associated with about a 2% decline in risk[18]; hence, the LDL changes induced by estrogen translate to a 29% reduction in CHD risk, and the HDL increase would mean a further 16.8% reduction in risk. Finally, these effects of estrogen appear to be similar for older women; Paganini-Hill and co-workers[19] studied elderly women (mean age 76 years) in an independent-living community situation (Leisure World, Laguna Hills, CA, USA) who were untreated (58%) or were receiving unopposed estrogen therapy (29%) or combination estrogen/progestin therapy (13%). A significant positive dose correlation for estrogen was seen for HDL cholesterol, while a significant inverse dose correlation was seen for total and LDL cholesterol levels. In that study, there was no strong evidence that addition of a progestin to the estrogen regimen would reduce the cardiovascular protective effect of estrogen.

Reduction of atherosclerosis

It is likely that estrogen exerts part of its protective effect through mechanisms other than lipids. In several randomized trials in monkeys, estrogen's influence on HDL and LDL levels also appeared to be only part of its benefits. In a randomized trial of ovariectomized monkeys fed a moderately atherogenic diet, Adams and colleagues reported that the extent of coronary atherosclerosis in monkeys given conjugated equine estrogens was half as great as in those given placebo[20], despite only modest changes in lipid levels. Similarly, Wagner and co-workers[21] observed that ovariectomized monkeys fed an atherogenic diet, and randomized to conjugated equine estrogens, had a 70% reduction in LDL uptake in the coronary arteries compared to monkeys given placebo, despite only modest differences in plasma lipids. This important finding suggests that estrogen may reduce atherosclerosis by preventing modification of LDL and, thereby, decreasing the avidity of its uptake in the vessel wall to form atherosclerotic lesions. In addition, cholesterol-fed female rabbits treated with hormones had one-third the aortic accumulation of cholesterol of untreated rabbits, which could only partly be explained by differences in cholesterol levels[22].

Hemodynamic parameters

Increasing evidence, from both animal and human studies, demonstrates that estrogen improves blood flow. In one experiment, Williams and associates[23] infused the coronary arteries of ovariectomized monkeys with acetylcholine. This caused arterial constriction in the monkeys with no estrogen supplementation, but minimal dilatation of the arteries was observed in those given conjugated equine estrogens. Similarly, decreased systemic vascular resistance was found when estrogen was administered to ewes[24], and estrogen led to a hyperpolarization of the coronary vascular smooth muscle membrane in dogs[25].

Postmenopausal women treated with estradiol had reduced arterial impedance and decreased vascular tone in uterine arteries[26]. Sarrel and colleagues[27] found increased hyperemic response after estrogen treatment in postmenopausal women; this response correlated with an expanded vasodilator reserve. Pines and co-workers[28] performed Doppler echocardiography on the aortas of postmenopausal women and found that central and peripheral hemodynamic parameters, including peak flow velocity, mean acceleration and ejection time, improved significantly after estrogen therapy. Gangar and associates used Doppler ultrasound to measure the pulsatility index, or impedance to blood flow, in the internal carotid artery of women treated with transdermal estradiol[29]; a significant reduction in impedance was observed after 9 weeks of estrogen treatment. Gilligan and colleagues[4] demonstrated greater coronary flow, lower coronary resistance and prevention of coronary artery constriction with acetylcholine infusion in 20 postmenopausal women after treatment with 17 β-estradiol. Interestingly, the same results were not found in men; acetylcholine caused coronary artery constriction both before and after estradiol administration in seven men[30]. The mechanism by which these changes occur in women is not yet established, although they may be a direct result of estrogen therapy, as estrogen receptors have been found in the muscularis of arteries in cardiovascular tissue[31]; in addition, recent studies indicate that estrogen can upregulate the transcription of nitric oxide synthase in non-vascular tissue[32] and increase plasma levels of nitric oxide in postmenopausal women[33]. The beneficial effects on blood flow and vasodilatation may explain the findings from a placebo-controlled trial that acute administration of estrogen can prolong treadmill time and decrease symptoms in women with coronary artery disease[34].

Antioxidant activity

Peroxidation of plasma lipids may represent an initial as well as a continuing step in the process of atherogenesis. The effect of estrogen administration on lipid peroxidation has been investigated in humans by Wilcox and co-workers[35] in a prospective, randomized cross-over study. Data were obtained from eight healthy postmenopausal women who received, in a random sequence, each of three estrogen compounds orally for 30 days. Levels of oxidized LDL in plasma were reduced with all of the estrogen compounds.

Mosca and colleagues[36] conducted a randomized, placebo-controlled study in 49 postmenopausal women to determine the susceptibility of LDL to oxidation after the women had been treated for 3 months with estrogen or micronized estradiol alone or either drug combined with medroxyprogesterone acetate (MPA). Unopposed estrogen proved to be the most effective agent for prevention of lipid peroxidation; addition of a progestin appears to attenuate this effect. Subbiah and associates[37] found that the conjugated equine estrogens were more potent than estradiol and estrone in terms of protection against oxidation of LDL.

Cholesterol, atherosclerosis and hemodynamic parameters in studies of estrogen among subjects with coronary disease

A variety of experiments in monkeys and rats with induced vascular disease have demonstrated substantial beneficial effects of estrogen on markers of disease progression. In a 30-month trial of ovariectomized monkeys with diet-induced atherosclerosis, Williams and colleagues provided one group with no treatment, one group with a lipid-lowering diet only, a third group with the diet and conjugated equine estrogens, and the fourth group with the diet and estrogen plus MPA[38]. Plaque size did not change in any of the groups, although coronary artery lumen size increased in all three treated groups, with the largest increase for the monkeys given estrogen with progestin. In addition, all treated groups had improved total cholesterol/HDL ratios and both hormone groups had a lowering in LDL molecular weights. Oparil and colleagues[39] treated rats with 17 β-estradiol, MPA, estrogen and MPA, and placebo followed by balloon injury of the carotid artery; 2 weeks later, rats given estradiol had substantially less neointima formation, and intimal area was reduced by more than 70%, compared to untreated rats, although, in rats given estrogen with progestin, the damaged intimal area was similar in the treatment and placebo groups. Similarly, Krasinski and associates[40] implanted 17β-estradiol or placebo pellets in rats and performed balloon injury. Re-endothelialization and functional endothelial recovery (nitric oxide production) were enhanced in the estrogen group and neointimal thickening was reduced. Williams and colleagues[38] also examined several indicators of blood flow in atherosclerotic monkeys, and found that diet treatment as well as diet plus hormone treatment improved dilator responses in the coronary artery, and that coronary flow reserve was greater in the monkeys given estrogen than in the other groups, although the addition of progestin diminished this benefit.

Studies in women with established CVD have also demonstrated favorable physiological changes with estrogen use. In a randomized cross-over trial of 11 postmenopausal women with coronary artery disease (≥ 70% stenosis of one or more coronary arteries), estrogen administration (1 mg Estrace®) 40 min before a treadmill test increased total exercise time and time to ST depression, and reduced symptoms on exertion in the women taking estrogen compared to those given placebo[34]. In women with hypertension, cardiac morphology and left ventricular function was improved after estrogen therapy[41]; compared to controls, left ventricular cavity dimensions and mass were smaller, and resting aortic blood flow velocity and acceleration increased after 6 months taking 0.625 mg of Premarin® or 2 mg estradiol. Espeland and co-workers[42] studied 186 postmenopausal women with evidence of early or subclinical carotid artery atherosclerosis who participated in a trial of lipid-lowering medication; during 4 years of follow-up, intimal media thickness progressed (mean 0.014 mm/year) in women taking placebo who never used estrogen, but regressed in women taking either estrogen alone (mean −0.009 mm/year), medication alone (mean −0.010 mm/year), or estrogen and medication (mean −0.015 mm/year). In 204 women who had had either atherectomy or angioplasty, the rate of restenosis (> 50% stenosis) after 6 months was lower in estrogen users (41%) than non-users (50%), especially among the women who had received atherectomy[43].

CONCLUSIONS

In summary, the evidence clearly supports a clinically important protection against heart disease for postmenopausal women who use estrogen. In addition, the available data strongly suggest that hormone use decreases the risk of second events in women with diagnosed cardiovascular disease. Furthermore, there is no reason to believe that hormone therapy should not provide similar benefits for secondary as for primary prevention of cardiovascular disease.

Other factors related to heart disease, including lipid lowering and aspirin use, have proven generally equivalent for both primary and secondary prevention. Thus, based on the limited evidence available, hormone use appears to decrease the risk of cardiovascular disease and increase survival in women with established coronary artery disease.

References

1. Stampfer MJ, Colditz GA, Willett WC. Menopause and heart disease: a review. *Ann NY Acad Sci* 1990;592:193–203
2. Grodstein F, Stampfer MJ. The epidemiology of coronary heart disease and estrogen replacement in postmenopausal women. *Prog Cardiovasc Dis* 1995;38:199–210
3. Postmenopausal Estrogen/Progestin Interventions Trial Writing Group. Effects of estrogen/progestin regimens on heart disease risk factors in postmenopausal women. *J Am Med Assoc* 1995;273:199–208
4. Gilligan DM, Quyyumi AA, Cannon RO. Effects of physiological levels of estrogen on coronary vasomotor function in postmenopausal women. *Circulation* 1994;89:2545–51
5. O'Keefe JH, Kim SC, Hall RR, et al. Estrogen replacement therapy after coronary angioplasty in women. *J Am Coll Cardiol* 1997;29:1–5
6. Kim SC, O'Keefe JH, Ligon RW, et al. Estrogen improves long-term outcome after coronary angioplasty (abstract). *Circulation* 1995;92(Suppl 1):674
7. Sullivan JM, El-Zeky F, Vander Zwaag R, et al. Estrogen replacement therapy after coronary artery bypass surgery: effect on survival. *J Am Coll Cardiol* 1994;23:49A
8. Henderson BE, Paganini-Hill A, Ross RK. Decreased mortality in users of estrogen replacement therapy. *Arch Intern Med* 1991;151:75–8
9. Bush TL, Barrett-Connor E, Cowan LD, et al. Cardiovascular mortality and noncontraceptive use of estrogen in women: results from the Lipid Research Clinics Program Follow-up Study. *Circulation* 1987;75:1102–9
10. Sullivan JM, van der Zwaag R, Hughes JP, et al. Estrogen replacement and coronary artery disease: effect on survival in postmenopausal women. *Arch Intern Med* 1990;150:2557–62
11. Newton KM, LaCroix AZ, McKnight B, et al. Estrogen replacement therapy and prognosis after first myocardial infarction. *Am J Epidemiol* 1997;145:269–77
12. Grodstein F, Stampfer MJ, Manson JE, et al. Postmenopausal estrogen and progestin use and the risk of cardiovascular disease. *N Engl J Med* 1996;335:453–61
13. Barrett-Connor E. Postmenopausal estrogen and prevention bias. *Ann Intern Med* 1991;115:455–6
14. Cauley JA, Cummings SR, Black DM, et al. Prevalence and determinants of estrogen replacement therapy in elderly women. *Am J Obstet Gynecol* 1990;163:1438–44
15. Matthews KA, Kuller LH, Wing RR, et al. Are users of estrogen replacement therapy healthier prior to use than are nonusers? *Am J Epidemiol* 1996;143:971–8
16. Bush TL, Miller VT. Effects of pharmacologic agents used during menopause. Impact on lipids and lipoproteins. In Mishell D, ed. *Menopause: Physiology and Pharmacology*. Chicago: Year Book Medical Publishers, 1986:187–208
17. Walsh BW, Schiff I, Rosner B, et al. Effects of postmenopausal estrogen replacement on the concentration and metabolism of plasma lipoproteins. *N Engl J Med* 1991;325:1196–204
18. Gordon DJ, Probstfield JL, Garrison RJ, et al. High-density lipoprotein cholesterol and cardiovascular disease. Four prospective American studies. *Circulation* 1989;79:8–15
19. Paganini-Hill A, Dworsky R, Krauss RM. Hormone replacement therapy, hormone levels, and lipoprotein cholesterol concentrations in elderly women. *Am J Obstet Gynecol* 1996;174:897–902
20. Adams MR, Kaplan JR, Manuck SB, et al. Inhibition of coronary artery atherosclerosis by 17-β-estradiol in ovariectomized monkeys. Lack of an effect of added progesterone. *Arteriosclerosis* 1990;10:1051–7
21. Wagner JD, Clarkson TB, St Clair RW, et al. Estrogen and progesterone replacement therapy reduces low density lipoprotein accumulation in the coronary arteries of surgically postmenopausal cynomolgus monkeys. *J Clin Invest* 1991;88:1995–2002
22. Haarbo J, Leth-Espensen P, Stender S, et al. Estrogen monotherapy and combined estrogen-progestogen replacement therapy attenuate aortic accumulation of cholesterol in ovariectomized cholesterol-fed rabbits. *J Clin Invest* 1991;87:1274–1279
23. Williams JK, Adams MR, Klopfenstein HS. Estrogen modulates responses of atherosclerotic coronary arteries. *Circulation* 1990;81:1680–7

24. Magness RR, Rosenfeld CR. Local and systemic estradiol-17-β: effects on uterine and systemic vasodilation. *Am J Physiol* 1989;256:536–42
25. Harder DR, Coulson PB. Estrogen receptors and effects of estrogen on membrane electrical properties of coronary vascular smooth muscle. *J Cell Physiol* 1979;100:375–82
26. Bourne T, Hillard TC, Whitehead MI, et al. Oestrogens, arterial status, and postmenopausal women. *Lancet* 1990;335:1470–1
27. Sarrel PM, Lindsay D, Rosano GMC, et al. Angina and normal coronary arteries in women: gynecologic findings. *Am J Obstet Gynecol* 1992;167:467–72
28. Pines A, Fisman EZ, Levo Y, et al. The effects of hormone replacement therapy in normal postmenopausal women: measurements of Doppler-derived parameters of aortic flow. *Am J Obstet Gynecol* 1991;164:806–12
29. Gangar KF, Vyas S, Whitehead M, et al. Pulsatility index in internal carotid artery in relation to transdermal oestradiol and time since menopause. *Lancet* 1991;338:839–42
30. Collins P, Rosano GMC, Sarrel PM, et al. 17-β-estradiol attenuates acetylcholine-induced coronary arterial constriction in women but not men with coronary heart disease. *Circulation* 1995;92:24–30
31. McGill HC. Sex steroid hormone receptors in the cardiovascular system. *Postgrad Med* 1989;64–8
32. Weiner CP, Lizasoain I, Baylis SA, et al. Induction of calcium-dependent nitric oxide synthases by sex hormones. *Proc Natl Acad Sci USA* 1994;91:5212–16
33. Cicinelli E, Matteo G, Ignarro LJ, et al. Acute effects of transdermal estradiol administration on plasma levels of nitric oxide in postmenopausal women. *Fertil Steril* 1997;67:63–6
34. Rosano GMC, Sarrel PM, Poole-Wilson PA, et al. Beneficial effect of estrogen on exercise-induced ischaemia in women with coronary artery disease. *Lancet* 1993;342:133–6
35. Wilcox JG, Sevanian A, Hwang J, et al. Cardioprotective effects of individual conjugated estrogens through their possible modulation of insulin resistance and oxidation of low-density lipoprotein. *Fertil Steril* 1997;67:57–62
36. Mosca L, Rubenfire M, Tsai A, et al. The benefit of estrogen replacement therapy on the susceptibility of low density lipoprotein (LDL) to oxidation in postmenopausal women and the effect of added progestin. Presented at the *4th International Conference on Preventive Cardiology*, Montreal, Canada, June 1997; abstr.
37. Subbiah MTR, Kessel B, Agrawal M, et al. Antioxidant potential of specific estrogens on lipid peroxidation. *J Clin Endocrinol Metab* 1993;77:1095–7
38. Williams JK, Anthony MS, Honore EK, et al. Regression of atherosclerosis in female monkeys. *Arterioscler Thromb Vasc Biol* 1995;15:827–36
39. Oparil S, Levine RL, Chen SJ, et al. Sexually dimorphic response of the balloon-injured rat carotid artery to hormone treatment. *Circulation* 1997;95:1301–7
40. Krasinski K, Spyridopoulos I, Asahara T, et al. Estradiol accelerates functional endothelial recovery after arterial injury. *Circulation* 1997;95:1768–72
41. Pines A, Risman EZ, Shapira I, et al. Exercise echocardiography in postmenopausal hormone users with mild systemic hypertension. *Am J Cardiol* 1996;78:1385–9
42. Espeland MA, Applegate W, Furberg CD, et al. Estrogen replacement therapy and progression of intimal–medial thickness in the carotid arteries of postmenopausal women. *Am J Epidemiol* 1995;142:1011–19
43. O'Brien JE, Peterson ED, Keeler GP, et al. Relation between estrogen replacement therapy and restenosis after percutaneous coronary interventions. *J Am Coll Cardiol* 1996;28:1111–18

23
Estrogen therapy after coronary artery thrombosis

J. M. Sullivan

A number of factors associated with increased risk of cardiovascular disease, among them tobacco smoke, diabetes mellitus, hypertension, hypercholesterolemia and estrogen deficiency, have been found to impair endothelial function. Part of this process involves the induction of adhesion molecules which appear on the surface of the endothelial cell, e.g. vascular cell adhesion molecule (VCAM), intercellular adhesion molecule (ICAM) and E-selectin. This allows white blood cells to adhere, travel beneath the endothelium, imbibe oxidized low-density lipoprotein (LDL) cholesterol and become lipid-laden macrophages that necrose and form a lipid core that is eventually covered by a thin fibrous cap. With the release of growth factors from endothelial cells and macrophages, vascular smooth muscle cells migrate into the area of atheroma formation and proliferate. Platelets adhere to the surface of the atheromatous plaque, initiating thrombi that become incorporated into the growing atheroma. Eventually, the surface of the plaque becomes unstable and a fissure develops, usually at the shoulders of the fibrous cap. This process prompts formation of a larger thrombus that can occlude the vessel and cause ischemic damage or infarction.

Quantitative angiographic studies have demonstrated that it is possible to retard the growth of atherosclerotic plaques and, at times, to promote regression of the atherosclerotic lesions[1]. Although the reduction in the size of the plaque is relatively little, several studies have shown that this is associated with a reduction of cardiac events of about 50%. These observations are the basis for the concept of atherosclerotic plaque stabilization, which requires meticulous control of cardiovascular risk factors.

Epidemiological studies have observed that cardiovascular risk increases after menopause, quadrupling after surgical menopause and approximately doubling after natural menopause[2]. Because several important studies concerning the relationship of estrogen and cardiovascular disease have been published recently, this chapter will serve to update a previous review[3].

ESTROGEN REPLACEMENT AND RISK OF CORONARY EVENTS

More than 35 observational studies have examined the effect of estrogen replacement therapy on the incidence of cardiovascular disease in postmenopausal women[4]. Ten of 13 case–control studies found that women who received estrogen replacement had fewer cardiovascular events than those who did not use estrogen. However, only one study reached statistical significance[5]. Seventeen cohort studies of postmenopausal women examined the incidence of cardiovascular events and total mortality relative to estrogen use. Sixteen studies linked estrogen use with a decreased cardiovascular event rate. Recently, 16-year follow-up data from the 59 337 participants of the Nurses' Health Study showed that the relative risk for major coronary heart disease was 0.60 (95% confidence interval (CI), 0.43–0.83) when women who used estrogen were compared with women who did not receive hormone replacement therapy[6]. Possible explanations for these conflicting results could have been differences in patient characteristics or trial endpoints. For example, certain trials used chest pain to indicate the presence of coronary artery disease. It is now accepted that the anginal syndrome can occur in persons who have no coronary atherosclerosis. Inclusion of such patients would bias the results of a study of atherosclerosis endpoints. These observational studies have been criticized also for selection bias: women who opt for estrogen replacement therapy might also be those who change their lifestyles in other ways that prevent cardiovascular disease.

Four laboratories have used coronary arteriography for cross-sectional studies of estrogen replacement therapy in postmenopausal patients[7-10]. All have found less extensive coronary atherosclerosis in women who took estrogen. Because there were differences other than estrogen use between patients with and without coronary disease, all studies used logistic regression analysis to identify estrogen replacement therapy as the variable independently and significantly associated with the absence of coronary disease.

There are few studies of estrogen replacement after coronary artery thrombosis. The first was the Coronary Drug Project[11], which randomized male survivors of acute myocardial infarction into several therapeutic arms, two of which involved conjugated equine estrogens in daily doses of 2.5 or 5.0 mg. The men receiving 5 mg per day experienced more cardiovascular events than those who received placebo; definite non-fatal myocardial infarction occurred in 6.2% of estrogen-treated men, but in only 3.2% of those receiving placebo. There was a statistically significant increase (3.5% vs. 1.3%) in incidence of definite pulmonary embolism or thrombophlebitis in the estrogen-treated men. Although the men receiving 2.5 mg per day of estrogens did not experience a statistically significant increase in heart attacks, this part of the study was stopped when malignancy was found more often in the estrogen-supplemented men than in those receiving placebo[12].

Because of the increased incidence of myocardial infarction seen in women over 35 years of age who smoked cigarettes and use oral contraceptives, which contained relatively high doses of estrogens and progestins, physicians have been reluctant to recommend the use of these agents to women who had, or were at increased risk for, cardiovascular disease. It is now appreciated that large doses of estrogen stimulate hepatic production of clotting factors, thus inducing a hypercoagulable state, which could be disastrous in the presence of extensive atherosclerosis.

EFFECTS OF ESTROGEN IN WOMEN WITH PREVIOUS CARDIOVASCULAR DISEASE

Two large, long-term observational studies[13,14] included women known to have cardiovascular disease at the time that they joined the study. Both found that estrogen replacement conveyed a greater survival benefit in the group at greater risk than in women who initially lacked historical or clinical evidence of cardiovascular disease. The Lipid Research Clinics Program[13] included a cohort of 2270 women who were followed for an average of 8.5 years. In women free of cardiovascular disease, the mortality rate was 12.8/10 000 in estrogen users and 30.2/10 000 in non-users, a decline of 58%. In women with cardiovascular disease, the cardiovascular death rate was 13.8/10 000 in estrogen users and 66.3/10 000 in non-users, a decrease of 79%.

The Leisure World Study[14] included 8881 postmenopausal women who were followed for 7.5 years. In women with no history of angina or myocardial infarction, all-cause mortality was 21.8/1000 in estrogen users and 26.7/1000 in non-users, 18% less. In women with a positive history, all-cause mortality was 27.5/1000 in estrogen users and 41.7/1000 in non-users, 34% less.

The effect of estrogen replacement on survival in patients with angiographically documented coronary artery disease was studied in 2268 women undergoing cardiac catheterization[15]. Actuarial methods were used to examine survival over 10 years. Patients who were free of coronary artery disease at baseline had 10-year survival rates greater than 90% regardless of estrogen use. In patients with mild to moderate coronary lesions at baseline, 10-year survival was significantly better among estrogen users than in non-users. Among those who never took estrogen, 85% were still alive, compared with 96% in those who were taking estrogen ($p = 0.027$). The difference in survival was greatest in patients with severely stenotic lesions: 60% of those who never used estrogen were alive at 10 years, compared with 98% of those who had ever taken estrogen ($p = 0.007$).

The Cox stepwise proportional hazards analysis was used to determine which factors had a statistically significant independent effect on total mortality. The most powerful determinants were the number of coronary arteries involved, the severity of cardiac functional impairment, age and disease of the left main coronary artery. The only significant factor predicting improved survival was estrogen use. Relative risk equalled 0.16 with a 95% confidence interval of 0.04–0.66.

The relationship between postmenopausal estrogen use and survival has also been studied in women who underwent coronary artery bypass surgery[16]. Life-table analysis was used to compare postsurgical survival in women who received estrogen replacement therapy with those who did not.

The 10-year survival rate was 81.4% in the estrogen users and 65.1% in the non-users ($p = 0.0001$). A Cox proportional hazards model selected the number of vessels diseased, estrogen use, left main coronary stenosis and diabetes mellitus as significant independent predictors of survival.

Two studies have examined the effect of estrogen on outcome after percutaneous transluminal coronary arterioplasty. In a study of 293 women, 100 received estrogen replacement[17]. Their subsequent myocardial infarction rate was 5% and their 7-year survival rate was 93%. In contrast, in the 193 women who did not receive estrogen, the infarction rate was 8% and 7-year survival was 75% ($p = 0.001$). A smaller study, involving 23 estrogen users and 84 non-users, found no differences in the rate of restenosis by angiographic study at 6 months, 48% vs. 50%[18]. The same study observed a 57% restenosis rate after coronary atherectomy in 79 women who did not use estrogen and a lower rate of 27% in 18 estrogen users ($p = 0.038$).

Only one study has examined the effect of estrogen replacement on the outcome of female survivors of acute myocardial infarction. Newton and colleagues[19] examined the experiences of 726 women of the Group Health Cooperative of Puget Sound. They observed a relative risk of second myocardial infarction of 0.64 (95% CI, 0.32–1.30) and of all-cause mortality of 0.50 (0.25–1.00) in current users of estrogen. The reduction of relative risk in past users was not significant.

The Nurses' Health Study also supports the concept that those women who are at the greatest risk of cardiovascular disease benefit most from estrogen replacement[20]. In women with one or more cardiovascular risk factors, the relative risk of survival was 0.51 (0.45–0.57), while in those without cardiovascular risk factors, the relative risk was 0.83 (0.62–1.28).

Recent data indicate that estrogen replacement increases the risk of deep vein thrombosis and pulmonary embolism. In a British study involving 103 cases of idiopathic venous thrombolism and 178 women controls, current users were found to have an odds ration of 3.5 (95% CI, 1.8–7.0) compared to those who did not use hormone replacement[21]. In a similar case–control study, the Group Health Cooperative of Puget Sound found a relative risk of 3.2 (95% CI, 1.5–6.8) comparing current users with non-users[22]. The Nurses' Health Study observed a twofold increase in the risk of pulmonary embolism among current postmenopausal estrogen users[23]. Although the three studies found that estrogen use was associated with an increase in the relative risk of venous thromboembolism, the absolute risk was low as venous thrombolism occurred infrequently. When weighed against a 44% reduction in cardiovascular disease, a highly prevalent disorder, the increased risk of venous thromboembolism does not contraindicate estrogen replacement but does point out the need for attention to a prior history of idiopathic thrombosis.

MECHANISMS OF CARDIOPROTECTION BY ESTROGEN

Epidemiological and experimental studies suggest that the effect of estrogen replacement therapy on serum lipids accounts for about 25–50% of its cardioprotective effect. Before menopause, women have higher high-density lipoprotein (HDL) levels than men. After menopause, LDL levels rise while HDL levels decline slightly or remain unchanged. Estrogen decreases LDL and total cholesterol levels and increases levels of HDL cholesterol and triglycerides[24].

Estrogen replacement is usually given in combination with a progestin. There are relatively few data concerning a possible cardioprotective effect of combined hormone replacement therapy. The PEPI Trial[25] found that conjugated estrogens, with or without progestins, lowered LDL by 14.5–17.2 mg/dl. Estrogen alone raised HDL by 5.6 mg/dl. The addition of a progestin attenuated the HDL rise to 1.2–1.5 mg/dl and micronized progesterone raised HDL by 4.2 mg/dl.

In a study involving surgically menopausal non-human primates, both estrogen alone and estrogen with progesterone reduced the extent of aortic atherosclerosis, even though combination therapy reduced HDL levels[26]. Combination therapy reduced LDL cholesterol uptake by arterial walls to the same extent as estrogen.

In long-term human cohort studies, HDL levels did not differ significantly between those taking estrogen or combination hormone replacement therapy[27]. The Uppsala Study[28] showed that estrogen or combination replacement therapy equivalently reduced the risk of first myocardial infarction (MI) or stroke. Nachtigall and colleagues[29], in the only randomized trial of estrogen–progestin therapy, showed a reduction in the rate of MI in 84 pairs of hospitalized women. Their results, however, did not achieve statistical significance.

The Puget Sound Area Health Group study provided supporting evidence that combination therapy reduced cardiovascular risk as well as estrogen alone. The relative risk of first myocardial infarction was 0.69 (95% CI, 0.54–1.25) in estrogen users and 0.53 (0.30–0.87) in estrogen–progestin users[30].

The 16-year follow-up of the Nurses' Health Study has provided valuable observations about combined hormone replacement[31]. In this study of 59 337 women, the relative risk of coronary heart disease in women who took estrogen with progestin was 0.39 (0.19–0.78) compared with that in women who did not take hormone replacement. The relative risk in women who took estrogen alone was 0.60 (0.43–0.83).

Thus, despite experimental and clinical data suggesting that progestin might reduce the observed cardiovascular benefit of estrogen replacement, the few observational studies and one controlled trial completed to date suggest otherwise.

EFFECTS OF ESTROGEN ON VASCULAR ENDOTHELIUM

In addition to their effect on lipids, estrogens have a direct effect on vascular reactivity that may influence the balance of myocardial oxygen supply and demand. The endothelium plays an important role in the modulation of blood vessel tone. Furchgott and Zawadzk[32] demonstrated that removing endothelium altered the way in which arterial strips responded to acetylcholine. Intact strips relaxed. After removal of the endothelium, acetylcholine caused constriction. Later research led to the discovery that acetylcholine stimulates the release of endothelial-derived relaxing factor, a vasodilating compound[33]. Relaxing factor was subsequently identified as nitric oxide, formed from L-arginine. Release of nitric oxide activates guanalyte cyclase. This triggers synthesis of cyclic guanosine monophosphate (GMP), which in turn alters calcium movement, causing vasodilatation.

Impaired endothelial function has been found in the elderly, in patients with hypertension, hypercholesterolemia or diabetes, in cigarette smokers and in estrogen-deficient women[34,35]. Studies in experimental animals[36] and in humans show that estrogen improves endothelium-dependent vasodilatation and increases release of nitric oxide[37–40]. Certain evidence suggests that estrogen induces nitric oxide synthase, but the data are contradictory[41]. Oxygen-derived free radicals inactivate nitric oxide. Estrogen has recently been shown to reduce the generation of oxygen free radicals, thus increasing the effect of nitric oxide[41]. Estrogen also modifies the release and effect of endothelin-1, a potent vasoconstrictor released by the endothelium[42].

The expression of adhesion molecules by injured endothelial cells is one of the first events in the formation of an atherosclerotic plaque. Molecules such as E-selectin, VCAM and ICAM cause monocytes to adhere to endothelium prior to migrating into the subendothelial space and become macrophages. Estradiol has been found to inhibit the expression of these adhesion molecules[43].

Estradiol has also been found to stimulate endothelial cell proliferation[44], to increase the ability of the endothelium to spread and cover defects[44,45] and to form tubes, i.e. vascular collateral channels[44]. There is one report that estradiol inhibits apoptosis, or programmed cell death, in endothelial cells exposed to tumor necrosis factor-α[46].

Ludmer and co-workers[47] demonstrated that infusion of acetylcholine into normal human coronary arteries caused vasodilatation, but infusion in an artery with an atherosclerotic lesion produced vasoconstriction of the stenotic and adjacent areas. This suggested that atherosclerotic involvement of the vessel wall impairs endothelial function. Williams and his colleagues[36] demonstrated that acetylcholine causes constriction when infused into coronary vessels of oophorectomized monkeys fed a high-lipid diet, suggesting loss of endothelial function. When the monkeys received estrogen replacement therapy, acetylcholine produced a more normal response.

Four recent studies have made similar observations in women with coronary disease, but the same results were not seen in men[37–40]. The other evidence that estrogen replacement therapy alters blood vessel function includes studies showing the presence of estrogen receptors in blood vessel walls[48], the ability of estrogen to act as a vasodilator, and the calcium channel blocking and potassium channel opening properties of estrogen. In addition, estrogen stimulates the production of prostacyclin and reduces production of thromboxane A_2[49].

In addition to being actively involved in regulating vascular tone through the production of vasorelaxing and vasoconstricting factors, healthy endothelial cells prevent white blood cells from adhering to blood vessel walls, an early event in the formation of atherosclerotic plaques. The endothelium also: regulates the growth of vascular smooth muscle, an important component in the growth of atherosclerotic plaques; limits the passage of LDL cholesterol into the blood vessel wall, which in turn retards the growth of the atherosclerotic plaque; and helps the metabolism of triglycerides through the action of cell membrane lipoprotein lipase[34].

IMPORTANCE OF OTHER CORONARY RISK FACTORS IN WOMEN

A National Center for Health Statistics survey[50] found that 29% of adult American women smoke cigarettes. Eighty-four per cent of women under age 50 with a history of acute MI are cigarette smokers[51]. Epidemiological studies suggest that cigarette smoking and oral contraceptives act synergistically as coronary risk factors in women over age 35 years[52].

In the United States, 30% of white women and 50% of black women weigh 20% more than their ideal body weight.

Twenty-three per cent of American women are hypertensive[53]. With aging, the prevalence of hypertension rises to 35% in white women and 55% in black women. These figures continue to increase with each decade of age. However, the recent NHANES III[54] survey indicates a definite decline in the prevalence of hypertension in the general population over the past decade.

The importance of hypertension as a coronary risk factor in women is controversial[55]. The prognosis appears more benign in women than in men, which may explain the apparent lack of benefit from antihypertensive therapy in three clinical trials. The Hypertension Detection and Follow-Up Program[56] found that effective treatment of mild hypertension reduced cardiovascular mortality. Analysis of the outcome in younger white women in this trial suggested no benefit. The relatively small number of white women in this trial, their low event rate and the trial's 5-year duration may have made it impossible to demonstrate a benefit of therapy.

The British Medical Research Council trial[57] included 8000 women, aged 35–64 years. Antihypertensive treatment reduced cardiovascular events by 25% and strokes by 48%. The Systolic Hypertension in the Elderly Program[58] reported a 36% reduction in strokes and a decline in coronary heart disease. A meta-analysis of randomized drug treatment trials, in which 47% of participants were women, showed a 42% decrease in stroke and a 14% decline in coronary disease. Based on these trials, women with systolic blood pressure over 160 mmHg and diastolic pressure over 90 mmHg should change lifestyle to reduce weight, lower sodium and alcohol intake, and increase exercise. Pharmacological treatment should be added[59] when lifestyle changes fail to lower blood pressure adequately.

A relationship between hyperlipidemia and coronary heart disease is found in both sexes, although epidemiological studies have found that the various lipid subfractions affect age groups differently. The Lipid Research Clinics Program Follow-up Study[60] followed 2270 women for an average of 8.5 years, and found no association between total or LDL cholesterol and cardiovascular death. Triglycerides were found to be a significant risk factor for cardiovascular death in women and HDL cholesterol was found to be protective. The Framingham study[61] reported that total and LDL cholesterol are definite risk factors for coronary disease in women in their fifth, sixth and seventh decades of life. The Framingham study[62] also found that, although the relative risk of coronary events for each increment in serum cholesterol was as high in women as in men, the absolute risk was half as great. Each 1% increase in total cholesterol was accompanied by a 2% increase in coronary disease in women. For each 10 mg/dl change in HDL, there was a 40–50% change in coronary risk.

Two randomized trials[63,64] on the effects of dietary and drug intervention on atherosclerosis involved cohorts containing 52% women. These studies showed that lowering LDL and increasing HDL slowed the progression of atherosclerosis in men and women. However, data were insufficient to show reduction of coronary events. The results of one primary prevention trial and six secondary prevention trials[65] suggested that women and men both benefit from lipid lowering. However, the small number of women (4%) present in these trials prevented a definitive conclusion. It is now reasonable to propose that lowering cholesterol is beneficial for women, based on the available data.

Evidence that diabetes mellitus is a very powerful predictor of cardiovascular risk for women is compelling. Several studies, including autopsy series, death certificate reviews and one prospective investigation have shown a stronger association between glucose intolerance and risk of coronary heart disease in women than in men[66–68]. In premenopausal women, diabetes mellitus increases cardiovascular risk to that of comparably aged men.

Regular aerobic exercise is frequently recommended for prevention and management of coronary heart disease. One possible mechanism of cardioprotection is through an effect on lipoproteins, particularly an elevation of HDL. Such a beneficial effect of exercise on HDL cholesterol has not been convincingly demonstrated in women, except for those who participate in endurance training[69,70].

Daily low-dose aspirin therapy has been shown to significantly reduce the incidence of heart attack and stroke in studies with predominantly male cohorts. The US Nurses' Health Study[71] also found that women who took 1–6 aspirin tablets a week had 32% fewer first episodes of MI. Women who took the most vitamin E for over 2 years had a 44% lower rate of coronary artery disease compared with others. Intake of betacarotene did not have a cardioprotective effect.

CONCLUSION

Treatment of cardiovascular risk factors can slow or prevent the growth of atherosclerotic plaque in many patients and can reduce the size of lesions in some. Although the change in the size of atherosclerotic lesions with cholesterol-lowering agents is unimpressive, the reduction in subsequent cardiovascular events is encouraging. An atherosclerotic plaque can be stabilized, reducing the likelihood that its surface will fissure or erode and allow formation of an occlusive thrombus. Estrogen replacement therapy, through an effect on serum lipids and an effect on the blood vessel wall, appears to play an important role in this process. Other important interventions include: antithrombotic therapy (aspirin) to reduce platelet adhesion; reduction of blood pressure to prevent endothelial damage; smoking cessation; and precise control of diabetes mellitus to prevent vascular damage. Antioxidants help by preventing the oxidation of LDL cholesterol, thereby reducing its uptake into the blood vessel wall and into atherosclerotic plaques. Antioxidants also contribute to the preservation of endothelial function.

References

1. Brown E, Albers JJ, Fisher LD, et al. Regression of coronary artery disease as a result of intensive lipid lowering therapy in men with high levels of apolipoprotein B. *N Engl J Med* 1990;323:1289–98
2. Kannel WB, Hjortland MC, McNamara PM, et al. Menopause and the risk of cardiovascular disease. The Framingham Study. *Ann Intern Med* 1976;85:447–52
3. Sullivan JM. Practical aspects of preventing and managing atherosclerotic disease in postmenopausal women. *Eur Heart J* 1996;17(Suppl.D):32–7
4. Stampfer MJ, Graham AC. Estrogen replacement therapy and coronary heart disease: a quantitative assessment of the epidemiologic evidence. *Pre Med* 1991;20:47–63
5. Ross RK, Paganini-Hill A, Mack T, et al. Menopausal oestrogen therapy and protection from death from ischemic heart disease. *Lancet* 1981;1:858–60
6. Grodstein F, Stampfer MJ, Manson JE, et al. Postmenopausal estrogen and progestin use and the risk of cardiovascular disease. *N Engl J Med* 1996;335:453–61
7. Sullivan JM, Vander Zwagg R, Lemp GF, et al. Post menopausal estrogen use and coronary atherosclerosis. *Ann Intern Med* 1988;108:358–63
8. Gruchow HW, Anderson AJ, Barboriak JJ, et al. Postmenopausal use of estrogen and occlusion of coronary arteries. *Am Heart J* 1988;115:954–63
9. McFarland KF, Boniface ME, Hornung CA, et al. Risk factors and noncontraceptive estrogen use in women with and without coronary disease. *Am Heart J* 1989;117:1209–14
10. Hong MK, Romm PA, Reagan K, et al. Effects of estrogen replacement therapy on serum lipid values and angiographically defined coronary artery disease in postmenopausal women. *Am J Cardiol* 1992;69:176–8
11. The Coronary Drug Project Research Group. The Coronary Drug Project. Initial findings leading to modifications of its research protocol. *J Am Med Assoc* 1970;214:1303–13
12. The Coronary Drug Project Research Group. The Coronary Drug Project. Findings leading to discontinuation of the 2.5-mg/day estrogen group. *J Am Med Assoc* 1973;226:652–7
13. Bush TL, Barrett-Connor E, Cowan LD, et al. Cardiovascular mortality and noncontraceptive use of estrogen in women: results from the Lipid Research Clinics Program Follow-up Study. *Circulation* 1987;75:1102–9
14. Henderson BE, Paganini-Hill A, Ross RK. Decreased mortality in users of estrogen replacement therapy. *Arch Intern Med* 1991;151:75–8
15. Sullivan JM, Vander Zwagg R, Hughes JP, et al. Estrogen replacement and coronary artery disease: effect on survival in postmenopausal women. *Arch Intern Med* 1990;150:2557–62
16. Sullivan JM, El-Zeky F, Vander Zwagg R, et al. Estrogen replacement therapy after coronary artery bypass surgery: effect on survival. *J Am Coll Cardiol* 1994;23:49A
17. O'Keefe JH Jr, Kim SC, Hall RR, et al. Estrogen replacement therapy after coronary angioplasty in women. *J Am Coll Cardiol* 1997;29:1–5
18. O'Brien JE, Peterson ED, Keeler GP, et al. Relation between estrogen replacement therapy and

restenosis after percutaneous coronary interventions. *J Am Coll Cardiol* 1996;28:1111–18
19. Newton KM, LaCroix AZ, McKnight B, *et al.* Estrogen replacement therapy and prognosis after first myocardial infarction. *Am J Epidemiol* 1997;145:269–77
20. Grodstein F, Stampfer MJ, Colditz GA, *et al.* Postmenopausal hormone therapy and mortality. *N Engl J Med* 1997;336:1769–75
21. Daly E, Vessey MP, Hawkins MM, *et al.* Increased risk of venous thromboembolism in hormone replacement therapy users. *Lancet* 1996;348:977–80
22. Jick H, Derby LF, Myers MW, *et al.* Risk of hospital admission for idiopathic venous thrombolism among users of postmenopausal estrogens. *Lancet* 1996;348:981–3
23. Grodstein F, Stampfer MJ, Goldhaber SZ, *et al.* A prospective study of exogenous hormones and risk of pumonary embolism in women. *Lancet* 1996;348:983–7
24. Walsh BW, Schiff I, Rosner B, *et al.* Effects of postmenopausal estrogen replacement on the concentrations and metabolism of plasma lipoproteins. *N Engl J Med* 1991;325:1196–204
25. The Writing Group for the PEPI Trial. Effects of estrogen or estrogen/progestin regimens on heart disease risk factors in postmenopausal women. The Postmenopausal Estrogen/Progestin Interventions (PEPI) Trial. *J Am Med Assoc* 1995;273:199–208
26. Clarkson TB, Shively CA, Morgan T, *et al.* Oral contraceptives and coronary artery atherosclerosis of cynomolgus monkeys. *Obstet Gynecol* 1990;75:217–22
27. Nabulsi AA, Folsom AR, White A, *et al.* Association of hormone-replacement therapy with various cardiovascular risk factors in postmenopausal women. *N Engl J Med* 1993;328:1069–75
28. Falkeborn M, Persson I, Adami HO, *et al.* The risk of acute myocardial infarction after oestrogen and oestrogen–progestogen replacement. *Br J Obstet Gynaecol* 1992;99:821–8
29. Nachtigall LE, Nachtigall RH, Nachtigall RD, *et al.* Estrogen replacement therapy II: a prospective study in the relationship to carcinoma and cardiovascular and metabolic problems. *Obstet Gynecol* 1979;54:74–9
30. Psaty BM, Heckbert SR, Atkins D, *et al.* The risk of myocardial infarction associated with the combined use of estrogens and progestins in postmenopausal women. *Arch Intern Med* 1994;154:1333–9
31. Grodstein F, Stampfer MJ, Manson JE, *et al.* Postmenopausal estrogen and progestin use and the risk of cardiovascular disease. *N Engl J Med* 1996;335:453–61
32. Furchgott RF, Zawadzk JV. The obligatory role of endothelial cells in the relaxation of arterial smooth muscle by acetylcholine. *Nature (London)* 1980;288:373–6
33. Ignarro LJ, Byrns RE, Buga GM, *et al.* Endothelium-derived relaxing factor (EDRF) released from artery and vein appears to be nitric oxide (NO) or a closely related radical species. *Fed Proc* 1987;46:644
34. Dzau VJ. Atherosclerosis and hypertension: mechanisms and interrelationships. *J Cardiovasc Pharmacol* 1990;15(Suppl.5):S59–84
35. Taddei S, Virdis A, Ghiadoni L, *et al.* Menopause is associated with endothelial dysfunction in women. *Hypertension* 1996;28:576–82
36. Williams JK, Adams MR, Klopfenstein HS. Estrogen modulates responses of atherosclerotic coronary arteries. *Circulation* 1990;81:1680–7
37. Herrington DM, Braden GA, Williams JK, *et al.* Endothelial-dependent coronary vasomotor responsiveness in postmenopausal women with and without estrogen replacement therapy. *Am J Cardiol* 1994;73:951–2
38. Reis SE, Gloth ST, Blumenthal RS, *et al.* Ethinyl estradiol acutely attenuates abnormal coronary vasomotor responses to acetylcholine in postmenopausal women. *Circulation* 1994;89:52–60
39. Gilligan DM, Quyyumi AA, Cannon RO III, *et al.* Effects of physiological levels of estrogen on coronary vasomotor function in postmenopausal women. *Circulation* 1994;89:2545–51
40. Collins P, Rosano GMC, Sarrel PM, *et al.* 17β-estradiol attenuates acetylcholine-induced coronary arterial constriction in women but not men with coronary heart disease. *Circulation* 1995;92:24–30
41. Arnal JF, Clamens S, Pechet C, *et al.* Ethinylestradiol does not enhance the expression of nitric oxide synthase in bovine endothelial cells but increases the release of bioactive nitric oxide by inhibiting superoxide anion production. *Proc Natl Acad Sci USA* 1996;93:4108–13
42. Jiang C, Sarrel PM, Poole-Wilson PA, *et al.* Acute effect of 17β-estradiol on rabbit coronary artery contractile responses to endothelin-1. *Am J Physiol* 1992;263:H271–5
43. Caulin-Glaser T, Watson CA, Pardi R, *et al.* Effects of 17β-estrodiol on cytokine-induced endothelial cell adhesion molecule expression. *J Clin Invest* 1996;98:36–42
44. Morales DE, McGowan KA, Grant DS, *et al.* Estrogen promotes angiogenic activity in human umbilical vein endothelial cells *in vitro* and in a murine model. *Circulation* 1995;91:755–63
45. Krasinaki K, Spyridopoulos I, Asahara T, *et al.* Estradiol accelerates functional endothelial recovery after arterial injury. *Circulation* 1997;95:1768–72

46. Spyridopoulos I, Sullivan AB, Kearney M, et al. Estrogen-receptor-mediated inhibition of human endothelial cell apoptosis. Estradiol as a survival factor. Circulation 1997;95:1505–14
47. Ludmer PL, Selwyn AP, Shook TL, et al. Paradoxical vasoconstriction induced by acetylcholine in atherosclerotic coronary arteries. N Engl J Med 1986;315:1046–51
48. Losordo DW, Kearney M, Kim EA, et al. Variable expression of the estrogen receptor in normal and atherosclerotic coronary arteries of premenopausal women. Circulation 1994;89:1501–10
49. Fogelberg M, Vesterquist O, Dicfalusy U, et al. Experimental athero-sclerosis: effects of estrogen and atherosclerosis on thromboxane and prostacyclin formation. Eur J Clin Invest 1990;20:105–10
50. Department of Health and Human Services. *Reducing the Health Consequences of Smoking: 25 Years of Progress.* Washington DC: Government Printing Office, 1989. DHHS publication (CDC) 89–8411
51. Rosenberg L, Miller DR, Kaufman DW, et al. Myocardial infarction in women under 50 years of age. J Am Med Assoc 1983;250:2801–6
52. Russell-Briefel R, Ezzati T, Fulwood R, et al. - Cardiovascular risk status and oral contraceptive use: United States, 1976–1980. Prev Med 1986;15:352–62
53. Drizd T, Dannenberg AL, Engel A. Blood pressure levels in persons 18–74 years of age in 1976–1980, and trends in blood pressure from 1960 to 1980 in the United States. PHS publication No. 86–1684. Washington DC: National Center for Health Statistics, July 1986
54. Burt VL, Whelton P, Roccella EJ, et al. Prevalence of hypertension in the US adult population. Results from the Third National Health and Nutrition Examination Survey, 1988–1991. Hypertension 1995;25:305–13
55. Kaplan N. Primary hypertension natural history, special populations and evaluations. *Clinical Hypertension,* 6th edn. Baltimore: Williams and Wilkins, 1994:109–43
56. HDFP Cooperative Group. Five-year findings of the Hypertension Detection and Follow-Up Program: II. Mortality by race, sex, and age. J Am Med Assoc 1979;242:2572–7
57. MRC Working Party. MRC trial of treatment of mild hypertension: principal results. Br Med J 1985;29–104
58. SHEP Cooperative Research Group. Prevention of stroke by antihypertensive drug treatment in older persons with isolated systolic hypertension: final results of the Systolic Hypertension in the Elderly Program (SHEP). J Am Med Assoc 1991;265:3255–64
59. Dannenberg AL, Drizd T, Horam MJ, et al. Progress in the battle against hypertension: changes in blood pressure levels in the United States from 1960–1980. Hypertension 1987;10:226–33
60. Bush TL, Barrett-Connor E, Cowan LD, et al. Cardiovascular mortality and noncontraceptive use of estrogen in women: results from the Lipid Research Clinics Program Follow-up Study. Circulation 1987;75:1102–9
61. Kannel WB, Castelli WP, Gordon T. Serum cholesterol, lipoproteins, and the risk of coronary heart disease. Ann Intern Med 1971;74:1–12
62. Kannel WB, Wilson PWF. Risk factors that attenuate the female coronary disease advantage. Arch Intern Med 1995;155:57–61
63. Kane JP, Malloy MJ, Ports TA, et al. Regression of coronary atherosclerosis during treatment of familial hypercholesterolemia with combined drug regimens. J Am Med Assoc 1990;264:3007–12
64. Levy RI, Brensike JF, Epstein SE, et al. The influence of changes in lipid values induced by cholestyramine and diet on progression of coronary artery disease: results of the NHLBI Type II Coronary Intervention Study. Circulation 1984;69:325–7
65. Rich-Edwards JW, Manson JE, Hennekens CH, et al. The primary prevention of coronary heart disease in women. N Engl J Med 1995;332:1758–66
66. Clawson BJ, Bell ET. Incidence of fatal coronary disease in nondiabetic and in diabetic patients. Arch Pathol 1949;48:105–6
67. Kessler II, Mortality experience of diabetic patients. A twenty-six year follow-up study. Am J Med 1971;51:715–24
68. Kannel WB, McGee DL. Diabetes and glucose tolerance as risk factors for cardiovascular disease: The Framingham Study. Diabetes Care 1979;2:120–6
69. Frey MAB, Doerr BM, Laubach LL, et al. Exercise does not change high-density lipoprotein cholesterol levels in women after ten weeks of training. Metabolism 1982;31:1142–6
70. Rotkis TC, Boyden TW, Stanforth PR, et al. Increased high-density lipoprotein cholesterol and lean weight in endurance-trained women runners. J Cardiac Rehabil 1984;4:62–6
71. Manson JE, Stampfer MJ, Colditz GA, et al. A prospective study of aspirin use and primary prevention of cardiovascular disease in women. J Am Med Assoc 1991;266:521–7

24

Hormone replacement therapy and diabetes mellitus

A. A. Oladipo, I. F. Godsland and J. C. Stevenson

INTRODUCTION

Hormone replacement therapy (HRT) is used for the relief of climacteric symptoms, prevention and treatment of osteoporosis, protection from coronary heart disease (CHD) and improvement of well-being. Women with diabetes mellitus may be deterred from taking HRT by their doctors or by cautions written in HRT package inserts. This stems from the observed adverse side-effects of the oral contraceptive estrogens on glucose tolerance. Diabetic women receive prescriptions for HRT 50% less frequently than their non-diabetic counterparts[1]. In contrast, women with hypertension are prescribed HRT much more frequently than women with diabetes. Oral contraceptive therapy and HRT are often regarded as similar because they both involve the administration of estrogen. They are entirely different, however, in that HRT requires modest doses of natural estrogen to rectify a state of hormone deficiency. Contraceptive therapy involves the administration of supraphysiological doses of synthetic estrogen to ensure effective contraception.

EFFECTS OF MENOPAUSE ON CARBOHYDRATE METABOLISM

Estrogen deficiency may well be associated with an increase in the incidence of diabetes mellitus. Siege and Hevelke reported such a relationship at the 6th Symposium of the German Endocrinological Society in 1959, in a study of 1455 diabetic women[2]. National surveys in the USA have shown that the incidence of diabetes increases dramatically in women over 50 years of age. When compared with men of similar age, this increase is greater for women. The prevalence of diabetes in white women aged between 50 and 65 years is 62% higher than in men of similar age[3].

In general, the transition to menopause has not been shown to cause an increase in fasting plasma glucose levels[4,5]. Neither is it apparently associated with an increase in 2-h oral glucose tolerance test (OGTT) plasma glucose or plasma insulin levels[6]. In a study of the relationship between the menopause and insulin response to glucose during intravenous glucose tolerance tests (IVGTTs), 66 premenopausal women were compared with 92 postmenopausal women[7,8]. The menopause did not cause a change in the plasma insulin response, but there was a significant decrease (15%) in the pancreatic insulin response. This was associated with an increase in plasma insulin half-life, which corrected for the deficiency in insulin secretion. The premenopausal women were studied in the luteal phase of the menstrual cycle when there could have been some increase in insulin resistance. No effect of the menopause *per se* was observed on insulin resistance, but further analysis revealed a progressive increase in insulin resistance with increasing time since menopause. Two other studies have demonstrated a progressive increase in circulating levels of insulin relating to time since menopause rather than chronological age[9,10]. This accords with increasing insulin resistance.

EFFECTS OF ESTROGEN ON CARBOHYDRATE METABOLISM

The menopause appears to be associated with a decrease in pancreatic insulin secretion, an increase in plasma insulin half-life and no effect on plasma insulin response during the IVGTT. Studies of estrogen administration and carbohydrate metabolism, therefore, would be expected to show opposite effects.

The natural estrogen, 17β-estradiol, is associated with improved insulin sensitivity[11]. Cagnacci and colleagues studied the effects of transdermal estradiol on plasma glucose, insulin and pancreatic insulin response during the OGTT in 15 postmenopausal women[12]. There was no change in glucose response, insulin response fell slightly and C-peptide response increased significantly. The increase in C-peptide response with no change in glucose response suggests an improved sensitivity of pancreatic insulin to glucose; the increase in C-peptide response with no increase in insulin response suggests an improvement in insulin elimination. The reduction in insulin response with no change in glucose response suggests a reduction in insulin resistance. Thus, each effect of estradiol was the opposite of the effect of the menopause.

The improvement in pancreatic insulin response with the administration of estrogen has been documented as far back as the late 1940s. Rodriguez showed that the incidence of diabetes in partially pancreatomized rats was reduced by 60% with the administration of estrogen[13]. In other animal studies of islets of Langerhans isolated from oophorectomized animals, there was a significant increase in pancreatic insulin response to glucose in animals treated with estrogen compared to untreated animals[14–16]. Furthermore, Manson in 1992, in a large prospective study of 21 028 postmenopausal non-diabetic women, showed reduced incidence of diabetes in HRT users over a 12-year period of follow-up[17].

Studies of carbohydrate metabolism with conjugated equine estrogens are few. The lower dose of 0.625 mg/day appears to have an improved or neutral effect on carbohydrate

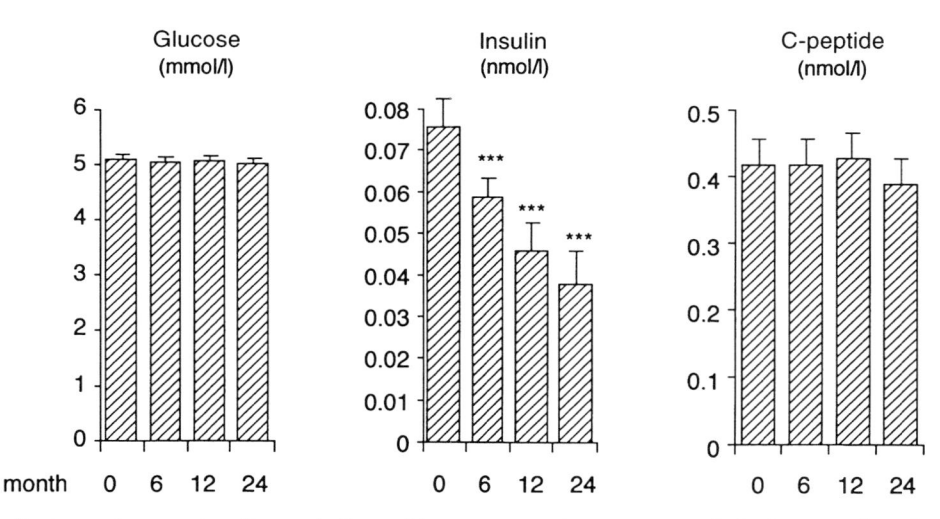

Figure 1 Fasting glucose, insulin and C-peptide concentrations measured during combined phase of treatment in women taking hormone replacement therapy (HRT) for 2 years with oral 17β-estradiol and cyclical dydrogesterone. ***$p < 0.001$. Adapted from reference 23

metabolism, while a higher dose of 1.25 mg/day causes a significant deterioration in glucose tolerance and insulin resistance[18–20].

The potent alkylated estrogens, ethinylestradiol and mestranol, are generally associated with changes consistent with increased insulin resistance[11]. This is possibly related to the secondary effects of these high-potency estrogens on glucocorticoid activity.

EFFECTS OF OPPOSED HRT ON CARBOHYDRATE METABOLISM

Estrogen replacement is administered alone to women without a uterus. For women with an intact uterus, an estrogen–progestogen combined HRT will be required for endometrial protection. Such a combination may be advisable in women who have had a subtotal hysterectomy, as residual endometrial tissue present on the cervical stump will respond to estrogen stimulation.

The effects of opposed HRT on carbohydrate metabolism are a consequence of the types of estrogen and progestogen used in that particular combination. Norethisterone acetate (NETA), levonorgestrel and medroxyprogesterone acetate are progestogens commonly used in combined HRT. Studies of their effects on carbohydrate metabolism suggest that NETA is entirely neutral[21,22]. However, the two other progestogens induce insulin resistance[18,21], and are associated with a deterioration in glucose tolerance[19–21]. Dydrogesterone, another progestogen increasingly used in HRT combinations, retains most of the beneficial effects of estradiol on glucose and insulin metabolism[23] (Figure 1).

HRT AND COMPLICATIONS OF DIABETES

Osteoporosis

Osteoporosis may be defined as a reduction in bone mass per unit volume such that fractures may occur with minimal trauma. It is the most common metabolic disease in the Western world. It has been reported in diabetes, particularly affecting cortical bone[24]. Trabecular bone predominates in the vertebral bodies and to a lesser extent in the posterior calcaneus, lower end of radius and proximal femur. These are the most common sites of osteoporotic fractures. Cortical bone predominates elsewhere in the skeleton, constituting 80% of the total skeleton.

Bone mass is normally maintained by a balance between bone formation (osteoblastic activity) and bone resorption (osteoclastic activity). In diabetes, bone formation is slowed; the osteons take between two and eight times longer to develop than in non-diabetics[25]. Diabetic osteopenia appears to be a low bone-turnover state with reduced osteoblastic activity, rather than increased bone resorption[26]. The exact mechanism by which this occurs is unknown, and may be related to the lack of insulin[27] (Figure 2). Insulin is an anabolic hormone[28,29]. It stimulates nucleotide synthesis by osteoblasts *in vitro*, promotes the intracellular accumulation of amino acids in membranous bone and restores levels of circulating somatomedin in experimental studies[30].

Patients with insulin-dependent diabetes mellitus (IDDM), who are insulin deficient and who also have an increased tendency to reduced body mass, have an increased risk of osteoporosis. However, patients with non-insulin-dependent diabetes mellitus (NIDDM), with insulin resistance and hyperinsulinemia who are frequently overweight, are reported to have an increased rather than a decreased bone mass[31].

Evidence regarding osteoporosis in diabetic patients is conflicting, however. In premenopausal women with IDDM, there is increased bone turnover, and they may be at increased risk of osteoporosis, therefore, after the menopause[32]. Postmenopausal women with IDDM have been shown to have lower spinal bone mineral density (BMD) when compared to age-matched controls or to postmenopausal women with NIDDM[33].

McNair measured BMD in insulin-treated diabetic adults matched for age and sex, and found it to be significantly reduced by 9.8%[34].

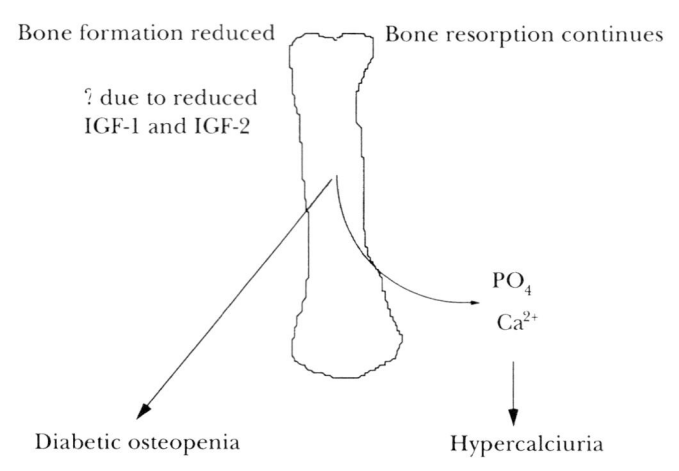

Figure 2 Bone formation is reduced while resorption continues at its normal rate. This 'uncoupling' liberates mineral from skeleton, resulting in hypercalciuria and diabetic osteopenia. IGF, insulin-like growth factor. Adapted from reference 27

Similar results have been reported in children[35]. The rate of bone loss is maximal at, or soon after, diagnosis of diabetes and has been shown to be negatively correlated with endogenous insulin levels[34]. The relationship between the degree of metabolic control in patients with IDDM and degree of osteopenia is as yet poorly understood.

Patients with NIDDM are theoretically protected from bone loss owing to their increased tendency for obesity and hyperinsulinemia. Increased adipose tissue yields metabolically active estrogen and insulin-like growth factor which stimulate bone formation. Mean BMD in women with NIDDM is similar to mean BMD matched for age and weight in controls[31]. Bone mineral content in the distal radius of pre- and postmenopausal women with NIDDM is not different from age-matched controls. In addition, in NIDDM, there is no relationship between glycemic control and bone mineral content[36].

Studies of NIDDM by other investigators have produced conflicting evidence[27]. Wakasugi and colleagues[37] showed that BMD is decreased in NIDDM and that the decrease correlates with duration of the disease and deficit in insulin secretion.

Bone density decreases with age. The menopause is the single most important cause of bone loss and osteoporosis[38]. In the Western world, the average life expectancy for women is 82 years. Jensen and co-workers have shown that, by the age of 70 years, one out of every two women will have sustained at least one osteoporotic fracture[39].

Of this number of women who are otherwise healthy, one out of every five women who sustains a hip fracture will die as a result, and many more will suffer prolonged pain and immobility[40]. Hormone replacement is the most effective therapy for the prevention and treatment of postmenopausal bone loss[41]. Commenced early in the menopause and continued for at least 5 years, HRT would halve the incidence of osteoporotic fractures[42]. There is no reason to suggest that this benefit is lost in women with diabetes who may already have accelerated bone loss premenopausally.

The diabetic complications of retinopathy, neuropathy and osteopathy may increase the incidence of fractures independent of bone mass[43]. These complications will greatly increase morbidity and mortality of osteoporotic fractures in postmenopausal diabetic women.

The increasing availability of non-invasive and sensitive measurements of bone density will allow these at-risk women to be screened; HRT can then be advised, as in non-diabetic postmenopausal women, for bone protection.

Hypertension

Hypertension in diabetes represents an important health problem, as the two diseases commonly occur together. The presence of one disease predisposes to the other, and hypertension is commonly found in diabetics[44]. It is present almost twice as much in diabetics than in the general population. As much as one-third to one-half of European diabetics over the age of 35 years may be affected. The prevalence is much higher in women and Afro-Caribbeans[45,46]. Women with diabetes and hypertension are at increased risk of dying from CHD and stroke when compared to male diabetics and normotensive diabetics. Current advice cautions on the use of HRT in women with hypertension with or without diabetes[47]. This is based on studies with oral contraceptive estrogens. In premenopausal women, oral contraceptive estrogens are known to cause an increase in systolic and diastolic blood pressure[48]. In normotensive postmenopausal women, the use of HRT does not appear to be associated with an increase in blood pressure[49]. There is accumulating evidence to show that HRT in hypertensive patients is not associated with a worsening of blood pressure control[50].

There is an age-related increase in blood pressure. The menopause is also associated with an increase in blood pressure which is entirely independent of age[51]. The mechanism of hypertension in postmenopausal diabetic women, thus, is multifactorial and is complicated by the effects of microvascular disease and nephropathy.

Feher and colleagues have demonstrated no significant changes in blood pressure in the short term in stable NIDDM in women on oral HRT[52]. Lip and associates, in 1994, demonstrated no change in mean blood pressure over 18 months in hypertensive postmenopausal women on HRT[50]. The route of estrogen administration did not significantly affect blood pressure. Other studies of hypertensive postmenopausal women on oral HRT have shown a fall in blood pressure[53,54].

The exact mechanism by which HRT may affect blood pressure is unknown. Studies investigating the effects of estradiol on the renin–angiotensin system in normotensive and hypertensive women did not show a change in plasma concentration of renin, angiotensin II and aldosterone[53]. There was no change in blood pressure over 6 months in normotensive women. Systolic blood pressure fell in hypertensive women during this treatment.

It would appear that diabetic women who are also hypertensive may be treated with oral or transdermal HRT, at least in the short term, as it does not have adverse effects on blood pressure control. The same indications in normotensive women would apply to this group of women.

The effect of long-term administration of HRT in hypertensive diabetic women needs to be investigated further with controlled clinical trials.

Diabetic dyslipidemia

Diabetes mellitus is associated with abnormal lipid and lipoprotein profiles. These dyslipidemias are well documented. Hypertriglyceridemia is the most common lipid abnormality. This is caused by reduced clearance of triglycerides by lipoprotein-lipase, which is insulin-dependent, and increased supply of non-esterified fatty acids to the liver. Very low-density lipoprotein (VLDL) and low-density lipoprotein (LDL) cholesterol levels are also increased. The high-density lipoprotein (HDL) cholesterol levels is decreased in IDDM and more significantly reduced in NIDDM[55]. Low levels of HDL and increased levels of triglycerides are both risk markers of atherosclerosis and coronary heart disease in women[56]. Coronary heart disease is the principal cause of death in diabetics, and women appear to be particularly susceptible[57]. Women with diabetes have significantly higher levels of triglycerides and lower levels of HDL than their male diabetic counterparts[58].

Lipoprotein(a) originates in the liver. Its function is not yet fully understood. It may compete with plasminogen for binding sites on endothelial cells and monocytes, thus inhibiting fibrinolysis and promoting thrombus formation. High levels of lipoprotein(a) are an independent marker of accelerated atherosclerotic disease.

Conflicting evidence exists in the literature about the levels of lipoprotein(a) in diabetes. Normal, reduced and increased levels have all been described[59]. The CHD risk profile in diabetes may be further worsened when lipoprotein(a) is elevated.

The menopause is associated with changes in the lipid profile which are unfavorable for CHD[60]. High-density lipoprotein cholesterol is reduced and total cholesterol, triglycerides and LDL cholesterol are increased. The onset of the menopause in diabetic women could impose a greater risk of CHD. There is well-established evidence in the literature that HRT lowers total cholesterol, independent of route of administration[61]. The increase in HDL associated with oral estrogen appears to be greater than that associated with transdermal estrogen[62]. Estrogen inhibits hepatic lipase activity, thereby increasing HDL cholesterol, especially the HDL-2 subfraction which is thought to protect against atherogenesis[63]. Estrogen reduces LDL cholesterol mainly through upregulation of apolipoprotein B 100 receptors. Hormone replacement therapy may increase the proportion of smaller, denser LDL particles[64], but it also reduces the oxidation of these particles rendering them less atherogenic[65]. The effect of estrogen on triglycerides is dependent on the type of estrogen and route of administration. Oral conjugated estrogens cause a significant increase in the level of triglycerides owing to the hepatic first-pass effect[62]. Oral estradiol causes a less marked increase in triglycerides.

Transdermal estradiol, on the other hand, causes a reduction in triglycerides[62]. This is of particular importance in deciding on the type of HRT to prescribe to diabetics who commonly have hypertriglyceridemia.

The effects of progestogens on lipids and lipoproteins differ depending on their androgenicity. Androgenic progestogens, e.g. norgestrel, derived from testosterone, negate the HDL-raising effect of estrogen because they increase hepatic lipase activity[62]. However, they cause a decrease in triglycerides[62] and lipoprotein(a)[66-68]. The less androgenic C-21 progestogens, in contrast, do not reverse the beneficial effect of estrogen on HDL cholesterol to any great extent. Dydrogesterone, in particular, does not appear to negate the effects of estradiol on HDL[23].

Evidence is accumulating to show that the beneficial effects of non-contraceptive estrogens are not lost in postmenopausal diabetic women[69]. Robinson and colleagues have shown that diabetic women on HRT have higher levels of HDL compared to those not on HRT[70]. They have shown that LDL cholesterol and apolipoprotein B levels are lower, and that apolipoprotein A levels are higher with HRT, to a similar degree in diabetic as in non-diabetic women. Administration of HRT to postmenopausal diabetic women appears to result in a less atherogenic lipid profile in this group of women who are at risk of CHD because of their abnormal lipid profile.

Coronary heart disease

Coronary heart disease (CHD) is the single most common cause of death in diabetes. It is not often appreciated that CHD is the major cause of death in women, and that CHD is associated with a worse prognosis in females than in males. In population studies, female diabetic patients have four times as much and male diabetics twice the cardiovascular mortality rate of age- and sex-matched non-diabetic controls[71]. In patients with established CHD, surgical and non-surgical revascularization procedures are less successful in females than in males[72,73]. The pathogenesis of CHD in diabetes is multifactorial and includes hyperinsulinemia, hypertension, abnormal lipid profile, arterial disease and nephropathy. Estrogen administration has been shown to have beneficial effects on most of these parameters.

There is substantial epidemiological evidence to show that non-diabetic postmenopausal women on HRT are protected from CHD[74-76]. The protection may be as much as 30–50%. In a population study of Swedish women receiving HRT, the addition of cyclical progestogens to estrogen therapy did not negate the protective effect of estrogen on cardiovascular morbidity[77]. Henderson and colleagues showed a decrease in mortality from acute myocardial infarction in users of HRT; this reduction was maintained in the presence of known risk factors for CHD[76]. Postmenopausal estrogen use protects against CHD even in current smokers[78].

McFarland and co-workers evaluated the risk factors for CHD in women with angiographically proven heart disease. The risk of severe CHD was significantly reduced by the use of non-contraceptive estrogen[79]. A reduced risk in CHD mortality of up to 87% has been reported in women with established CHD using estrogen[80].

The presence of diabetes does not appear to negate the beneficial effect of HRT on the heart: HRT reduces the risk of non-fatal myocardial infarction in the presence of diabetes and known risk factors for CHD[81,82]. The cardioprotective effects of HRT may prove to be the most important benefit of HRT in diabetic and non-diabetic women. The exact extent and mechanism of CHD reduction in diabetes are unknown. Long-term randomized clinical trials need to be carried out to evaluate this issue.

CONCLUSION

The benefits of HRT on the skeletal system and cardiovascular system are clear. Diabetic women constitute a high-risk group of women, and the complications arising from the disease itself are a major health concern. There have been few studies into the effects of HRT on diabetes. Estrogen does not appear to worsen the morbidity and mortality associated with diabetes. In prescribing HRT to diabetics, there is little scientific justification at present to routinely recommend more intense monitoring of these patients. The potential impact of HRT on cardiovascular morbidity and mortality in diabetes is overwhelming, and needs to be clarified by randomized clinical trials. Hormone replacement therapy may yet occupy a place in the primary prevention of CHD in women, particularly those at high risk of CHD, such as diabetics.

References

1. Feher MD, Isaacs AJ. Is hormone replacement therapy prescribed for diabetic women? *Br J Clin Pract* 1996;50:431–2
2. Siege K, Hevelke G. The effect of female gonadal function on the manifestation and frequency of diabetes mellitus. In *6th Symposium of the German Endocrinological Society: Modern Developments in Progestagenic Hormones in Veterinary Medicine*. Kiel: Springer-Verlag, 1959:274–9
3. Harris MI, Hadden WC, Knowler WC, Bennett PH. Prevalence of diabetes and impaired glucose tolerance and plasma glucose levels in the US population aged 20–74 years. *Diabetes* 1987;36:523–34
4. Hjortland MC, McNamara PM, Kannel WB. Some atherogenic concomitants of the menopause: the Framingham study. *Am J Epidemiol* 1976;103:304–11
5. Bonithon-Kopp C, Scarabin P, Darne B, *et al.* Menopause related changes in lipoproteins and some other cardiovascular risk factors. *Int J Epidemiol* 1990;19:42–8
6. Mathews K, Meilahn E, Kuller L, *et al.* Menopause and risk factors for coronary heart disease. *N Engl J Med* 1989;321:641–6
7. Godsland IF, Walton C, Stevenson JC. Impact of menopause on metabolism. In Diamond MP, Naftolin F, eds. *Metabolism in the Female Life Cycle*. Rome: Serono Symposia, 1993:171–89
8. Walton C, Godsland I, Proudler A, Wynn V, Stevenson J. The effects of the menopause on insulin sensitivity, secretion and elimination in nonobese, healthy women. *Eur J Clin Invest* 1993;23:466–73
9. Proudler A, Felton C, Stevenson J. Ageing and the response of plasma insulin, glucose and C-peptide concentrations to intravenous glucose in postmenopausal women. *Clin Sci* 1992;83:489–94
10. Godsland IF, Crook D, Stevenson JC, *et al.* The insulin resistance syndrome in postmenopausal women with cardiological syndrome X. *Br Heart J* 1995;74:47–52
11. Godsland IF. The influence of female sex steroids on glucose metabolism and insulin action. *J Intern Med* 1996;240(Suppl):1–60

12. Cagnacci A, Soldani R, Carriero P, *et al.* Effects of low doses of transdermal 17β-estradiol on carbohydrate metabolism in postmenopausal women. *J Clin Endocrinol Metab* 1992;74:1396–400
13. Rodriguez R. Influence of estrogens and androgens on the production and prevention of diabetes. In Leibel B, Wrenshall G, eds. *On the Nature and Treatment of Diabetes.* New York: Excerpta Medica; 1965:288–307
14. Bailey C, Ahmed-Sorour H. Role of ovarian hormones in the long-term control of glucose homeostasis. *Diabetologia* 1980;19:475–81
15. El Seifi S, Green I, Perrin D. Insulin release and steriod-hormone binding in isolated islets of Langerhans in the rat: effects of ovariectomy. *J Endocrinol* 1981;90:59–67
16. Faure A, Haourari M, Sutter B-C-J. Insulin secretion and biosynthesis after oestradiol treatment. *Horm Metab Res* 1985;17:378
17. Manson JE. A prospective study of postmenopausal oestrogen therapy and subsequent incidence of non-insulin dependent diabetes mellitus. *Ann Epidemiol* 1992;2:665–73
18. Lindheim SR, Presser SC, Ditkoff EC, *et al.* A possible bimodal effect of estrogen on insulin sensitivity in postmenopausal women and the attenuating effect of added progestin. *Fertil Steril* 1993;60:664–7
19. Lobo RA, Pickar JH, Wild RA, *et al.* Metabolic impact of adding medroxyprogesterone acetate to conjugated estrogen therapy in postmenopausal women. *Obstet Gynecol* 1994;84:987–95
20. The Writing Group for the PEPI Trial. Effects of estrogen or estrogen/progestin regimens on heart disease risk factors in postmenopausal women: the Postmenopausal Estrogen/Progestin Interventions (PEPI) Trial. *J Am Med Assoc* 1995;273:199–208
21. Godsland I, Gangar K, Walton C, *et al.* Insulin resistance, secretion and elimination in postmenopausal women receiving oral or transdermal hormone replacement therapy. *Metabolism* 1993;42:846–53
22. Luotola H, Loikkaanen M. Effects of natural oestrogen/progestogen substitution therapy on carbohydrate and lipid metabolism in postmenopausal women. *Maturitas* 1986;8:245–53
23. Crook D, Godsland IF, Hull J, *et al.* Hormone replacement therapy with dydrogesterone and 17β-oestradiol: effects on serum lipoproteins and glucose tolerance during 24 month follow-up. *Br J Obstet Gynaecol* 1997;104: 298–304
24. McNair P, Madsbad S, Christensen MS. Bone mineral loss in insulin treated diabetes mellitus; studies in pathology. *Acta Endocrinol* 1979;90: 463–72
25. Takeheshi H, Frost HM. The kinetics of the resorption process in osteonal remodelling of diabetic rib. *Henry Ford Med Bull* 1964;12:537–45
26. Silberg R. The skeleton in diabetes mellitus: a review of the literature. *Diabetes Res* 1986;3: 329–38
27. Bruce R, Stevenson JC. Bone and mineral metabolism in diabetes. In Pickup JC, Williams G, eds. *Chronic Complications of Diabetes.* Oxford: Blackwell Scientific Publications. 1994:269–72
28. Puche RC. The effect of insulin on bone resorption. *Calcif Tissue Res* 1973;12:8–15
29. Hahn TJ. Insulin effect of amino-acid transport in bone: dependence on protein synthesis and sodium. *Am J Physiol* 1971;220:1717–23
30. Phillip LS. Diabetic control, somatomedin and growth in rats. *Diabetes* 1977;26:864–9
31. Winstock RS, Goland RS. Bone mineral density in women with type II diabetes. *J Bone Miner Res* 1989;4:97–101
32. Gallacher SJ, Fenner JA, Fisher BM, *et al.* An evaluation of bone density and turnover in premenopausal women with type 1 diabetes mellitus. *Diabetic Med* 1993;10:129–33
33. Saneshigie S. Spinal bone mineral density in the female diabetic population. *Jpn J Geriatr* 1992;29: 864–73
34. McNair P. Osteopenia in insulin dependent diabetes mellitus: relation to age at onset, sex and duration of disease. *Diabetologie* 1978;15:87–9
35. Shore RM. Osteopenia in juvenile diabetes. *Calcif Tissue Int* 1981;33:455–7
36. Giacci A, Fassina A. Bone mineral density in diabetes mellitus. *Bone* 1988;9:29–36
37. Wakasugi M, Wakao R, Tawata M, *et al.* Bone mineral density as measured by dual energy X-ray absorptiometry in patients with non insulin dependent diabetes mellitus. *Bone* 1993;14: 29–33
38. Stevenson JC, Banks LM, Spinks TJ, *et al.* Regional and total skeletal measurements in the early menopause. *J Clin Invest* 1987;80:258–62
39. Jensen GF, Christiansen C, Boesen J, *et al.* Epidemiology of spinal and long bone fractures: a unifying approach to postmenopausal osteoporosis. *J Orthop Res* 1982; 166:75–81
40. Stevenson JC, Whitehead MI. Postmenopausal osteoporosis. *Br Med J* 1982;285:585–8
41. Consensus Development Conference. Prophylaxis and treatment of osteoporosis. *Br Med J* 1987;295:15
42. Stevenson JC, Lees B, Davenport M, *et al.* Determinants of bone density in normal women: risk factors for future osteoporosis? *Br Med J* 1989;298:924–8
43. Ziegler R. Diabetes mellitus and bone metabolism. *Horm Metab Res* 1992;26(Suppl):90–4

44. World Health Organization Multinational Study. Prevalence of small vessel and large vessel disease in diabetic patients from 14 centres. *Diabetologia* 1985;28:(Suppl):615–40
45. Drury PL. Hypertension. *Baillière's Clin Endocrinol Metab* 1988;2:375–89
46. Simson DC. Aetiology and prevalence of hypertension in diabetic patients. *Diabetes Care* 1988;11:821–7
47. Drife JO. Hormone replacement therapy. *Prescribers J* 1989;29:131–8
48. Khaw KT, Peart WS. Blood pressure and contraceptive use. *Br Med J* 1982;285:403–7
49. Perry I, Beevers M, Beevers DG, et al. Oestrogens and cardiovascular disease. *Br Med J* 1988;297:1127
50. Lip GYH, Beevers M, Churchill D, et al. Hormone replacement therapy and blood pressure in hypertensive women. *J Hum Hyperten* 1994;8:491–4
51. Staessen J, Bulpitt CJ, Fagard R, et al. The influence of menopause on blood pressure. *J Hum Hypertens* 1989;3:427–33
52. Feher MD, Cox A, Levy A, et al. Short term blood pressure and metabolic effects of tibolone in postmenopausal women with non-insulin dependent diabetes. *Br J Obstet Gynaecol* 1996;103:281–3
53. Jespersen CM, Arnung K, Hagan C, et al. Effects of natural oestrogen therapy on blood pressure and renin–angiotensin system in normotensive and hypertensive menopausal women. *J Hypertens* 1983;1:361–4
54. Pfeffer RI, Kurosaki TT, Charlton SK. Oestrogen use and blood pressure in later life. *Am J Epidemiol* 1979;110:469–78
55. Billingham MS, Leatherdale BA, Hall RA, et al. High density lipoprotein cholesterol and apolipoprotein a-1 concentrations in non-insulin dependent diabetes treated by diet and chlorpropamide. *Diabetes Metab* 1982;8:229–33
56. Miller Bass K, Newschaffer CJ, Klag MJ, et al. Plasma lipoprotein levels as predictors of cardiovascular death in women. *Arch Intern Med* 1993;153:2209–16
57. Barrett-Connor EL, Cohn BA, Wingard DL, et al. Why is diabetes mellitus a stronger risk factor for fatal ischaemic heart disease in women than in men? The Rancho Bernardo Study. *J Am Med Assoc* 1991;265:627–31
58. Walden C, Knopp R, Wahl P. Sex differences in the effect of diabetes mellitus on lipoprotein triglyceride and cholesterol concentrations. *N Engl J Med* 1984;311:953–9
59. Westerhuis LW, Venekamp WJ. Serum lipoprotein-a levels and glyco-metabolic control in insulin and non-insulin dependent diabetes mellitus. *Clin Biochem* 1996;29:255–9
60. Stevenson JC, Crook D, Godsland IF. Influence of age and menopause on serum lipids and lipoproteins in healthy women. *Atherosclerosis* 1993;98:83–90
61. Whitcroft SI, Crook D, Marsh MS, et al. Long-term effects of transdermal and oral hormone replacement therapies on serum lipid and lipoprotein concentrations. *Obstet Gynecol* 1994;84:222–6
62. Crook D, Cust MP, Ganger KF, et al. Comparison of oral and transdermal oestrogen/progestin hormone replacement therapy: effects on serum lipids and lipoproteins. *Am J Obstet Gynecol* 1992;166:950–5
63. Crook D, Stevenson JC, Whitehead MI. Estrogen replacement therapy and cardiovascular disease: effects on plasma lipid risk markers. In Swartz DP, ed. *Hormone Replacement Therapy*. Baltimore: Williams and Wilkins, 1992:139–70
64. Van der Mooren MJ, de Graf J, Demacker PN, et al. Changes in the low density lipoprotein profile during 17β-oestradiol/dydrogesterone therapy in post menopausal women. *Metabolism* 1994;43:799–802
65. Sack MN, Rader DJ, Cannon RO. Oestrogen and inhibition of oxidation low-density lipoproteins in post menopausal women. *Lancet* 1994;343:269–70
66. Farrish E, Rolton HA, Barnes JF, et al. Lipoprotein(a) concentrations in postmenopausal women taking norethisterone. *Br Med J* 1991;303:694
67. Rymer J, Crook D, Sidhu M, et al. Effects of tibolone on serum concentrations of lipoprotein(a) in post menopausal women. *Acta Endocrinol* 1993;128:259–62
68. Marsh MS, Crook D, Whitcroft SIJ, et al. Effect of continuous combined oestrogen and desogestrel hormone replacement therapy on serum lipids and lipoproteins. *Obstet Gynecol* 1994;83:19–23
69. Brussard HE, Gevers-Leuven JA, Kluft C, et al. Effect of 17β-oestradiol on plasma lipids in postmenopausal women with type-II diabetes mellitus. *Arterioscler Thromb Vasc Biol* 1997;17:324–30
70. Robinson JC, Folsom AR, Nabulsi AA, et al. Can postmenopausal hormone replacement therapy improve plasma lipids in women with diabetes? *Diabetes Care* 1996;19:480–5
71. Jarret RJ. The epidemiology of CHD and related factors in the context of diabetes mellitus and impaired glucose tolerance. In Jarret R, ed. *Diabetes and Heart Disease*. Amsterdam: Elsevier Science, 1984:1–23
72. Tofler GH, Stone PH, Muller JE, et al. Effects of gender and race on prognosis after myocardial infarction: adverse prognosis for women,

particularly black women. *J Am Coll Cardiol* 1987; 9:473–82
73. Cowley MJ, Mullin SM, Kelsey SF, *et al.* Sex differences in early and long-term results of coronary angioplasty in National Heart and Lung Institute PTCA registry. *Circulation* 1985;71:90–7
74. Bush TL, Barrett-Connor E, Cowan LD, *et al.* Cardiovascular mortality and noncontraceptive use of estrogen in women: results from the Lipid Research Clinics Program Follow-up Study. *Circulation* 1987;75:1102–9
75. Hunt K, Vessey M, McPherson K, *et al.* Long term surveillance of mortality and cancer incidence in women receiving hormone replacement therapy. *Br J Obstet Gynaecol* 1987;94:620–35
76. Henderson BE, Paganini-Hill A, Ross RK. Oestrogen replacement therapy and protection from acute myocardial infarction. *Am J Obstet Gynecol* 1988;159:312–17
77. Falkeborn M, Persson I, Adami HO, *et al.* The risk of acute myocardial infarction after oestrogen and oestrogen/progestogen replacement. *Br J Obstet Gynaecol* 1992;97:821–8
78. Criqui MH, Suarez L, Barrett-Connor E, *et al.* Post menopausal oestrogen use and mortality. Results from a prospective study in a defined, homogeneous community. *Am J Epidemiol* 1988; 128:606–14
79. McFarland KF, Boniface ME, Hornung CA, *et al.* Risk factors and noncontraceptive oestrogen use in women with and without coronary disease. *Am Heart J* 1989; 117:1209–14
80. Hong MK, Romm PA, Reagan K, *et al.* Effects of oestrogen replacement therapy on serum lipids values and angiographically defined coronary artery disease in postmenopausal women. *Am J Cardiol* 1992;69:176–8
81. Stampfer MJ, Willett WC, Colditz GA, *et al.* A prospective study of postmenopausal oestrogen therapy and coronary heart disease. *N Engl J Med* 1985;313:1044–9
82. Hernandez-Avila M, Walker AM, Jick H. Use of replacement oestrogens and the risk of myocardial infarction. *Epidemiology* 1990;1:128–33

25
Treatment of progestogen intolerance

N. Panay and J. Studd

INTRODUCTION

Progestogens are necessary for non-hysterectomized women on estrogen therapy, to maintain a secretory or atrophic endometrium and to prevent hyperplasia[1]. Unfortunately, intolerance of progestogenic side-effects and progestogen-related bleeding problems are the main reasons for the poor compliance with hormone replacement therapy (HRT)[2,3]. This leads to high discontinuation rates[4] and reduces the cost-effectiveness of therapy[5]. There has also been anxiety that progestogens may produce metabolic disturbances, for instance in cardiovascular risk markers, and that there may be an adverse effect on the risk of breast cancer. It is vital to be able to treat progestogen intolerance effectively to maximize the benefits of estrogen therapy and aid compliance. To achieve this goal, it is necessary to have a good understanding of the pathogenesis of progestogenic side-effects. Through this, effective treatment regimens to reduce progestogen intolerance can be instituted to either deal with the side-effects directly or alter the progestogen regimen. This chapter aims to provide the reader with current and possible future management options for dealing with progestogen intolerance.

MANAGEMENT OF ADVERSE PROGESTOGENIC EFFECTS

The effect common to all progestogens is that of inducing a secretory phase in the estrogen-primed endometrium. However, depending on their derivation and dosage, progestogens may have androgenic and/or estrogenic or anti-androgenic and/or antiestrogenic effects. Progestogens may also have mineralocorticoid and glucocorticoid-type effects (Table 1). All these effects are instrumental in determining the pathophysiology of adverse progestogenic effects. Figure 1 shows a classification of the

Table 1 Summary of psychological, physical and metabolic effects of progestogens

Psychological	*Metabolic*	*Physical*
Anxiety	adverse lipid changes	acne
Irritability	increased insulin resistance	greasy skin
Aggression	increased vascular resistance	abdominal cramps/bloating
Restlessness		fluid retention
Panic attacks		weakness
Depressed mood		headaches
Poor concentration		dizziness
Forgetfulness		breast tenderness
Lethargy		??breast cancer
Emotional lability		

Progesterone

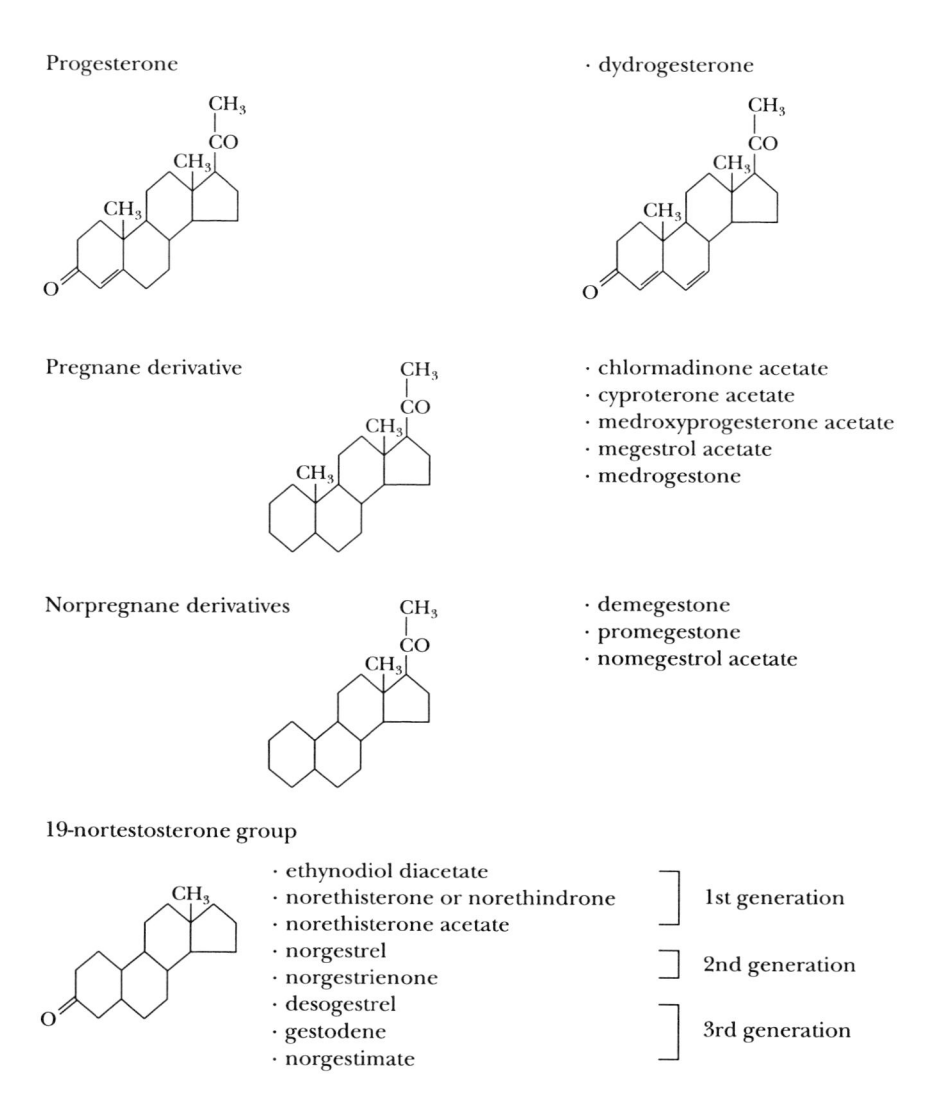

· dydrogesterone

Pregnane derivative
- chlormadinone acetate
- cyproterone acetate
- medroxyprogesterone acetate
- megestrol acetate
- medrogestone

Norpregnane derivatives
- demegestone
- promegestone
- nomegestrol acetate

19-nortestosterone group
- ethynodiol diacetate
- norethisterone or norethindrone   ⎤ 1st generation
- norethisterone acetate
- norgestrel
- norgestrienone   ⎤ 2nd generation
- desogestrel
- gestodene   ⎤ 3rd generation
- norgestimate

Figure 1 Chemical classification of progestogens

various types of progestogens and their derivation from progesterone.

Bleeding problems

Pathogenesis of bleeding problems

The effect of progestogens on the endometrium is mediated via a decrease in estrogen receptors and an increase in the 17α-oxoreductase activity that converts estradiol to estrone. Progestogens inhibit mitotic activity as shown by the decrease in the number of mitoses in both the glandular epithelium and stroma. They induce secretory transformation, with production of stromal edema, pseudodecidualization and glandular suppression. After a few weeks of progestogenic exposure, areas of superficial focal necrosis become apparent and, in the long term, the endometrium develops very suppressed glandular development, thin atrophic stroma and more generalized necrotic areas.

Progestogens are protective to the endometrium in a dose- and duration-dependent manner. The incidence of endometrial hyperplasia is reduced to 4% with 7 days of progestogen treatment, 2% with 10 days and 0% with 12 days of progestogen if prescribed at an adequate daily dosage[1,6]. Despite these effects, the exact relationship between progestogens in HRT and bleeding patterns remains largely unknown. This is because of considerable interindividual variability[7], complex estrogen–progestogen interactions[8] and the absence of an appropriate animal model. These factors and the different plasma estradiol levels with different doses or routes of administration explain why some patients experience problems with heavy, prolonged periods and endometrial hyperplasia, whereas the same duration, dose and type of progestogen would produce atrophy in another patient. A recent study has demonstrated that, broadly speaking, there appear to be two endometrial bleeding responses to sequential HRT: one with a mean cycle length of 29 days (late bleeders) and another with a cycle of shorter duration (early bleeders). The latter group appear to have less variability in cycle length and bleeding of shorter duration. No significant differences were demonstrable between the two groups in terms of past history or physical characteristics, except that early bleeders included more smokers. It was postulated that smoking could lead to bleeding problems as a result of a hypoestrogenic state[9].

Prevention and treatment of bleeding problems

Dose and duration of progestogen Manipulation of the dosage and duration of progestogen in sequential HRT is of value and has been practiced for many years. If heavy/prolonged bleeding occurs on sequential therapy and pathology has been excluded, it may be necessary to use a longer duration and/or more androgenic progestogen to control the bleeding. It is of more value to increase the duration of progestogen than the dosage in controlling bleeding problems. These increases will need to be balanced according to the physical/psychological side-effects produced by the progestogen. If cystic hyperplasia does occur with estrogen therapy, it can be resolved with three courses of 21 days of progestogen in virtually all cases[10].

Continuous combined regimens A smaller dosage of progestogen given on a daily basis should theoretically produce amenonorrhea with an atrophic endometrium, which should be more acceptable to postmenopausal women[11,12]. Irregular vaginal bleeding occurs in approximately 40% of women during the first 3 months of treatment leading to high drop-out rates. Those who continue treatment over 6–9 months can expect high rates of amenorrhea with minimal side-effects and good rates of compliance (Figure 2). Three oral preparations of continuous combined therapy are now available, which can be used if bleeding is not desired by the woman, assuming that it has been at least 1 year since the last menstrual period or if HRT has been used for at least a year.

Quarterly regimens Long-cycle HRT reduces to a minimum the number of progestogenic episodes and withdrawal bleeds. Despite there

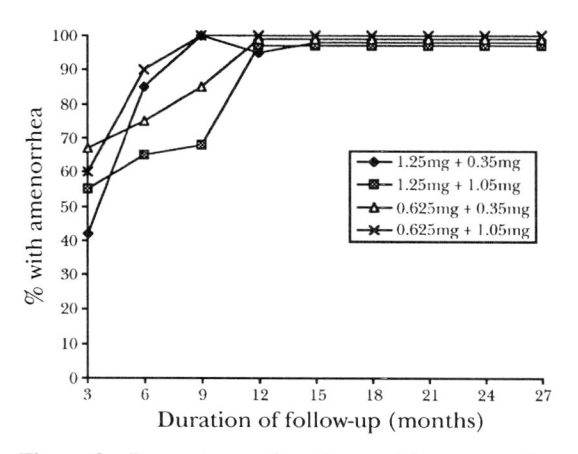

Figure 2 Percentage of patients with amenorrhea in women receiving oral conjugated estrogens (0.625–1.25 mg) and low-dose progestogen (norethisterone 0.35–1.05 mg) continuously. Adapted from reference 11

being only four cycles per year, the rates of endometrial hyperplasia appear to be comparable with those of sequential regimens after 1 year of treatment[13]. The disadvantage of this regimen is that, when the progestogenic episode does occur, it can be associated with heavy and/or prolonged withdrawal bleeding.

Hormone releasing intrauterine systems The *levonorgestrel intrauterine system* (LNG IUS) (Figure 3) consists of a plastic T-shaped frame with a steroid reservoir around the vertical stem of polydimethylsiloxane containing 52 mg of levonorgestrel released at a rate of 20 µg per day. It has been shown to be effective at controlling endometrial hypertrophy by suppressing endometrial growth[14]. After a few weeks, the endometrial glands atrophy, the stroma becomes swollen and decidual, the mucosa thins and the epithelium becomes inactive. As a result of the suppression caused by the local release of hormone, also mediated by the regulatory action of high local levels of progestogen on endometrial estrogen receptors, the endometrium becomes unresponsive to estrogen[15]. In the past few years, workers have also shown that the LNG IUS can prevent endometrial proliferation and reduces bleeding in perimenopausal women using oral or transdermal estradiol[16–18]. Work recently completed in the present authors' unit showed that severity of bleeding was reduced to a minimum when patients using mainly estradiol implants, even with relatively high serum estradiol levels, were switched from oral progestogens to the LNG IUS. Endometrial suppression was uniform, with no cases of endometrial proliferation or hyperplasia at 1 year, and a greater than 50% rate of amenorrhea at this time[19] (Figures 4a and b).

The LNG IUS is licensed for use as progestogenic opposition in HRT in Finland but it is only licensed in the UK for contraception at present. Its use in the HRT context, therefore, should be restricted to hospitals for now, where monitoring of the endometrium can be carried out with scans and biopsies.

The *Progestasert® intrauterine progesterone system* (PIPS) (Figure 3) consists of a polymeric T-shaped platform with a reservoir containing 38 mg of progesterone released at a rate of 65 µg per day. Results of two recent studies[20,21] indicate that the PIPS also suppresses endometrial proliferation in postmenopausal women taking 0.625 mg oral conjugated estrogen daily. Shoupe and colleagues reported a progestational effect of the system on the endometrium after 12 months; prior to the study, biopsy had shown a proliferative endometrium. Although progestogenic side-effects are rare, irregular

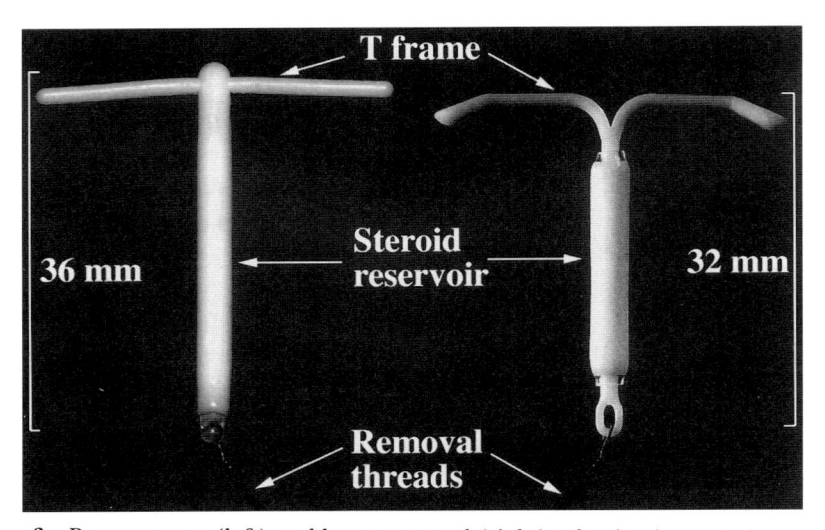

Figure 3 Progesterone (left) and levonorgestrel (right) releasing intrauterine systems

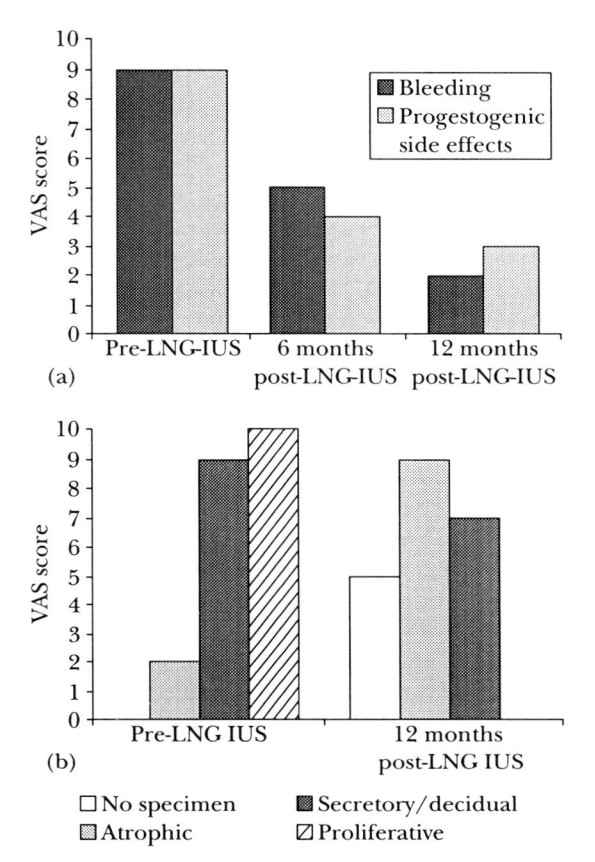

Figure 4 (a) Visual analog scale (VAS) scores of global progestogenic side-effects and bleeding severity in women using estrogens with levonorgestrel intrauterine system (LNG IUS) for progestogenic opposition; (b) effect of LNG IUS on endometrium after 1 year. Adapted from reference 19

bleeding is common in the first 3–6 months of usage. As the progesterone in the system only lasts for 18 months, the LNG IUS should be the first choice if heavy bleeding is the specific problem, as it appears to be quicker and superior in controlling bleeding and lasts for 5 years.

Physical and psychological progestogenic side-effects

Pathogenesis of physical progestogenic side-effects

Mineralocorticoid activity Most of the physical symptoms associated with progestogen intolerance such as edema, weight gain, bloating and migraine may be due to the mineralocorticoid-like effect of progestogens. It was originally thought that progestogens acted like progesterone, which enhances the renin–aldosterone cascade by acting as a precursor[22]. However, it may be that progestogens actually compete for the mineralocorticoid receptor. This effect can lead to retention of sodium and fluid gain during the progestogenic phase.

Androgenic effects on skin Effects such as acne, greasy skin and darkening of facial hair tend to occur mainly with the 19-nortestosterone derivatives which can have androgenic effects owing to their relatively strong binding affinity for the androgen receptor. Progesterone and dydrogesterone and norpregnane derivatives have no androgenic effects. Pregnane progestogens, particularly medroxyprogesterone, have mild androgenic effects, as their binding for the androgen receptor is a little higher than that of progesterone[23].

Breast cancer The effect of progestogens on breast cancer risk is still controversial and the data are incomplete. Some workers claim that they may have a beneficial effect and others claim an adverse effect. Progestogens do seem to enhance the mitotic activity of normal breast epithelial cells[24]. However, in the latest update of the Nurses' Health Study of 725 550 women with 1935 newly diagnosed cases of breast cancer, there was no difference in the relative risk of breast cancer in those using estrogen alone, estrogens and progestogens, or progestogens alone[25]. It is clear that more long-term data are needed to obtain conclusions about the effects of progestogens on breast cancer risk.

Pathogenesis of psychological progestogenic side-effects

Progesterone receptors are found in the caudate, cerebellum, cortex, habenula, hippocampus, hypothalamus, olfactory lobe, lamina terminalis and area postrema[26]. Limbic system functions, which subserve emotion and behavior, can be influenced, therefore, by circulating reproductive steroids such as progesterone and progestogens. There is evidence that progesterone and progesterone metabolites affect a number of central nervous system (CNS) transmitter systems to bring about mood changes, and these effects can be extrapolated to the progestogens in HRT[27].

Progesterone metabolites and the γ-aminobutyric acid A (GABA$_A$) receptor The GABA$_A$ receptor usually has antianxiolytic properties. It has been suggested that pregnenolone sulfate, a progesterone metabolite, may have antagonistic properties leading to inhibition of the GABA$_A$ receptor, thus producing negative mood effects.

Progesterone on monoamine turnover and metabolism Progesterone and progestogens have been shown to increase metabolism and turnover of monoamines in the rat brain. Also, platelet monoamine oxidase activity has been shown to decrease in the luteal phase. These effects could theoretically produce negative mood changes.

Serotonin (5HT) system Studies have shown that the 5HT uptake and content of platelets is significantly lower in the premenstrual phase in patients diagnosed with premenstrual syndrome (PMS) compared to controls. There is also evidence for the beneficial effects of serotonin reuptake inhibitors in PMS symptoms. It is possible, therefore, that symptoms related to the progestogenic component of HRT are, in part, due to actions on the serotonin system.

Other transmitter systems Pregnenolone sulfate appears to have an action at the *N*-methyl-D-aspartate (NMDA) receptor which is part of the CNS excitatory system, but the role of the receptor in the hormonal effects on mood is still unclear.

The times in a woman's life when the estrogen levels are low, i.e. postpartum and in the perimenopause, or when progesterone levels are high, i.e. premenstrually, are when the greatest excesses of depression occur. There are indications that it is the high luteal-phase progesterone levels which exacerbate PMS symptoms such as depression and mood swings. This is supported by the fact that abolition of ovulation with gonadotropin releasing hormone (GnRH) analogs or percutaneous estrogens alleviates symptoms. Certain women appear to be sensitive to the production of negative mood changes by progestogens. Cullberg[28] showed that women who had previously suffered from PMS reacted badly when taking oral contraceptives. This suggests that women with PMS are more sensitive to hormonal provocation than women without. There are also some endocrine indications that the hypothalamo-pituitary unit is more sensitive to ovarian hormones in women with PMS than in controls[29]. This is important as it suggests that it would be possible to predict which patients would experience negative mood changes during oral contraceptive use and HRT.

There are reports relating negative mood changes during HRT to the addition of progestogens in sequential therapy. The symptoms occur soon after progestogens are commenced and last for a couple of days after progestogens are ceased[30]. Holst and colleagues[31] showed that the progestogen component of combined preparations can have negative mood effects, especially depression, anxiety and cognitive impairment. Magos and co-workers[32] demonstrated the psychological PMS-type effects of norethisterone in postmenopausal women and showed that these changes appear to be dose-dependent, with the 5-mg dose causing more severe symptoms than the 2.5-mg dose (Figure 5). The authors regarded the addition of cyclical progestogen to continuous estrogen therapy as 'a model for the etiology of PMS'. The similarity of progestogenic side-effects to PMS symptoms was confirmed by Smith and associates[33]. In contrast to all these studies, Marslew and colleagues[34] found that two types of 19-nortestosterone and hydroxyprogesterone progestogens caused only mild adverse effects, but the only negative mood effect assessed was that of irritability.

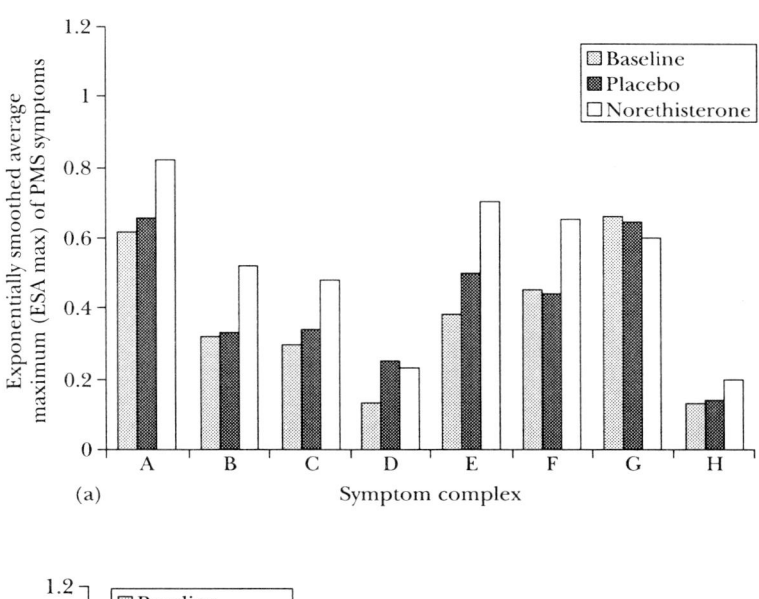

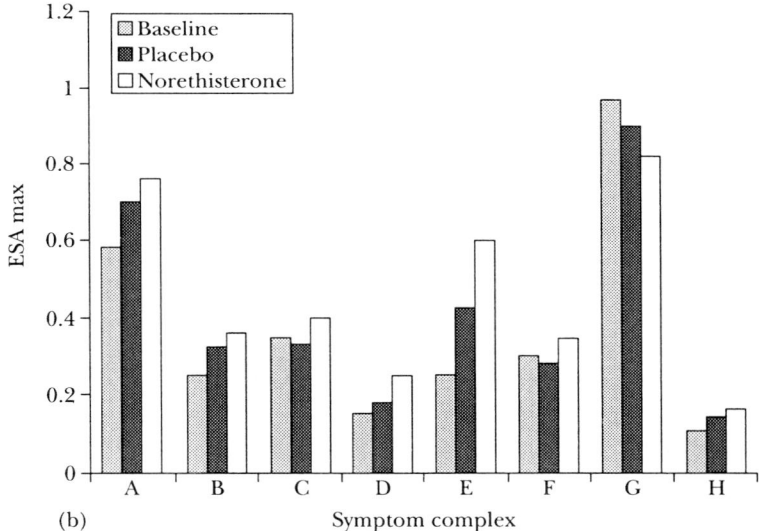

Figure 5 Production of premenstrual syndrome (PMS) type symptoms in women without a uterus receiving cyclical placebo and (a) 5 mg and (b) 2.5 mg norethisterone each month. Adapted from reference 32. Symptom clusters A–H represent groups of Moos premenstrual distress questionnaire: A, pain; B, concentration; C, behavioral change; D, autonomic reactions; E, water retention; F, negative affect; G, arousal; H, control

Prevention and treatment of physical and psychological progestogenic side-effects

Direct treatment of physical symptoms Most practitioners commence HRT with a proprietary sequential regimen, usually oral. About 20% of women will have significant progestogen intolerance with about half this number having serious side-effects which will prevent them from continuing with treatment. Many progestogen-induced side-effects will resolve within a reasonable trial period of 2–3 months. Therefore, patients should be counselled appropriately and given encouragement if dropout rates are to be improved[35]. Low continuation rates with HRT could be caused by a lack of interest of practitioners in finding a suitable progestogenic regimen for their patients. A recent survey showed that ever-use of HRT was as high as 55% in menopausal female doctors[36], which suggests that lack of interest may be greater in male doctors.

If symptoms do not resolve, or are severe, a number of possible actions may be taken to deal with the side-effects directly. Side-effects related to fluid retention, such as edema and bloating, may respond to a mild diuretic such as 25 mg of either spironolactone or hydrochlorothiazide[37]. The diuretic should be given in the last week of added progestogen. In the future, it may be possible to substitute an antimineralocorticoid-type progestogen such as drospirenone[38] to counteract fluid retention problems. Breast tenderness may be either aggravated or relieved with added progestogen. If it is aggravated, the addition of an androgen (e.g. a 100-mg testosterone implant every 6 months) may occasionally ameliorate breast tenderness. Headaches are unlikely to occur if estrogens are used continuously but, if they do occur during the progestogenic phase, they may be improved by the addition of a mild diuretic or of androgen. It must not be forgotten that nuisance progestogenic side-effects such as bloating or breast tenderness and headaches will be better tolerated if the physician prepares the woman, offers a solution and helps to put the problem into perspective.

Dose and duration of progestogen In the 'Consensus statement on progestin use in postmenopausal women'[39] in Florida, it was deemed important to individualize the length of progestogen treatment because of potential side-effects and symptomatic complaints (Table 2). Negative mood effects and physical symptoms may develop *de novo* while a patient is receiving progestogens. Also, it may be felt that patients are predisposed to developing negative mood effects because of a past history of severe PMS or a bad reaction to the pill. The minimum recommended duration of progestogen required to prevent endometrial hyperplasia completely is 12 days[1]. However, if a patient is psychologically and/or physically progestogen-intolerant, the duration of progestogen can be reduced to 10 or even 7 days per month. This will increase the risk of endometrial hyperplasia, particularly if implants are being used, so it will be necessary to have a lower threshold for endometrial sampling should there be any suspicious bleeding. Heavy/prolonged bleeding may also be a problem with the shorter duration of progestogen.

Table 2 Minimum doses of progestogen given orally in hormone replacement therapy (HRT) as endometrial protection (taken for 12 days per month)

Progestogen type	Dose (mg/day) *
Micronized progesterone	200
Dydrogesterone	10
Medroxyprogesterone	5
Norethisterone	1
Norgestrel	150 µg
Cyproterone	1

*Unless otherwise stated

Continuous combined/gonadomimetic therapy For patients experiencing negative mood effects or physical symptoms while taking sequential therapy, continuous combined therapy may be used to reduce the daily dose of progestogen, but this may produce constant low-grade PMS-type symptoms. The gonadomimetic, tibolone, seems to produce fewer psychological progestogenic side-effects but, unfortunately, has some androgenic physical side-effects in some patients.

Quarterly regimens Long-cycle HRT reduces to four per annum the number of progestogenic episodes. The disadvantage of this regimen is that the relatively high dosage of progestogen required per progestogenic episode can lead to severe physical and/or psychological progestogenic symptoms when the episode does occur. Nevertheless, this provides an effective regimen for some patients, as the prolonged unopposed estrogenic phase allows for the beneficial effects of unopposed estrogen on the CNS without the possible attenuating effects of progestogen. It is possible that this regimen may be useful in depressed perimenopausal women who are progesterone/progestogen-intolerant.

Intrauterine systems The plasma concentrations achieved by the LNG IUS are lower than those seen with oral progestogens, the levonorgestrel implant, the combined oral contraceptive or the mini-pill[40–42]. Also, unlike with oral contraceptives, the levels with the LNG IUS do not display peaks and troughs. It is postulated, therefore, that using the LNG IUS rather than an oral progestogen, to prevent endometrial hyperplasia, would be an ideal way of avoiding both physical and psychological progestogenic side-effects in women being treated with estrogens for the menopause.

Even with the lower, more constant, levels of progestogen released by the LNG IUS, some women still seem to experience adverse physical and psychological progestogenic side-effects such as edema, headache, breast tenderness, acne and mood swings[43]. These effects have been shown to subside after the first few months of usage[44]. Work in the present authors' unit showed that adverse progestogenic effects were reduced to a minimum when patients who were progestogen-intolerant were switched from oral progestogens to the LNG IUS (see Figure 4a). The PIPS, releasing natural progesterone rather than a progestogen, should be an even better method than the LNG IUS of avoiding adverse physical and psychological progestogenic effects in women being treated with estrogen replacement therapy. Studies are currently being conducted to confirm this hypothesis and the PIPS is only available on a trial basis in a few centers at present.

Progesterone vaginal gel Studies have recently confirmed the safety of progesterone vaginal gel for use as progestogenic opposition for estrogen replacement therapy, for example the study by Casanas-Roux and colleagues[45]. This product, now available on the UK market, should be an ideal way of avoiding physical and psychological progestogenic effects. Endometrial suppression is achieved by vaginal administration on an alternate-day basis for 14 days per month. There is a 'uterine first-pass effect' which allows the targeted receptors in the uterus to be contacted before the drug enters the systemic circulation. This leads to a high uterine-to-plasma gradient, low circulating progesterone metabolites and, therefore, minimal systemic side-effects. The gel provides a good alternative in oral progesterone-intolerant women who have no objection to using a vaginal preparation.

Transdermal progestogens The avoidance of first-pass metabolism should, in theory, produce fewer adverse physical effects, particularly if natural progesterone is used. Unfortunately, the steroid mass required for endometrial transformation would necessitate an unacceptably large patch. The existing progestogen patches using norethisterone provide satisfactory secretory transformation. Studies of the combination patch show it to be well tolerated with only minimal differences in the physical, psychological and metabolic scores measured in the estradiol-only and estradiol–norethisterone treatment phases[46].

Subcutaneous/injectable progestogens In theory, levonorgestrel silastic implants and injectable depot progestogens could also be used as progestogenic opposition to avoid the hepatic first-pass effect. From the experience of family planning, these progestogens are usually well tolerated. However, endometrial monitoring would have to be carried out to ensure suppression. It is astonishing that so little work has been done on the value of these much used preparations in HRT menopause regimens.

Alternative progestogens and progesterone Depending on their derivation, progestogens may have various physical and psychological effects. Non-androgenic progestogens and progesterone have the best physical effects although they are not devoid of psychological effects.

Oral micronized *progesterone* has been developed to overcome absorption problems which meant that, in the past, it had to be given by injection, vaginally or rectally. Unlike many oral progestogens, side-effects are uncommon with progesterone administration. Dalton[47], using low-dose progesterone for the treatment of PMS, claims not to have detected any adverse effects in 40 women treated over 10 years for PMS. Oral micronized progesterone, 300 mg per day for 12 days each month or progesterone suppositories, 25 mg twice daily for 12 days can be used as progestogenic opposition.

Recently, interest has been generated into exploring the potential of natural progesterone cream derived from plant sources, including wild yam, where it is found in its precursor form, diosgenin. Nutritionists and some doctors claim that it is sufficient in itself to provide relief of short- and long-term menopausal problems including reversal of osteoporosis. Unfortunately, the bone data are only from a few uncontrolled cases. It certainly does appear to have minimal adverse effects and, anecdotally, some patients do seem to derive benefits of increased energy, libido and improved skin. However, prospective, randomized placebo-controlled studies are necessary to confirm the claims of its benefits; these have not yet been performed. It would be interesting to see whether it could be used as progestogenic opposition for estrogen therapy.

The *pregnane*, cyproterone acetate (CPA), has recently been incorporated into HRT regimens because of its low incidence of side-effects. In a study by Koninckx and colleagues[48], CPA 1 mg for 10 days per cycle proved to be the optimum dosage as a sequential regimen with estradiol valerate 2 mg, providing adequate endometrial protection and minimal adverse effects. The under-used *norpregnanes* such as promegestone and nomegestrol are devoid of androgenic side-effects and, being potent progestogens, provide satisfactory endometrial protection[23].

The *third-generation nortestosterone-derived progestogens*, e.g. desogestrel and gestodene, were developed in an attempt to minimize undesirable androgenic effects. These newer progestogens have a much higher selectivity ratio than the older ones. Some workers have demonstrated the beneficial effects of desogestrel as progestogenic opposition in terms of side-effects and effect on lipids[49]. However, recent data concerning use of these preparations in combination with ethinylestradiol in the combined pill suggested that users of the older second-generation pills had half the risk of thromboembolic disease. Although the data have been much criticized and are probably irrelevant to their usage in HRT, development of these progestogens for opposition in HRT has been suspended.

The antimineralocorticoid progestogens
Drospirenone, chemically related to 17α-spironolactone with approximately eight times its antimineralocorticoid activity, has recently been used in combination with ethinylestradiol. Unlike with traditional oral contraceptives, there was a small decrease in body weight and blood pressure[38]. In the future, progestogen-intolerant women using HRT who suffer from an increase in body weight, edema and breast tenderness may benefit from the development of antimineralocorticoid progestogens.

Metabolic side-effects

Pathogenesis of metabolic progestogenic side-effects

Lipids and lipoproteins There has been anxiety that the beneficial effects of estrogen replacement therapy on the risk of cardiovascular disease are attenuated by the need to add progestogen in non-hysterectomized women. This is partly from data reporting that the nortestosterone-derived C19 progestogens used in monotherapy lead to unfavorable lipid changes. In a study by Farish and colleagues[50], postmenopausal women treated with norethisterone 5 mg per day had a significant drop in high-density lipoprotein-2 (HDL-2) and HDL-3 levels. In contrast, the C21 progestogens appear to have no significant effects on lipoprotein metabolism when used in moderate or low dosages[51].

Insulin resistance The addition of progestogen to estrogen therapy may produce adverse effects on glucose and insulin metabolism. In a study by Godsland and co-workers[52] levonorgestrel addition to conjugated equine estrogens led to a decrease in insulin sensitivity.

Vascular effects The modifying effects of progestogens on the pulsatility index have been studied as an indication of cardiovascular risk. Hillard and associates[53] examined the effects of progestogens on resistance to flow in 12 postmenopausal women. The pulsatility index (PI) was higher during the estrogen–progestogen phase than during the estrogen-only phase, but remained lower than before treatment. Marsh and colleagues[54] also showed an increase in mean uterine artery PI by 30% during the norethisterone phase of combined therapy but that this change was short-lived, the PI falling within 4 days of the progestogen being stopped. Encouragingly, long-term studies on estrogen and progestogen comedication cannot demonstrate any marked decrease in blood flow in comparison with estrogen-only therapy[55].

Prevention and treatment of metabolic progestogenic side-effects

Anxieties about adverse lipid changes, increased vascular resistance and increased insulin resistance may particularly be an issue in the patient who has either pre-existing cardiovascular disease or who develops cardiovascular disease while receiving HRT. In these patients, it would be wise to use at the outset, or change to, progesterone itself or a less androgenic type of progestogen. Currently, therefore, these progestogens are being incorporated into HRT regimens wherever possible in preference to those which are more androgenic.

Dose, duration and type of progestogen Keeping the dose and duration of progestogen to the minimum required to protect the endometrium will minimize the adverse metabolic effects. The net result of estrogen and progestogen combinations in HRT appears to depend on the balance between these steroids as well as the type of progestogen used. Progesterone and dydrogesterone seem to have no effect[56], whereas medroxyprogesterone may have an effect depending on the dose of estrogen. The C19 progestogens such as norethisterone and levonorgestrel can oppose the increases in HDL[57], but Jensen and Christiansen[58] showed that increasing the dose of estrogen led to a dose-dependent rise in HDL. In the 3-year postmenopausal estrogen/progestin interventions (PEPI) trial[59], estrogen alone or in combination with a progestogen improved lipoprotein and lowered fibrinogen levels without detectable effects on post-challenge insulin levels or blood pressure. There were no long-term adverse effects of added progestogen, especially when adequate doses of estrogen were given. This may be most important in improving the lipid pattern to decrease the risk for cardiovascular disease. Recent data from the Nurses' Health Study have also shown that the addition of progestogen does not attenuate the cardiovascular benefits of estrogens[60].

Non-androgenic progestogens may avoid adverse changes of progestogens on insulin resistance. Work by Stevenson[61], using cyclical dydrogesterone with oral estradiol, suggested an improvement in insulin resistance. Such a regimen using a non-androgenic progestogen would be particularly indicated in women with diabetes mellitus.

Continuous combined/gonadomimetic therapy

Workers have been unable to demonstrate a metabolic advantage to using continuous combined therapy. To the contrary, there is some evidence to suggest that continuous progestogen, albeit low-dose, may have a more adverse metabolic effect than sequential therapy. The effect of tibolone on lipids is also inconsistent with an adverse, lowering effect on HDL cholesterol but a beneficial, lowering effect on total and low-density lipoprotein (LDL) cholesterol and lipoprotein(a)[62,63].

Quarterly regimens In theory, the prolonged unopposed estrogenic phase allows for the beneficial effects of unopposed estrogen on cardiovascular risk without the possible attenuating effects of progestogen. In practice, no significant difference has been demonstrated between sequential and quarterly HRT users, possibly because of the high level of progestogen when the episode does occur.

Intrauterine systems Even with the lower, more constant levels of progestogen released by the LNG IUS, some women still seem to experience adverse metabolic progestogenic effects such as decreased LDL levels[43]. From studies of plasma hormone levels, menstrual patterns and blood chemistry in various patient groups, Tillson and colleagues[64] and Wan and co-workers[65] found that the PIPS produced no significant systemic effects. Shoupe and associates[20] showed beneficial effects in that serum HDL increased by 22% and LDL decreased by 21% from baseline with the combined estrogen–PIPS regimen. Archer and colleagues[21] and Spellacy and co-workers[66] reported no change in total cholesterol levels. Surprisingly, Spellacy and co-workers detected an increase in insulin secretion suggesting that, even with the PIPS, there may be some systemic effects.

The PIPS, therefore, may be an even better method than the LNG IUS of avoiding adverse metabolic progestogenic effects in women being treated with estrogen replacement therapy. Studies are currently being conducted to confirm this hypothesis and the PIPS is only available on a trial basis in a few centers at present.

Progesterone vaginal gel The combination of the 'uterine first-pass effect', avoidance of the hepatic first-pass metabolism and low circulating progesterone metabolites results in a negligible effect on lipid, lipoprotein and insulin metabolism. Use of this product as progestogenic opposition, therefore, should maximize the cardioprotective benefits of estrogens.

Transdermal progestogens The avoidance of first-pass metabolism should, in theory, produce fewer adverse metabolic effects, particularly if natural progesterone is used. Unfortunately, the existing progestogen patches require a more androgenic and, hence, metabolically unfriendly progestogen to bring about secretory transformation in the endometrium. Work is currently being carried out to produce progestogen patches with C21 pregnane progestogens, which have a superior metabolic effect.

Alternative to progestogens/progesterone

Unopposed estrogens

There will be a few cases for which it will not be possible to find suitable progestogenic opposition. In these cases, the option of very-low-dose unopposed estrogens can be considered. For a non-hysterectomized woman, the risk of endometrial hyperplasia will be high, depending on the dose. Endometrial sampling, therefore, must be performed on a 6-monthly basis with a baseline sample to exclude initial pathology. If hyperplasia develops and progestogens are not tolerated, then treatment should be stopped, or a progestogen coil could be inserted, or even hysterectomy should be considered.

Tibolone

Tibolone, a synthetic gonadomimetic compound with estrogenic, progestogenic and androgenic properties, provides the user with bleed-free HRT. In the non-hysterectomized woman who cannot tolerate progestogens, particularly sequential, this compound may be better tolerated. Studies have demonstrated adequate relief of climacteric symptoms coupled with low rates of breakthrough bleeding and good endometrial suppression with this compound, over many years of follow-up[62,67,68].

Hysterectomy

Hysterectomy, with adequate estrogen replacement, may have to be considered if other actions fail and the woman wishes to continue using HRT[69]. This procedure should not be regarded as a last resort, because it provides the convenience of long-term uncomplicated HRT as well as curing any painful periods, PMS and menstrual migraine. Thus, compliance is excellent and, in a recent study of 209 consecutive hysterectomies, reviewed 2–5 years after surgery, 100% were still taking estrogens[70].

Bisphosphonates

The bisphosphonates provide an option for the progestogen-intolerant woman who wishes to have HRT solely for the benefit of treating osteoporosis.

Selective estrogen-receptor modulators (SERMs), e.g. droloxifene and raloxifene

Selective estrogen-receptor modulators possess both estrogenic and antiestrogenic properties. The aim is to develop one which is selectively estrogenic in the skeletal and cardiovascular systems, while possessing antiestrogenic effects in the breast and endometrium. Data are still not complete for all parameters in any of these drugs. Also, they currently appear to have no beneficial effects on vasomotor symptoms or on the central nervous system. However, in the future, a SERM which fulfills all the desirable criteria may well provide the answer to many of the problems associated with HRT in general, and of progestogen intolerance specifically.

CONCLUSION

Progestogen use is essential in the non-hysterectomized woman using anything but very-short-term estrogen replacement therapy. Intolerance of progestogenic side-effects remains a major obstacle to the maximization of patient compliance with hormone replacement therapy (HRT). This chapter has highlighted the adverse effects that progestogens can produce and discussed possible ways of preventing or treating these (Table 3). It must not be forgotten that sympathetic counselling may be all that is required, as many progestogenic side-effects and bleeding problems resolve after a few months. Premenstrual-type effects and bleeding problems often resolve after a few months and can often be dealt with by changing the type of progestogen, the dose or the duration. Metabolic and physical benefits are maximized by using C21 progestogens and aiming for as high an estrogen/progestogen dosage ratio as possible, without compromising endometrial safety.

Table 3 Clinical management of progestogen intolerance

Symptom/disturbance	Action
Heavy/prolonged bleeding	increase dose/duration progestogen
	use more androgenic progestogen
	long-cycle/continuous combined HRT
	progestogen IUS
Progestogenic side-effects (physical/psychological)	diuretics (fluid retention symptoms)
	androgens (breast/headaches/libido)
	decrease dose/duration progestogen
	less androgenic progestogen (physical)
	more androgenic progestogen (psychological)
	long-cycle HRT/gonadomimetic
	progestogen/progesterone IUS
	vaginal progesterone gel
	hysterectomy + unopposed estrogen
	unopposed estrogen + endometrial sampling
	?SERMs
Metabolic side-effects (lipids/insulin resistance, etc)	less androgenic progestogen
	?long-cycle HRT
	?progestogen/progesterone IUS
	?SERMs

HRT, hormone replacement therapy; IUS, intrauterine system; SERMs, selective estrogen-receptor modulators

Continuous combined and gonadomimetic preparations are useful alternatives to sequential therapy for the appropriate woman. Vaginal progesterone gel and intrauterine progestogen/progesterone systems will become more commonly used in HRT regimens. Hysterectomy remains an option for the severely progestogen-intolerant woman in whom other regimens have not succeeded. In the future, compliance could be maximized by development of the ultimate selective estrogen-receptor modulator, which would have estrogenic effects on vasomotor symptoms, the skin, skeletal, cardiovascular and central nervous systems and antiestrogenic effects on endometrial and breast tissue. For the present, research continues into the development of more selective progestogens, improved regimens and sophisticated delivery systems to be used with estrogen therapy.

References

1. Sturdee DW, Wade-Evans T, Paterson MEL, et al. Relations between bleeding pattern, endometrial histology and oestrogen treatment in menopausal women. Br Med J 1978;10:1575–7
2. Ferguson KJ, Hoegh C, Johnson S. Estrogen replacement therapy: a survey of women's knowledge and attitudes. Arch Int Med 1989;149:133
3. Studd JWW. Complications of hormone replacement therapy in post-menopausal women. J R Soc Med 1992;85:376–8
4. Barlow DH, Grosset KA, Hart H, et al. A study of the experience of Glasgow women in the climacteric years. Br J Obstet Gynaecol 1989;96: 1192–7
5. Cheung AP, Wren BG. A cost-effectiveness analysis of hormone replacement therapy. Med J Aust 1992;156:312–16
6. Paterson MEL, Wade-Evans T, Sturdee DW, et al. Endometrial disease after treatment with oestrogens and progestogens in the climacteric. Br Med J 1980;1:822–4
7. Lane G, Siddle NC, Ryder TA, et al. Dose dependent effects of oral progesterone on the oestrogenised postmenopausal endometrium. Acta Obstet Gynaecol Scand 1983;106:17–22
8. Henderson BE, Ross RK, Lobo RA, et al. Re-evaluating the role of progestogen therapy after the menopause. Fertil Steril 1988; 49:9S–15S
9. Habiba MA, Bell SC, Abrams K, et al. Endometrial responses to hormone replacement therapy. Hum Reprod 1996;11:503–8
10. Thom MH, White PJ, Williams RM, et al. Prevention and treatment of endometrial disease in climacteric women receiving oestrogen therapy. Lancet 1979;2:455–7
11. Magos AL, Brincat M, Studd JWW, et al. Amenorrhoea and endometrial atrophy with continuous oral oestrogen and progestogen therapy in postmenopausal women. Obstet Gynecol 1985;65: 496–9
12. MacLennan AH, MacLennan A, Wenzel S, et al. Continuous low-dose oestrogen and progestogen replacement therapy: a randomised trial. Med J Aust 1993;159: 102–6
13. Ettinger B, Selvy J, Citron JT, et al. Cyclic hormone replacement therapy using quarterly progestin. Obstet Gynecol 1994;83:693–700
14. Silverberg SG, Haukkamaa M, Arko H, et al. Endometrial morphology during long-term use of levonorgestrel-releasing intrauterine devices. Int J Gynaecol Pathol 1986;5:235–41
15. Luukkainen T, Allonen H, Haukkamaa M, et al. Five years' experience with levonorgestrel releasing IUDs. Contraception 1996;33:139–48
16. Andersson K, Mattsson L-A, Rybo G, et al. Intrauterine release of levonorgestrel – a new way of adding progestogen in hormone replacement therapy. Obstet Gynecol 1992;79:963–7
17. Suhonen SP, Holmstrom T, Allonen HO, et al. Intrauterine and sub-dermal progestin administration in postmenopausal hormone replacement therapy. Fertil Steril 1995;63:336–42
18. Raudaskoski TH, Lahti EI, Kauppila AJ, et al. Transdermal estrogen with a levonorgestrel-releasing intrauterine device for climacteric complaints: clinical and endometrial responses. Am J Obstet Gynecol 1995;172:114–19
19. Panay N, Studd JWW, Thomas A, et al. The levonorgestrel intrauterine system as progestogenic opposition for oestrogen replacement therapy. Presented at the Annual Meeting of the British Menopause Society, Exeter, UK, July 1996
20. Shoupe D, Meme D, Mezro G, et al. Prevention of intrauterine hyperplasia in postmenopausal women with intrauterine progesterone. N Engl J Med 1991;325:1811–12
21. Archer DF, Viniegra-Sibai A, Hsiu JG, et al. Endometrial histology, uterine bleeding and metabolic changes in postmenopausal women using

21. a progesterone-releasing intrauterine device and oral conjugated estrogens for hormone replacement therapy. *Menopause* 1994;1:109–16
22. Oelkers W, Schoneshofer M, Blumel A. Effects of progesterone and four synthetic progestogens on sodium balance and the renin–aldosterone system in man. *J Clin Endocrinol Metab* 1974;39: 882–90
23. Rozenbaum H. How to choose the correct progestogen. In Birkhauser MH, Rozenbaum H, eds. *Menopause. European Consensus Development Conference, Montreux, Switzerland.* Paris: Editions ESKA, 1996:243–56
24. Persson I. Possible adverse effects of progestins on breast cancer risk. In Birkhauser MH, Rozenbaum H, eds. *Menopause. European Consensus Development Conference, Montreux, Switzerland.* Paris: Editions ESKA, 1996:211–17
25. Colditz GA, Hankinson SE, Hunter DJ, *et al.* The use of estrogens and progestins and the risk of breast cancer in post-menopausal women. *N Engl J Med* 1995;332:1582–93
26. Maggi A, Perez J. Role of female gonadal hormones in the CNS: clinical and experimental aspects. *Life Sci* 1985;37:893–906
27. Backstrom T, Bixo M, Seipel L, *et al.* Progestins and behaviour. In Gennazzani AR, Petraglia F, Purdy RH, eds. *The Brain: Source and Target for Sex Steroid Hormones.* New York: Parthenon Publishing, 1996:277–91
28. Cullberg J. Mood changes and menstrual symptoms with different gestagen/estrogen combinations. A double blind comparison with placebo. *Acta Psychol Scand* 1972;236(Suppl):1–46
29. Backstrom T, Smith S, Lothian H, *et al.* Prolonged follicular phase and depressed gonadotrophins following hysterectomy and corpus luteectomy in women with premenstrual tension syndrome. *Clin Endocrinol* 1985;22:723–32
30. Hammarback S, Backstrom T, Holst J, *et al.* Cyclical mood changes as in the premenstrual tension syndrome during sequential estrogen–progestagen post-menopausal replacement therapy. *Acta Obstet Gynaecol Scand* 1985;64:393–7
31. Holst J, Backstrom T, Hammarback S, *et al.* Progestogen addition during oestrogen replacement therapy – effects on vasomotor symptoms and mood. *Maturitas* 1989;11:13–20
32. Magos AL, Brewster E, Singh R, *et al.* The effects of norethisterone in postmenopausal women on oestrogen replacement therapy: a model for premenstrual syndrome. *Br J Obstet Gynaecol* 1986;93:1290–6
33. Smith RNJ, Holland EFN, Studd JWW. The symptomatology of progestogen intolerance. *Maturitas* 1994;18:87–91
34. Marslew U, Riis B, Christiansen C. Progestogens: therapeutic and adverse effects in early postmenopausal women. *Maturitas* 1991;13:7–16
35. Nachtigall LE. Enhancing patient compliance with hormone replacement therapy at menopause. *Obstet Gynecol* 1990;75:(Suppl 4):77S–80S
36. Isaacs AJ, Britton AR, McPherson K. Utilisation of hormone replacement therapy by women doctors. *Br Med J* 1995;311:1399–401
37. Gambrell RD. Progestogens in estrogen replacement therapy. *Clin Obstet Gynaecol* 1995;38: 890–901
38. Oelkers W, Foidart JM, Domborvicz N, *et al.* Effects of a new oral contraceptive containing an antimineralocorticoid progestogen, drospirenone, on the renin–aldosterone system, body weight, blood pressure, glucose tolerance and lipid metabolism. *J Clin Endocrinol Metab* 1995;80:1816–21
39. Consensus statement on progestin use in postmenopausal women. *Maturitas* 1988;11:175–7
40. Diaz S, Pavez M, Miranda P, *et al.* Long term follow-up of women treated with Norplant® implants. *Contraception* 1987;35:551–67
41. Kuhnz W, Al-Yacoub G, Fuhrmister A. Pharmacokinetics of levonorgestrel and ethinylestradiol in nine women who received a low-dose oral contraceptive over a treatment period of 3 months, and, after a washout phase, a single oral administration of the same contraceptive formulation. *Contraception* 1992;46:455–69
42. Weiner E, Victor A, Johansson EDB. Plasma levels of D-norgestrel after oral administration. *Contraception* 1976;40:425–38
43. Raudaskoski TH, Tomas EI, Paakkari IA, *et al.* Serum lipids and lipoproteins in postmenopausal women receiving transdermal oestrogen in combination with a levenorgestrel intrauterine device. *Maturitas* 1995;22:47–53
44. Nilsson CG, Lahteenmaki PLA, Luukkainen T, *et al.* Sustained intrauterine release of levonorgestrel over 5 years. *Fertil Steril* 1986;45:805–7
45. Casanas-Roux F, Nisolle M, Marbaix E, *et al.* Morphometric, immunohistological and three-dimensional evaluation of the endometrium of menopausal women treated by oestrogen and Crinone, a new slow-release vaginal progesterone. *Hum Reprod* 1996;11: 357–63
46. Ellerington MC, Whitcroft SIJ, Whitehead MI. HRT: developments in therapy. *Br Med Bull* 1992; 48:401–25
47. Dalton K. *Premenstrual Syndrome and Progesterone Therapy.* London: Heinemann Press, 1977
48. Koninckx PR, Lauweryns JM, Cornille FJ. Endometrial effects during hormone replacement therapy with a sequential, oestradiol valerate/cyproterone acetate preparation. *Maturitas* 1993; 16:97–110

49. Saure A, Hirvonen E, Tikkanen MJ, *et al*. A novel oestradiol–desogestrel preparation for hormone replacement therapy: effects on hormones, lipids, bone, climacteric symptoms and endometrium. *Maturitas* 1993;16: 1–12
50. Farish E, Fletcher CD, Hart DM, *et al*. Lipoprotein and apoprotein levels in postmenopausal women during treatment with norethisterone. *Clin Chim Acta* 1986;159:147–51
51. Barnes RB, Roy S, Lobo RA. Comparison of lipid and androgen levels after conjugated estrogen or depo-medroxyprogesterone acetate in postmenopausal women. *Obstet Gynecol* 1985;66: 217–19
52. Godsland I, Gangar KF, Walton C, *et al*. Insulin resistance, secretion and elimination in postmenopausal women receiving oral or transdermal hormone replacement therapy. *Metabolism* 1993;42:846–53
53. Hillard TC, Bourne TH, Whitehead MI, *et al*. Differential effects of transdermal oestradiol and sequential progestogens on impedance to flow within the uterine arteries of postmenopausal women. *Fertil Steril* 1992;58:959–63
54. Marsh MS, Bourne TH, Whitehead MI, *et al*. The temporal effect of progestogen on the uterine artery pulsatility index in postmenopausal women receiving sequential hormone replacement therapy. *Fertil Steril* 1994;62:771–4
55. Samsioe G, Astedt B. Does progestogen co-medication attenuate the cardiovascular benefits of oestrogens? In Birkhauser MH, Rozenbaum H, eds. *Menopause. European Consensus Development Conference, Montreux, Switzerland*. Paris: Editions ESKA, 1996:175–83
56. Siddle NC, Jesinger DK, Whitehead MI. Effect on plasma lipids and lipoproteins of postmenopausal oestrogen therapy with added dydrogesterone. *Br J Obstet Gynaecol* 1990;97: 1093–100
57. Whitcroft SI, Crook D, Marsh MS, *et al*. Long term effects of oral and transdermal hormone replacement therapies on serum lipid and lipoprotein concentrations. *Obstet Gynecol* 1994; 84:1–5
58. Jensen J, Christiansen C. Dose–response effects on serum lipids and lipoproteins following combined oestrogen–progestogen therapy in postmenopausal women. *Maturitas* 1987;9:259–66
59. Miller VT, Bush T, Wood PD, *et al*. Effects of estrogen or estrogen/progestin regimens on heart disease risk factors in postmenopausal women: the postmenopausal estrogen/progestin interventions (PEPI) trial. *J Am Med Assoc* 1995;273:199
60. Grodstein F, Stampfer MJ, Manson JE, *et al*. Postmenopausal estrogen and progestin use and the risk of cardiovascular disease. *N Engl J Med* 1996; 335:453–61
61. Stevenson JC. Do we need different galenic forms of oestrogens and progestogens? In Birkhauser MH, Rozenbaum H, eds. *Menopause. European Consensus Development Conference, Montreux, Switzerland*. Paris: Editions ESKA, 1996:231–5
62. Rymer J, Fogelman I, Chapman MG. The incidence of vaginal bleeding with tibolone treatment. *Br J Obstet Gynaecol* 1993;101:53–6
63. Milner MH, Sinnott MM, Cooke TM, *et al*. A 2 year study of lipid and lipoprotein changes in postmenopausal women with tiblone and estrogen–progestin. *Obstet Gynecol* 1996;87:593–9
64. Tillson SA, Marian M, Hudson R, *et al*. The effect of intrauterine progesterone on the hypothalamic–hypophyseal–ovarian axis in humans. *Contraception* 1975;11:179–92
65. Wan LS, Ying-Chih H, Manik G, *et al*. Effects of the Progestasert® on the menstrual pattern, ovarian steroids and endometrium. *Contraception* 1977;16:417–34
66. Spellacy W, Buhi WC, Birk SA. Carbohydrate and lipid studies in women using the progesterone intrauterine device for 1 year. *Fertil Steril* 1979;31: 381–4
67. Genazzani AR, Benedek-Jaszmann LJ, Hart DM, *et al*. Org OD14 and the endometrium. *Maturitas* 1991; 13:243–51
68. Ginsberg J, Prelevic G, Butler D, *et al*. Clinical experience with tibolone (Livial) over 8 years. *Maturitas* 1995;21:71–6
69. Studd JWW. Shifting indications for hysterectomy. *Lancet* 1995;345:388
70. Khastgir G, Studd JWW. A survey of patient satisfaction and wellbeing following hysterectomy and bilateral salpinoophorectomy with oestrogen and testosterone implants. *Obstet Gynecol* 1998;submitted

26

Hormone replacement therapy after hysterectomy

J. Studd and G. Khastgir

INTRODUCTION

Hysterectomy is one of the most common gynecological operations, with over 60 000 cases being performed in the UK every year[1]. It is usually performed for symptom relief to improve the quality of life rather than as a life-saving procedure[2]. Thus, a patient's general well-being should not be hampered by any side-effect of hysterectomy, but ovarian hormone deficiency is one such consequence that results in both short- and long-term health problems. When compared to women after a natural menopause, the vasomotor symptoms are more frequent in hysterectomized women, who are also more likely to develop other less typical features of ovarian failure such as psychological symptoms and sexual problems[3]. As a result of long-term estrogen deficiency, the incidences of cardiovascular disease and osteoporosis are high following bilateral oophorectomy, but moderately increased even after hysterectomy with ovarian conservation[4–7].

Despite such a high prevalence of ovarian hormone deficiency after hysterectomy, few of these women actually receive hormone replacement therapy (HRT). Climacteric complaints are usually ignored in younger women with residual ovaries and, in the absence of menstruation, the diagnosis of ovarian failure is often missed[8]. There is rarely any protocol for regular follow-up to check hormone levels after hysterectomy. More worrying is the fact that, even after bilateral oophorectomy, HRT is often not advised and, when started, it is usually taken for a short period owing to lack of follow-up[9]. The low uptake and continuation rates are also partly due to widespread misconceptions among both women and their doctors about risks associated with HRT[10].

This chapter discusses different aspects of HRT following hysterectomy. The endocrinological changes following hysterectomy with or without oophorectomy emphasize the specific need for HRT. Unopposed estrogen replacement is adequate for the majority, but the case for testosterone supplementation is addressed. The hormonal need may be higher after hysterectomy in younger women than in those after a natural menopause. Thus, the role of different doses of HRT in both short-term symptom relief and long-term health protection is analyzed. Finally, a practical guideline is suggested regarding how health professionals can ensure that those women who would benefit most from HRT do receive the treatment.

ENDOCRINE CHANGES AFTER HYSTERECTOMY AND OOPHORECTOMY

Hysterectomy with ovarian conservation

After hysterectomy, there is an immediate but transient drop in the circulating estradiol level owing to an acute reduction in ovarian blood flow during surgical manipulation. The estradiol level otherwise remains unchanged in premenopausal women at least up to 12 months following hysterectomy. At that time, ovarian histology begins to demonstrate features of relative hypoxemia and diminished follicular reserve, but these early structural changes are not clinically evident owing to the large functional reserve[11]. Long-term follow-ups after at least 2 years of hysterectomy have shown that circulating gonadotropin levels in young women (< 44 years) are higher than in age-matched controls[12] (Figure 1). This is more common in those suffering from vasomotor symptoms and represents an impending ovarian failure. The circulating estradiol level may initially remain normal with raised gonadotropin levels, but subsequently falls in 25–50% of women. As the most likely cause of premature ovarian failure is decreased blood flow, it is likely to affect the ovarian stroma, resulting in a fall of the circulating testosterone level as well. These endocrinological changes are seen usually within 2–5 years of surgery, but are more liable to develop after longer intervals[13,14].

Hysterectomy and bilateral oophorectomy

In premenopausal women, the circulating estradiol level falls within 24 h of bilateral oophorectomy to 80% below the mean level of the follicular phase[15]. However, removal of the ovaries after a natural menopause results in an unaltered estradiol level, as it arises mainly from aromatization of adrenocortical androgens in the peripheral fat (Figure 2)[16]. Bilateral oophorectomy also causes a significant decrease in the circulating testosterone level owing to the loss of ovarian stroma. In premenopausal women, the circulating testosterone level falls by 30% to a level significantly lower than that after a natural menopause[15]. A relatively lower degree of fall in the testosterone level in comparison to that of estradiol is due to the extraovarian synthesis of testosterone in the adrenal cortex and body fat. In postmenopausal women, ovaries are not defunct endocrine organs, but contribute 50% of testosterone and 30% of androstenedione to the circulation[17]. Indeed, the ovarian stroma may increase with higher gonadotropin stimulation, resulting in a higher testosterone level than that before the menopause. Thus, when the ovaries of a postmenopausal woman are removed, there is a significant fall in the circulating level of testosterone (Figure 2)[17]. Testosterone replacement, therefore, should be considered following oophorectomy, irrespective of whether it is performed before or after the natural menopause.

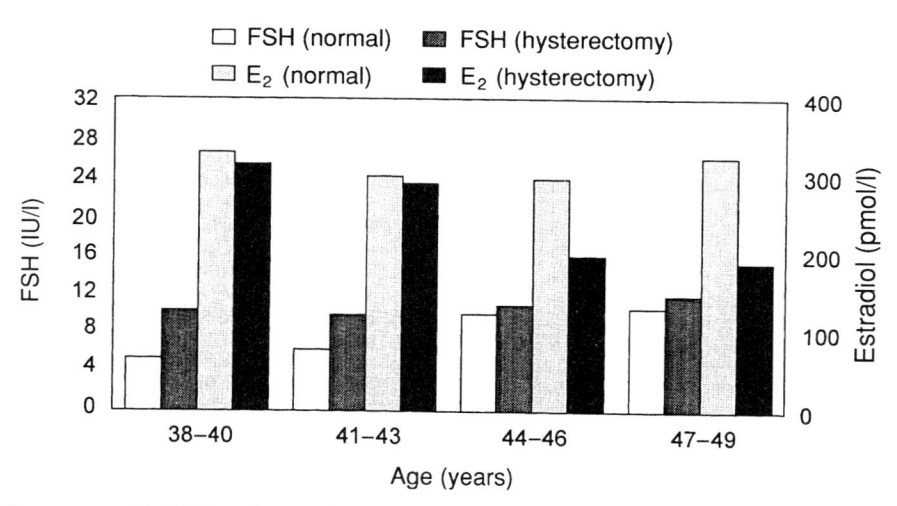

Figure 1 Plasma estradiol (E_2) and gonadotropin (follicle stimulating hormone, FSH) levels in normal and hysterectomized women of premenopausal age. Adapted from reference 12

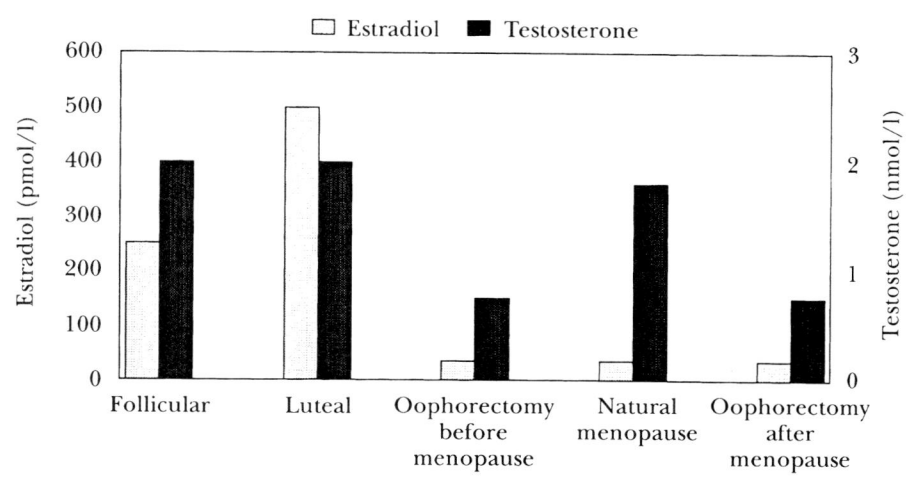

Figure 2 Plasma estradiol and testosterone levels before and after spontaneous menopause and bilateral oophorectomy. Adapted from references 15–17

INDICATIONS FOR HRT AFTER HYSTERECTOMY

Pre-existing ovarian failure

As hysterectomy is commonly performed in the age range 40–49 years, the decline in ovarian function often precedes the surgery[18]. These perimenopausal women usually have anovulatory cycles resulting in heavy periods, which are often prolonged, irregular and painful. The decline in ovarian function may not be suspected in the presence of menstrual periods and, even then, HRT is avoided because of the fear that the problem may become worse. Although hysterectomy relieves the period problems, it may be avoided in some perimenopausal women by treating the actual cause with HRT[8].

After hysterectomy, a further decline in the function of conserved ovaries results in worsening of cyclical symptoms, such as bloating, mastalgia, headache, irritability and depression. These symptoms are characteristic of premenstrual syndrome but are best called, in the absence of menstruation, the *ovarian cycle syndrome*[19]. The diagnosis is usually missed because, in the absence of menstruation, the cyclical pattern of these symptoms may not be recognized. Indeed, they tend to be referred as vague and inconsistent complaints probably due to an emotional setback following hysterectomy. However, even in the absence of climacteric symptoms, there is a strong case for considering HRT in all perimenopausal women who are at a higher risk of osteoporosis and cardiovascular disease following hysterectomy.

Premature ovarian failure following hysterectomy

The conservation of ovaries at hysterectomy is aimed at preventing the effects of hormonal deficiency, but there is accumulating evidence suggesting that retained ovaries may fail prematurely. The incidence of ovarian failure after hysterectomy varies between 25 and 50% and can develop at any time, but usually 2–5 years after surgery[13,14]. The age at hysterectomy seems to have no influence, but the average age of menopause is 4 years earlier than that of the control group[14]. The premature ovarian failure is independent of the indication for hysterectomy, implying that it is the surgery rather than the initial disease that leads to the endocrine changes. The type of hysterectomy is also irrelevant, but prior tubo-ovarian surgery, resection of ovarian lesions and suturing of the residual ovary are associated with a shortening in duration of future functioning.

The definite cause of ovarian failure is uncertain, but a compromised ovarian vascular supply resulting from the surgery is the most likely mechanism[13,14]. Ovaries receive a dual blood supply through the ovarian artery and the tubal branch of the uterine artery, with a considerable variation in their respective shares. After clamping of the uterine artery, the functioning of residual ovaries depends on the type of blood supply in that individual. The ovarian veins are devoid of valves and prone to the development of varicosity, which would contribute to the stagnation of ovarian venous flow due to loss of utero-ovarian anastomosis at hysterectomy[11].

There is rarely any practice of routine follow-up by the gynecologist or general practitioner to enable early diagnosis of this potential iatrogenic ovarian failure. With the assumption that the conserved ovaries function until the age of natural menopause, the climacteric symptoms are often dismissed or misdiagnosed as psychological illness as a result of hysterectomy. A survey from general practices has shown that, among those women who were not on HRT following hysterectomy, one-quarter had gonadotropin levels in the menopausal range despite ovarian conservation[8]. Without regular vigilance, such women may needlessly be exposed to the risk of cardiovascular disease and osteoporosis.

Bilateral oophorectomy with hysterectomy

Approximately 20% of women undergoing hysterectomy for benign conditions have bilateral oophorectomy at the same time[18]. The decision to remove the ovaries is influenced by the indication for hysterectomy and age at the time of surgery. In patients with endometriosis, pelvic congestion syndrome and premenstrual syndrome, oophorectomy is an essential adjunct to hysterectomy for achieving a permanent cure. With other indications for hysterectomy, following full discussion and consent, the ovaries may be removed prophylactically, usually after the age of 40. Apart from preventing ovarian cancer, it also avoids any residual ovarian pain and the ovarian cycle syndrome[19].

As the main argument against bilateral oophorectomy is the consequences of prolonged ovarian hormone deficiency, such an intervention indeed demands HRT postoperatively. No matter how beneficial the prophylactic effect, oophorectomy cannot be justified unless arrangements can be made for long-term HRT. Such a clear-cut need for HRT, in many ways, is preferable to the uncertainty or false assurance of continued function of the residual ovaries. However, in reality, a large number of women who undergo bilateral oophorectomy never take HRT or do so only for a short while after surgery. A survey of general practices in the UK has shown that HRT use in such women is only 30% even under the age of 40 years, and the mean duration of use is 2 years[8]. The apparent failure to provide long-term estrogen therapy in such an obvious high-risk population must be seen as a major practical problem surrounding prophylactic oophorectomy before the menopause.

IMMEDIATE BENEFITS OF HRT

Relief of climacteric symptoms

After hysterectomy with ovarian conservation, women report both higher frequency and increased severity of climacteric symptoms than do healthy women of a similar age (Figure 3)[3]. This results in frequent consultations with the doctors who should be alert to the presence of these complaints, especially in those who are considered to be *too young*. The early complaints are of vasomotor disturbances but, with a longer interval after surgery, other estrogen-deficiency symptoms such as depression, loss of libido and urinary symptoms become the predominant complaints[15] (Figure 4). However, these non-specific symptoms may be difficult to associate unless the presence of vasomotor disturbances is queried. In some patients, these symptoms precede hysterectomy and persist in the postoperative period, which indicates that declining ovarian function may remain undetected[20].

Estrogen is usually effective in relieving most climacteric symptoms. However, unlike during natural menopause, hysterectomized women may not respond to the lowest available

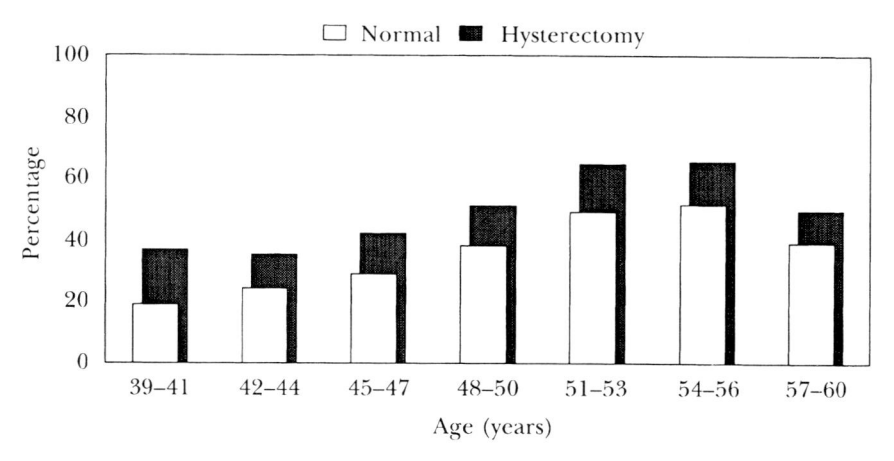

Figure 3 Incidence of climacteric symptoms in normal and hysterectomized women of perimenopausal age. Adapted from reference 3

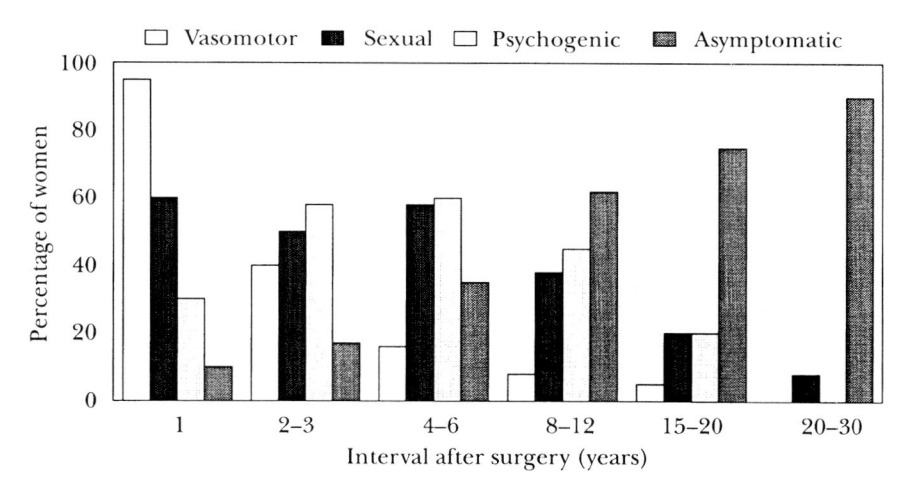

Figure 4 Incidence of climacteric symptoms in oophorectomized women in relation to time interval after surgery. Adapted from reference 15

therapeutic dose. In clinical practice, many younger patients who are started on lower doses of estrogen following bilateral oophorectomy still experience severe menopausal symptoms, and over 75% need a higher dose of HRT[20,21]. More than half of these women need to change the type and dose of HRT at least twice, and some up to seven times before achieving a satisfactory control. Symptom control is more likely to be effective with the transdermal patch or gel, or subcutaneous implant, where there is an option of increasing the dosage if necessary[22,23]. Testosterone replacement should be considered if symptoms such as lethargy, loss of libido, depression and headache persist despite an adequate dose of estrogen replacement. In randomized double-blind studies, the somatic symptom scores after bilateral oophorectomy were lower with combined estrogen–testosterone than with estrogen alone, but scores in both hormone groups were much lower than those in the placebo group (Figure 5)[24,25].

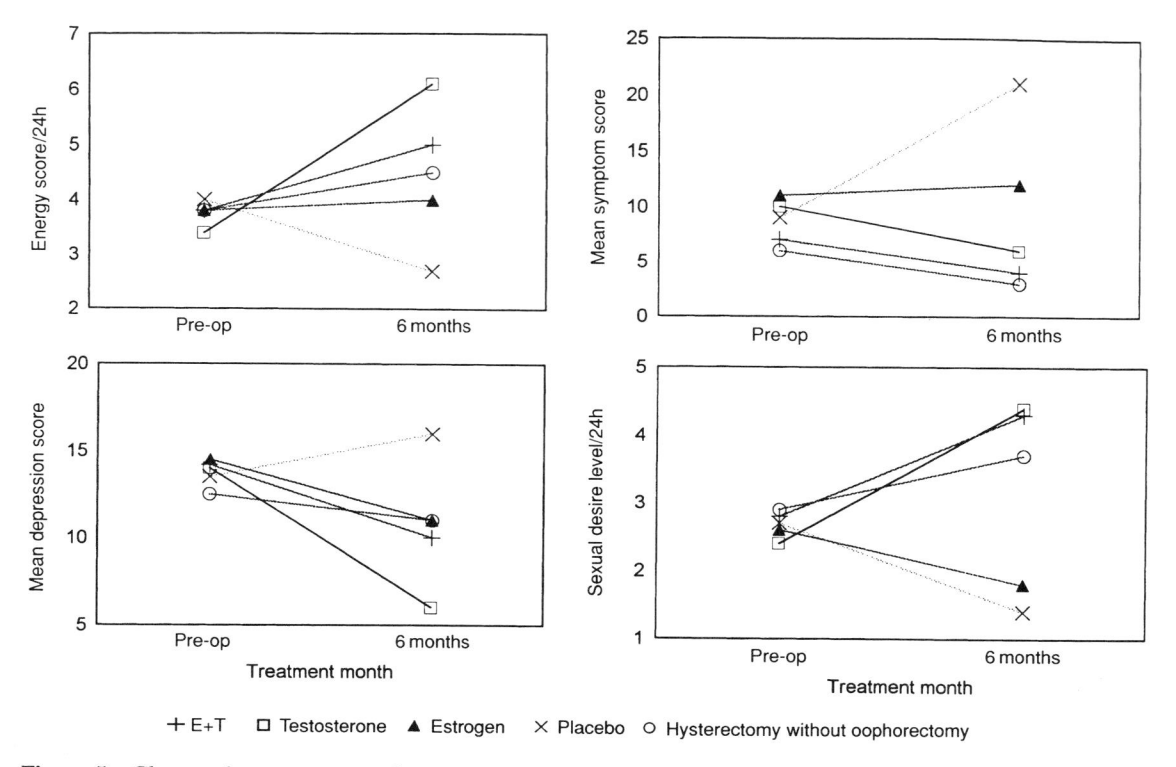

Figure 5 Changes in energy, somatic symptoms, mental state and sexual desire scores with different hormone replacement therapies (HRTs) following hysterectomy and bilateral oophorectomy. Adapted from references 25–27. E + T, estrogen and testosterone

Reduced psychological morbidity

Several prospective studies have shown that the incidence of depression is higher in women before hysterectomy but, postoperatively, the mood improves in the majority[28,29]. It should be no surprise that years of suffering with ineffective medical treatment for heavy periods, chronic pelvic pain, severe premenstrual syndrome and menstrual migraine make women depressed. The improvement in mood following hysterectomy is obviously due to permanent relief from these debilitating symptoms. However, in some women, depression may persist after hysterectomy or develop for the first time postoperatively. This depression is most probably a result of coexisting or subsequent ovarian failure following hysterectomy[20]. The causative role of declining estrogen is supported by the occurrence of psychological problems at other times of hormonal flux, such as postnatal depression and premenstrual syndrome. Androgens also have a role in behavior and mood that is likely to be affected with depletion of the endogenous source following bilateral oophorectomy[26].

Several double-blind placebo-controlled studies have shown that estrogen given by any route improves psychological scores and symptoms following hysterectomy with or without oophorectomy[30–32]. Estrogen may improve mood by correcting vasomotor instability, insomnia and dyspareunia in what is called a *domino effect*, but there is also a dose-dependent mental tonic effect irrespective of any symptoms. Evidently, the latter is caused by the excitatory effect of estrogen on the central nervous system, activating the neurons directly by altering the electrical activity and indirectly through the neurotransmitters, resulting in an antidepressant effect[33]. Testosterone replacement in addition to estrogen may be required to treat any residual depression, particularly following bilateral oophorectomy along with hysterectomy[24]. Thus, following hysterectomy and bilateral oophorectomy, the improvement of the psychological score with either combined estrogen and testosterone or testosterone alone was greater than that with estrogen alone[26] (Figure 5).

Improved sexual outcome

The influence of hysterectomy on sexual function may be variable, with improvement in some, no change in most of the others and deterioration in only a small minority[32,34]. An improvement is expected in women whose sexual life has been affected by heavy periods or pelvic pain, which are relieved after hysterectomy. If sexual function is normal before hysterectomy, it is most likely to remain unchanged postoperatively. However, an associated ovarian failure can adversely affect sexuality, which may either precede hysterectomy or develop later. A positive sexual outcome immediately after hysterectomy followed by deterioration after 2 years also supports a hormonal etiology rather than a direct effect of surgery[35]. When bilateral oophorectomy is performed, poor sexual function is more common owing to an absence of testosterone along with estrogen[32,36]. The changes in libido in these women correlate with plasma testosterone levels rather than estrogen levels, but coital and orgasmic frequencies are unrelated to the changing levels of circulating hormones.

Estrogen deficiency causes vaginal dryness and impairs peripheral sensory perception, both of which result in dyspareunia. This reduces sexual frequency and satisfaction which may lead to secondary loss of libido. Estrogen replacement, therefore, enhances sexual activity following hysterectomy by relieving vaginal symptoms without any direct influence on libido. However, the positive effect of estrogen on sexuality is partly due to an improvement in mood and as a result of the relief of menopausal symptoms[37]. Testosterone is involved in the modulation of sex drive and, with the decline or loss of ovarian production, there may be a primary loss of libido. Testosterone replacement, either alone or with estrogen, enhances sexual motivation with a minimum effect on coitus frequency and orgasmic response (Figure 5)[24,27]. However, the added effect of testosterone over estrogen may not always be evident in the absence of loss of libido as a specific complaint[38].

Improved general health, well-being and quality of life

General health and well-being improve significantly in the majority of patients after hysterectomy[20,28,29]. These are a result of a marked recovery from fatigue, depression and sexual dysfunction, in addition to the relief of heavy periods and pelvic pain for which the surgery was indicated. The changes are observed within 3 months and sustained at 1 year, resulting in overall improvement in quality of life. In about 20% of patients, poor general health and well-being persist after hysterectomy owing to pre-existing ovarian failure, rather than the indication for surgery[20]. Similarly, premature ovarian failure following hysterectomy is likely to hamper long-term well-being despite initial complete relief of gynecological symptoms[3,39].

Estrogen replacement therapy can prevent ovarian failure-related deterioration of general health and well-being. Addition of testosterone has a significant effect in improving appetite, well-being and energy levels, especially if these symptoms persist after estrogen replacement[24,25]. In a prospective study monitoring the effects of estrogen and testosterone following hysterectomy and bilateral oophorectomy, those on combined estrogen–testosterone or testosterone alone experienced increased well-being, improved appetite and higher energy than the estrogen-alone and placebo-treated groups (Figure 5)[25]. The differential effect is a reflection of the anabolic and energizing properties of androgen. Routine use of estrogen and testosterone implants following hysterectomy and bilateral oophorectomy results in better long-term general health and well-being[40].

LONG-TERM BENEFITS OF HRT

Cardiovascular protection

Hysterectomy in premenopausal women is associated with a three-fold increased risk of coronary heart disease (CHD), and the deleterious effect has been demonstrated even with ovarian conservation[4,41]. During the 10 years following a hysterectomy, it is claimed that there is a 4% probability of developing CHD and a 0.4% chance of dying from myocardial infarction[4]. However, others have suggested that CHD occurs predominantly when the ovaries are removed at hysterectomy without any postoperative HRT[5]. The risk increases with decreasing age at surgery so, at the age of 35 years, the risk is seven-fold higher than for age-matched premenopausal women. It is the early loss of ovarian function that is responsible for the higher incidence of cardiovascular problems. Estrogen deficiency-induced cardiovascular damage is multifaceted and includes adverse changes in circulating lipid and lipoprotein profile, alterations in insulin resistance, increased body fat in the adverse androgenic distribution, changes in hemostatic factors and increase in arterial resistance[42,43]. Hypertension, a known risk factor for CHD, is twice as common in women following hysterectomy with ovarian conservation than in non-hysterectomized controls of similar age[44].

There is overwhelming evidence that estrogen replacement reduces the risk of coronary heart disease but the beneficial effect is proportional to the duration of therapy[42,45]. In women with a premature menopause, the current use of estrogen replacement nullifies the risk of CHD but, when estrogen is discontinued, the risk increases by 20%[46]. After the age of 50, the reduction in the risk of CHD among those who are current HRT users is 50% and that among former users is 20%, compared to age-matched individuals never on HRT[47]. The impact of estrogen is as great, if not greater, in women with high risk factors for cardiovascular disease. The benefit in terms of survival is maximum in women with established coronary heart disease and there is 80% risk reduction in current HRT users[48].

The beneficial effects of estrogen on the cardiovascular system are not dose-dependent. Most of these changes are also independent of the route of estrogen administration, except for the plasma lipoprotein profile which changes more favorably with the oral route. The preoperative lipid values remain unchanged in premenopausal women if estrogen replacement is started immediately after hysterectomy and bilateral oophorectomy[49]. Addition of oral testosterone has an adverse impact on the circulating lipids and reduces the beneficial effect of estrogen[50], but such hepatic response may be bypassed by using testosterone injection or implant[51].

Prevention of osteoporosis

Premenopausal women undergoing hysterectomy are more likely to develop osteoporosis owing to an earlier onset of accelerated bone loss as a result of postoperative decline in ovarian function[6]. The problem is often overlooked, as the residual ovaries may produce enough estrogen to avoid vasomotor symptoms but not sufficient to protect the skeleton[7]. The bone density in these women has been reported to be significantly less than in age-matched healthy women, irrespective of their menopausal status[6,7]. In premenopausal women who have had a bilateral oophorectomy, the bone density is even lower, as the rate of bone loss is faster owing to an abrupt decline in the circulating hormones (Figure 6)[52]. However, such enhanced bone loss is absent if the ovaries are removed after the natural menopause, which confirms that estrogen deficiency is the most important single causative factor for the bone loss.

Estrogen replacement therapy offers long-term protection against bone loss following hysterectomy. This has been confirmed by the fact that bone densities in both current and previous estrogen users are higher than in non-users[6]. A significant proportion of women continue to lose bone despite taking the recommended bone-sparing dose of estrogen[53]. It is recommended, therefore, either to monitor the

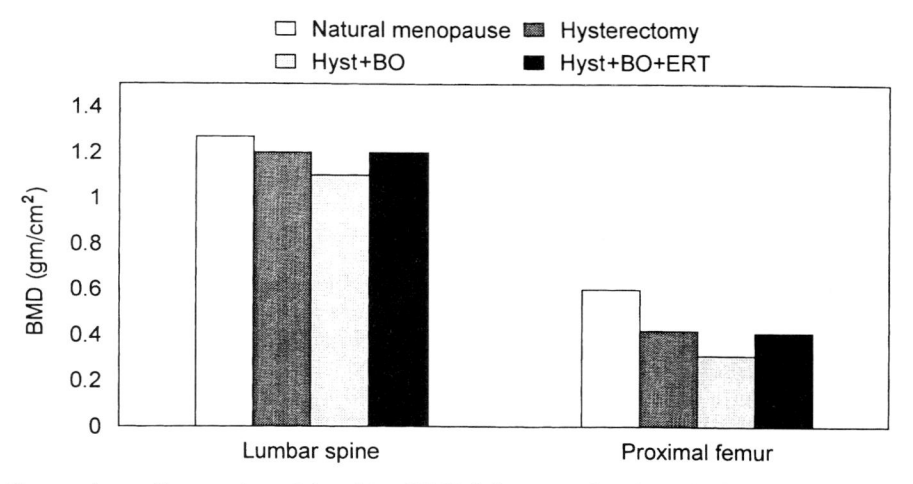

Figure 6 Comparison of bone mineral densities (BMDs) for natural and surgical menopauses with or without hormone replacement therapy (HRT). Adapted from reference 6. Hyst, hysterectomy; BO, bilateral oophorectomy; ERT, estrogen replacement therapy

response with bone density scans every 2–3 years or to start with a higher dose of estrogen from the beginning. Estrogen replacement not only prevents the bone loss but also increases the bone mass. The extent of improvement depends on the route and dose of replacement. There is an annual increase in bone density of 2% with oral estrogen, 2–3.5% with patches and 6–10% with implants. A significant correlation between the plasma estradiol levels and the percentage increase in bone density explains the dose-response of estrogen replacement[54]. Women who had a low bone density at baseline have a greater percentage increase with estrogen replacement. Therefore, there is no truth in the view that women over 60 or many years post-hysterectomy are *too old* or *too osteoporotic* for HRT[55].

It has been suggested that androgens have the potential of improving bone mass and bone mineral content mainly by a direct anabolic effect, but also by peripheral conversion to estrogen. This is supported by the fact that a higher circulating level of androgen is related to a lower incidence of osteoporotic fracture. Following hysterectomy and bilateral oophorectomy, a combined oral estrogen and testosterone replacement has resulted in a better response in bone density than that of estrogen alone[50]. With subcutaneous implants, the anabolic effect of testosterone on bone is more likely, but has not yet been convincingly demonstrated owing to the lack of long-term data[56].

COMPLIANCE WITH HRT AFTER HYSTERECTOMY

HRT indicated for the long term

In women with premature ovarian failure, HRT should be continued at least until the age of natural menopause. Following this essential period, they should be counselled about the benefits and risks of prophylactic long-term HRT and the decision to continue further will depend upon their own response. The compliance to long-term HRT following hysterectomy should be better in the absence of withdrawal bleeding and progestogenic side-effects, the two most common reasons for poor acceptance and discontinuation of the treatment[57].

Current practice of HRT after hysterectomy

An opinion poll organized by the UK National Osteoporosis Society has shown that HRT awareness is low among hysterectomized women. Of all the respondents who had a hysterectomy in the past 5 years, almost two-thirds claimed to have never received any advice about HRT at the time of surgery. Half of these women were not using HRT and 5% of them were not even aware whether their ovaries had been removed at the time of hysterectomy. There are sporadic reports of a compliance rate relatively higher (70%) than the national average, but even then 15–25% of patients did not receive HRT after bilateral oophorectomy[58,59]. In the tertiary setup of the gynecological endocrinology clinic, the long-term compliance with HRT following hysterectomy and bilateral oophorectomy has been over 90% in women under the age of 40 years[21]. In the present authors' own experience with routine use of estradiol and testosterone implants, the continuation rate is 96% after 5 years[40,57]. It is the rate of uptake rather than compliance which is more likely to affect the use of HRT following hysterectomy[59]. Patient satisfaction, which influences the compliance, has been reported to be higher if the follow-up is arranged in a dedicated HRT clinic, whether this is in the general practice or at the hospital[21,59].

Reasons for poor HRT compliance

Although there are very few absolute contraindications, ill-informed medical advice is one of the main reasons for not taking HRT[10]. With anxieties over safety, it may not be prescribed in women with ischemic heart disease, cerebrovascular accidents, diabetes and hypertension. It is well proven that estrogen is not only safe but also improves the prognoses of these diseases and the benefit is more than that for the average healthy woman. The presumed contraindications and side-effects of HRT have arisen because of the failure to discriminate between natural and synthetic estrogens in terms of potency and action, which has led to unfounded extrapolation of oral contraceptive-pill data to the HRT information sheets. This incorrect information is largely responsible for failure to prescribe HRT on the part of the doctor and for poor compliance by the patient.

A further reason for discontinuation of HRT is that there is often inadequate communication between the gynecologist, the patient and the general practitioner. The patients may be unaware of the importance of HRT following hysterectomy, and may not have been told or retained the information whether their ovaries have been removed at the time of surgery. The gynecologist usually discharges the patients 6 weeks after surgery expecting that the general practitioner will prescribe the HRT. The general practitioner may be under the impression that the patient is receiving HRT from the hospital or may even be uncertain whether an oophorectomy has been performed. As a result of such misunderstandings, the patients will not receive HRT after the initial postoperative dose.

With the obsession of many clinicians for using the lowest possible dose of oral estrogen, some women may suffer from climacteric symptoms following hysterectomy despite being on HRT[21,57]. Testosterone supplementation is often ignored, which results in refractory symptoms of headache, depression, poor libido and tiredness. The lack of efficacy owing to inadequate dose and inappropriate type of HRT may lead to dissatisfaction and discontinuation of the treatment[57]. It would seem prudent to use an effective higher dose of estrogen by a more effective route and addition of testosterone for complete symptom control, thereby improving the patient's confidence and compliance with HRT.

The main worry about long-term HRT is the possible increased risk of breast cancer. The concern is based on the issue that the factors leading to prolonged ovarian activity, such as early menarche, late menopause and nulliparity or late first pregnancy, are associated with an increase in the risk of breast cancer. Conversely, with premature menopause, the risk is reduced by minimizing the estrogenic stimulation of breast tissue. Thus, hysterectomy with or without bilateral oophorectomy in premenopausal women decreases the risk of breast cancer, possibly by curtailing ovarian function at a critical period. The use of HRT in these women up to the age of 50 may increase the risk slightly, but the risk is still lower than in those with normal ovarian function[60,61] (Figure 7). It is inappropriate, therefore, to extrapolate the risk of long-term HRT after natural menopause to relatively younger hysterectomized women with premature ovarian failure.

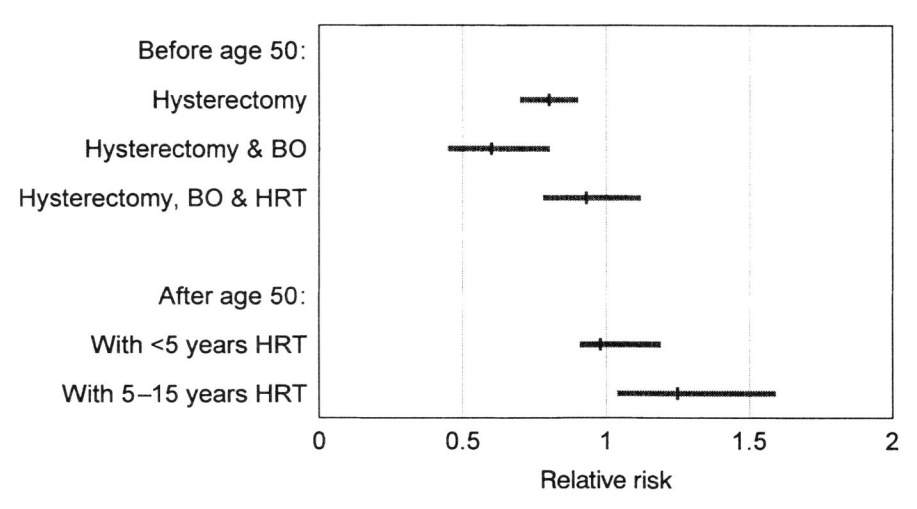

Figure 7 Relative risks of breast cancer following hysterectomy, bilateral oophorectomy (BO) and hormone replacement therapy (HRT). Adapted from references 60 and 61

Practical guidelines to improve HRT compliance

The need for long-term HRT following hysterectomy and bilateral oophorectomy should be emphasized at a stage when the decision for surgery is taken. Before discharging the patient from the hospital, the gynecologist must liaise with the general practitioner concerning the patient's follow-up for HRT. The patient should be reviewed every 6 months to ensure continued compliance. The dose, type and route of HRT should be altered in response to poor symptom control and side-effects. Those who continue to experience problems should be referred to a specialist menopause clinic for satisfactory stabilization. After this stage, the follow-up may be carried out by the general practitioner, but good communication and continued access to the specialist menopause clinic should be maintained if any problem develops in the future.

Health professionals should be extra vigilant about the possibility of premature failure of the residual ovaries when dealing with hysterectomized patients. Two blood tests at an interval of a fortnight are needed to avoid an incorrect diagnosis owing to low estradiol levels in the early follicular phase or high gonadotropin levels in mid-cycle. An abnormal hormonal profile confirming ovarian failure indicates HRT even in the absence of any climacteric symptoms. Many women experience their most severe symptoms owing to fluctuation in hormone levels, and should not be denied HRT on the basis of premenopausal hormone levels.

Ideally, following hysterectomy, all women should receive a reminder to attend the clinic annually for either a hormone screen or confirmation of HRT compliance. It is easy to identify hysterectomized women in a community, as they are the ones who are excluded from the cervical cancer screening list. The ovaries are removed in 20% of hysterectomies and, in a quarter of the remaining cases, the conserved ovaries fail prematurely. One in five women in the UK are likely to have a hysterectomy before the age of 60[1], and the prospect of ovarian hormone deficiency in nearly half of these women indicates the size of the problem. The task of identifying and arranging HRT for such a large population seems phenomenal but, in a general practice serving a population of 2000, there would be only 50–60 hysterectomized women.

CONCLUSIONS

If the ovaries are conserved at hysterectomy, there should not be a complacent view of continued function until the age of natural menopause. The residual ovaries may fail earlier, although it is still uncertain whether this is due to hysterectomy or whether the indication for the treatment is associated with declining ovarian function. It is important to recognize such patients either by their cyclical presentation of climacteric symptoms or by regular endocrine monitoring, in which case a high gonadotropin level is an earlier diagnostic finding than a low estradiol level. These women with ovarian failure require long-term estrogen replacement, which is more acceptable in the absence of withdrawal bleeding and progestogenic side-effects. A higher dose of estrogen and additional testosterone supplementation may be needed for total symptom control, particularly after bilateral oophorectomy. The short-term benefits of HRT, such as relief from climacteric symptoms, improvement in mental health, and unchanged or improved sexuality, influence patient satisfaction following hysterectomy. An appropriate selection of effective HRT and a routine follow-up may help to improve the long-term compliance that is needed for preventing cardiovascular disease and osteoporosis. Risk–benefit analysis of HRT has confirmed that the potential to improve quality and length of life is more applicable following hysterectomy. In spite of these well-established benefits, the majority of patients either do not receive or fail to continue using HRT. Thus, correct advice on HRT-related misconceptions, proper selection of the type and dose of HRT, and organization of regular follow-ups are required for long-term compliance with HRT in this high-risk population.

References

1. Coulter A, McPherson K, Vessey M. Do British women have too many or too few hysterectomies? *Soc Sci Med* 1988;27:987–94
2. Studd JWW. Shifting the indications for hysterectomy. *Lancet* 1995;345:388–9
3. Oldenhave A, Jaszmann L, Everaerd W, et al. Hysterectomized women with ovarian conservation report more climacteric complaints than do normal climacteric women of similar age. *Am J Obstet Gynecol* 1993;168:765–71
4. Centerwall BS. Premenopausal hysterectomy and cardiovascular disease. *Am J Obstet Gynecol* 1981;139:58–61
5. Rosenburg L, Hennenkens CH, Rosner B, et al. Early menopause and the risk of myocardial infarction. *Am J Obstet Gynecol* 1981;139:47–51
6. Hreshchyshyn MM, Hopkins A, Zylstra S, et al. Effects of natural menopause, hysterectomy and oophorectomy on lumbar spine and femoral neck bone densities. *Obstet Gynecol* 1988;72:631–8
7. Watson N, Studd J, Garnett T, et al. Bone loss following hysterectomy with ovarian conservation. *Obstet Gynecol* 1995;86:72–7
8. Studd JWW. Hysterectomy and menorrhagia. *Bailliere's Clin Obstet Gynecol* 1989;3:415–24
9. Spector TD. Use of oestrogen replacement therapy in high risk groups in the United Kingdom. *Br Med J* 1989;299:1434–5
10. Norman SG, Studd JWW. A survey: views on hormone replacement therapy. *Br J Obstet Gynecol* 1994;101:879–87
11. Souza AZ, Fonseca AM, Izzo VM, et al. Ovarian histology and function after total abdominal hysterectomy. *Obstet Gynecol* 1986;68:847–9
12. Kaiser R, Kusche M, Wurz H. Hormone levels in women after hysterectomy. *Arch Gynecol Obstet* 1989;244:169–73
13. Riedel HH, Lehman-Willenbrock E, Semm K. Ovarian failure phenomenon after hysterectomy. *J Reprod Med* 1986;31:597–600
14. Siddle N, Sarrel P, Whitehead M. The effect of hysterectomy on the age at ovarian failure: identification of a subgroup of women with premature loss of ovarian function and literature review. *Fertil Steril* 1987;47:94–100
15. Chakravarti S, Collins WP, Newton JR, et al. Endocrine changes and symptomatology following oophorectomy in pre-menopausal women. *Br J Obstet Gynaecol* 1977;84:769–75
16. Vermeulen A. The hormonal activity of the postmenopausal ovary. *J Clin Endocrinol Med* 1976;42:247–53
17. Adashi EY. The climacteric ovary as a functional gonadotropin driven androgen producing gland. *Fertil Steril* 1994;62:20–7
18. Pokras R, Hufnagel V. Hysterectomy in the United States 1965–84. *Am J Publ Health* 1988;78:852–3

19. Studd JWW. Prophylactic oophorectomy. *Br J Obstet Gynaecol* 1989;96:506–9
20. Carlson KJ, Miller BA, Fowler FJ. The Maine women's health study: I. Outcomes of hysterectomy. *Obstet Gynecol* 1994;83:556–65
21. Reid BA, Ganger KF. Oophorectomy in young women: can it ever be justified? *Contemp Rev Obstet Gynaecol* 1994;6:41–5
22. Kamel EM, Maurer SA, Hochler MG, et al. Gonadotropin dynamics in women receiving immediate or delayed transdermal oestradiol after oophorectomy. *Obstet Gynecol* 1991;78:98–102
23. Anderson CHM, Raju SK, Forsling ML, et al. Oestrogen replacement after oophorectomy: comparison of patches and implants. *Br Med J* 1992;305:90–1
24. Brincat M, Magos AI, Studd JWW, et al. Subcutaneous hormone implants for the control of climacteric symptoms. A prospective study. *Lancet* 1984;1:16–18
25. Sherwin BB, Galfand MM. Differential symptom response to parenteral oestrogen and/or testosterone administration in the surgical menopause. *Am J Obstet Gynecol* 1985;151:153–60
26. Sherwin BB and Gelfand MM. Sex steroids and affect in the surgical menopause: a double-blind cross over study. *Psychoneuroendocrinology* 1985;10:325–35
27. Sherwin BB, Gelfand MM, Brender W. Androgen enhances sexual motivation in females: a prospective, crossover study of sex steroid administration in the surgical menopause. *Psychosom Med* 1985;47:339–50
28. Gath D, Cooper P, Day A. Hysterectomy and psychiatric disorder: I. Levels of psychiatric morbidity before and after hysterectomy. *Br J Psychiatry* 1982;140:335–42
29. Ryan MM, Dennerstein L, Peperell R. Psychological aspects of hysterectomy: a prospective study. *Br J Psychiatry* 1989;154:516–22
30. Dikoff EC, Crary WG, Christo M, et al. Oestrogen improves psychological function in postmenopausal women. *Obstet Gynecol* 1991;78:991–5
31. Best N, Rees M, Barlow D. Effect of oestradiol implant on nonadrenergic function and mood in menopausal patients. *Psychoneuroendocrinology* 1992;17:87–93
32. Nathorst-Boos J, von Schoultz B. Psychological reaction and sexual life after hysterectomy with and without oophorectomy. *Gynecol Obstet Invest* 1992;34:97–101
33. McEwen BS. Ovarian steroids have diverse effects on brain structure and function. In Berg G, Hammar M, eds. *The Modern Management of Menopause*. New York: Parthenon Publishing, 1993:269–78
34. Helstrom L, Lungberg PO, Sorbom D, et al. Sexuality after hysterectomy: a factor analysis of women's sexual lives before and after hysterectomy. *Obstet Gynecol* 1993;81:357–62
35. Bernhard LA. Consequence of hysterectomy in the lives of women. *Health Care Women Int* 1992;13:281–91
36. Studd JWW, Collin WP, Chakravarti S, et al. Oestradiol and testosterone implants in the treatment of psychosexual problems in the post-menopausal woman. *Br J Obstet Gynaecol* 1977;84:314–15
37. Dennerstein L, Burrows GD, Wood C, et al. Hormones and sexuality: effect of oestrogen and progestogen. *Obstet Gynecol* 1980;56:316–22
38. Burger H, Hailes J, Nelson J, et al. Effect of combined implants of oestradiol and testosterone on libido in postmenopausal women. *Br Med J* 1984;294:936–7
39. Schofield MJ, Bennett A, Redman S, et al. Self-reported long-term outcomes of hysterectomy. *Br J Obstet Gynaecol* 1991;98:1129–36
40. Khastgir G, Studd JWW. A survey of patients' attitude, experience and satisfaction with hysterectomy, oophorectomy and hormone replacement by oestradiol and testosterone implants. *Obstet Gynecol* 1997;submitted
41. Palmer JR, Rosenberg L, Shapiro S. Reproductive factors and risk of myocardial infarction. *Am J Epidemiol* 1992;131:408–16
42. Gruchow HW, Anderson AJ, Barboriak JJ, et al. Postmenopausal use of oestrogen and occlusion of coronary heart disease. *Am Heart J* 1988;115:954–63
43. Stampfer MJ, Colditz GA, Willett WC. Menopause and heart disease: a review. *Ann NY Acad Sci* 1990;592:193–203
44. Luoto R, Kaprio J, Reunanen A, et al. Cardiovascular morbidity in relation to ovarian function after hysterectomy. *Obstet Gynecol* 1995;85:515–22
45. Stampfer MJ, Colditz GA. Oestrogen replacement therapy and coronary heart disease: a quantitative assessment of the epidemiological evidence. *Prevent Med* 1991;20:47–63
46. Grady D, Rubin SM, Petitti DB, et al. Hormone therapy to prevent disease and prolong life in postmenopausal women. *Ann Intern Med* 1992;117:1016–37
47. Rosenburg L, Slone D, Shapiro S, et al. Noncontraceptive oestrogen and myocardial infarction. *J Am Med Assoc* 1980;244:339–42
48. Sullivan JM, Zwagg RV, Lemp GF, et al. Oestrogen replacement and coronary heart disease. *Arch Int Med* 1990;150:2557–62
49. Erenus M, Kutlay K, Kutlay L. Comparison of the impact of oral versus transdermal oestrogen on serum lipoproteins. *Fertil Steril* 1994;61:300–2

50. Watts NB, Notelovitz M, Timmons MC, et al. Comparison of oral oestrogen and oestrogen plus androgen on bone density and lipid–lipoprotein profiles in surgical menopause. *Obstet Gynecol* 1995;85:529–37
51. Sherwin BB, Gelfand MM, Schucher R, et al. Postmenopausal oestrogen and androgen replacement and lipoprotein lipid concentration. *Am J Obstet Gynecol* 1987;156:414–19
52. Pansini F, Bagni B, Bonaccorsi G, et al. Oophorectomy and spinal bone density: evidence of higher rate of bone loss in surgical compared with spontaneous menopause. *Menopause* 1995; 2:109–15
53. Bouillon B, Burckhardt P, Christiansen C, et al. Consensus development conference: prophylaxis and treatment of osteoporosis. *Am J Med* 1991;90:107–10
54. Studd JWW, Savvas M, Watson NR, et al. The relationship between plasma oestradiol and the increase in bone density in postmenopausal women after treatment with subcutaneous hormone implants. *Am J Obstet Gynecol* 1990;163: 1474–9
55. Studd JWW, Holland EFN, Leather AT, et al. The dose-response of percutaneous oestradiol implants on the skeletons of postmenopausal women. *Br J Obstet Gynaecol* 1994;101: 787–91
56. Garnet TJ, Studd JWW, Savvas M, et al. The effects of plasma oestradiol levels on the increase in vertebral and femoral bone density following oestradiol and testosterone implants. *Obstet Gynecol* 1992;79:768–72
57. Studd JWW. Continuation rates with cyclical and continuous regimens of oral oestrogen and progestogens. *Menopause* 1996;3:181–2
58. Seeley T. Oestrogen replacement therapy after hysterectomy. *Br Med J* 1992;305:811–12
59. Griffiths F, Convery B. Women's use of hormone replacement therapy for relief of menopausal symptoms, for prevention of osteoporosis and after hysterectomy. *Br J Gen Pract* 1995;45:355–8
60. Irwin KL, Lee NC, Peterson HB, et al. Hysterectomy, tubal sterilization and risk of breast cancer. *Am J Epidemiol* 1988;127:1192–201
61. Meijer WJ, van Lindert ACM. Prophylactic oophorectomy. *Eur J Obstet Gynecol Reprod Biol* 1992; 47:59–65

27
Efficacy of combined estrogen–androgen preparations in the postmenopause

B. B. Sherwin

During the past decade, findings from well-controlled studies have demonstrated unequivocally the protective effect of exogenous estrogen with respect to cardiovascular disease and osteoporosis in postmenopausal women. Despite the fact that the premenopausal ovary also produces one-third of all testosterone in women, there is still a paucity of studies on the benefits and risks of combined estrogen–androgen (E–A) replacement therapy following a natural or surgical menopause. However, interest in combined E–A regimens is increasing, probably as a result of heightened concern regarding quality-of-life issues among the current generation of 50-year-olds. The small but growing body of literature on combined E–A preparations currently available allows several conclusions regarding their effects and provides suggestions for future research.

ANDROGEN PRODUCTION IN WOMEN

In women, both the adrenal and the ovary contain the biosynthetic pathways necessary for androgen synthesis and secretion. It has been estimated that, in premenopausal women, 49% of testosterone, the most potent androgen, is of adrenal origin, 17% arises from peripheral conversion of other steroid precursors and 33% is produced by the ovary[1]. The ovary also produces approximately 60% of androstenedione and 20% of dehydroepiandrosterone (DHEA). After the menopause, the ovarian production of androstenedione decreases profoundly and secretion of testosterone also declines owing to atrophy of ovarian stromal tissue[2]. The fall in the secretion of androstenedione, a major source of testosterone, results in a further decline in circulating testosterone in most postmenopausal women.

In addition to the postmenopausal decrease in the ovarian production of testosterone, it is also important to consider that, in plasma, testosterone is largely bound to sex hormone-binding globulin (SHBG)[3], which is increased by estrogen and decreased by androgens[3]. Therefore, in postmenopausal women treated with estrogen alone, even less of the already diminished testosterone is able to exert biological activity because the exogenous estrogen will have increased SHBG production and, thereby, the amount of SHBG-bound testosterone. It is probable, therefore, that postmenopausal women treated with estrogen replacement therapy have less available free testosterone than untreated women.

Whether or not testosterone should also be replaced in postmenopausal women of course depends on the behavioral and biochemical effects of exogenous testosterone. At present, evidence is available to suggest that testosterone influences the central nervous system, bone metabolism and lipoprotein lipid metabolism. Each of these areas will be discussed in turn.

TESTOSTERONE AND THE CENTRAL NERVOUS SYSTEM

Autoradiographic studies have demonstrated that neurons containing specific receptors for testosterone are predominantly found in the preoptic area of the hypothalamus, with smaller concentrations in the limbic system (amygdala and hippocampus) and the cerebral cortex[4].

In male rats, there is evidence that serotonin receptor subtypes mediate androgen effects on sexual behavior. The type of androgen treatment which induces male sexual behavior increases 5HT1A receptor binding in the preoptic area and decreases 5HT3 receptors in the amygdala[5]. No such studies have been undertaken in female rats whose sexual behavior is largely under the control of estrogen and progesterone acting on the ventromedial nucleus. On the other hand, effects of testosterone on various components of mating behavior have been studied intensively in female non-human primates. On the whole, these studies show that the administration of testosterone to ovariectomized rhesus monkeys increased proceptive behavior (i.e. increased attempts to solicit mounts from the male). Implantation of minute amounts of testosterone into the anterior hypothalamus of estrogen-treated ovariectomized and adrenalectomized unreceptive female rhesus monkeys also resulted in restoration of their proceptivity without affecting other aspects of sexual behavior such as attractivity[6].

These studies on testosterone and sexual behavior in female non-human primates serve to underline two points. One is that there is a specificity of action of testosterone on components of sexual behavior such that it enhances proceptivity (the animal's motivation to engage in sexual behavior) but has no effect on its attractivity or its receptivity to males. Second, the fact that a very small dose of testosterone implanted in the hypothalamus was effective in restoring sexual desire in rhesus monkeys[6] suggests that testosterone exerts its effect on sexual desire in female rhesus directly on the brain and not by an influence on peripheral tissues.

TESTOSTERONE AND SEXUALITY IN THE POSTMENOPAUSE

Several correlational studies have tested the association between circulating levels of the sex steroids and aspects of sexual behavior in postmenopausal women. Leiblum and colleagues[7] reported that neither estradiol nor testosterone discriminated between sexually active and inactive untreated postmenopausal women, but sexually active women had less vaginal atrophy than the inactive women. In a longitudinal study of perimenopausal women, plasma testosterone levels were positively associated with coital frequency[8]. Moreover, a positive correlation occurred between testosterone levels and sexual desire and sexual arousal in premenopausal women over the age of 40 years[9]. Other epidemiological studies that have investigated changes in sexual functioning in peri- and postmenopausal women failed to measure circulating levels of hormones[10,11]. One recent population-based study in middle-aged women failed to find an association between testosterone levels and any aspect of sexual functioning[12].

Another and perhaps more powerful paradigm for investigating the role of testosterone in women involves administering hormone replacement therapy to women who have just undergone total abdominal hysterectomy (TAH) and bilateral salpingo-oophorectomy (BSO). When both ovaries are removed from premenopausal women, circulating testosterone levels decrease significantly within the first 24–48 h postoperatively[13]. The fact that these women are deprived of ovarian androgen production following this surgical procedure has provided a rationale for administering both estrogen and androgen as replacement therapy.

In Britain and Australia, subcutaneous implantation of pellets containing estradiol and testosterone has been used as a treatment for menopausal symptoms for several decades. This route of sex-steroid administration results in a slow constant release of the sex hormones over a period of at least 6 months. Women complaining of decreased libido despite treatment with estrogen received subcutaneous implants of 40 mg estradiol and 100 mg testosterone[14].

Patients reported a significant increase in libido by the third postimplantation month. These findings gained support from a double-blind study of women complaining of loss of libido despite treatment with oral estrogens[15]. They randomly received a subcutaneous implant containing either estrogen alone or estrogen plus testosterone. After 6 weeks, the loss of libido in the estrogen-alone implant group remained, whereas the combined estrogen–testosterone group showed significant symptomatic relief.

In a recent prospective, 2-year, single-blind randomized trial, 34 postmenopausal women received either estradiol 50 mg implants or estradiol 50 mg plus testosterone 50 mg implants administered every 3 months[16]. Women who received the combined implant had a significantly greater improvement compared with those receiving estrogen alone, in sexual activity, satisfaction, pleasure and orgasm.

During the past decade, several prospective, controlled studies of general and sexual effects of combined estrogen–androgen parenteral preparations in surgically menopausal women were carried out in our laboratory. These studies have shown that the addition of testosterone to an estrogen replacement regimen induces a greater sense of energy level and well-being and is associated with fewer somatic and psychological symptoms when compared with the administration of estrogen alone[17–19]. Furthermore, the intramuscular administration of testosterone, either alone or in combination with estradiol, increased motivational aspects of sexual behavior (such as desire and fantasies) compared with the administration of estrogen alone or a placebo[12]. Levels of sexual desire and interest covaried with plasma testosterone level throughout a treatment month as the intramuscular drug was being metabolized[17]. The androgenic enhancement of sexual motivation in women treated with the combined intramuscular drug has been shown to persist with long-term chronic administration of monthly injections that cause an initial surge in testosterone levels and metabolize slowly over a period of several weeks[18].

Taken together, the findings from the subcutaneous implant pellet studies and the prospective studies on oophorectomized women provide compelling evidence that testosterone acts to increase overall energy level and also to enhance sexual desire and arousal in women, although frequency of sexual activity and of orgasms are unaffected. These findings allow the conclusion that, in women, just as in men[20], testosterone has its major impact on the cognitive motivational, or libidinal aspects of sexual behavior such as desire and fantasies, and not on physiological responses. Moreover, studies on non-human primates suggest the likelihood that testosterone exerts this effect on sexual desire via mechanisms that impact directly on the brain rather than by an effect on peripheral tissues[6].

It has been recently established that exogenous testosterone has a positive influence on bone metabolism in postmenopausal women. Women randomly treated with subcutaneous implants of estrogen plus testosterone had a greater increase in bone mineral density in the hip and lumbar spine than those given estrogen-alone implants[21]. In a more recent, open-label study of postmenopausal women randomized to either oral estrogen plus methyltestosterone or estrogen alone, both therapies similarly reduced biochemical markers of bone resorption (deoxypyridinoline, pyridinoline, hydroxyproline), while only users of the combined therapy had increased markers for bone formation (bone-specific alkaline phosphatase, osteocalcin, C-terminal procollagen peptide)[22]. The weight of the evidence, therefore, suggests that while estrogen alone prevents bone loss in postmenopausal women, combined estrogen–testosterone regimens appear to actually increase bone mass by 2–4%.

POSSIBLE ADVERSE EFFECTS OF COMBINED ESTROGEN–TESTOSTERONE REGIMENS

Lipoprotein lipids and cardiovascular health

Meta-analyses of observational studies suggest a 50% reduction in heart disease risk in postmenopausal women taking estrogen[23].

Although the co-administration of a progestin either continuously or cyclicly attenuates the beneficial effect of estrogen on high-density lipoprotein (HDL) cholesterol, the lipid profile in hormone-treated women is preferable to that in placebo-treated women[24].

The addition of testosterone to an estrogen replacement therapy regimen may partially offset the beneficial effects of estrogen on risk factors for cardiovascular disease. Oral estrogen–androgen replacement reduced both total cholesterol and low-density lipoproteins (LDLs) more than oral estrogen alone[25]. However, the addition of testosterone to the regimen also decreased HDL levels relative to estrogen alone, thereby resulting in a detrimental increase in the ratio of HDL total cholesterol[25]. However, combined preparations also lower triglyceride levels compared to those with estrogen alone, which is thought to be beneficial[21].

Studies of non-oral routes of administration of estrogen–androgen drugs tell a somewhat different story. Subcutaneous implantation of estradiol 40 mg and testosterone 100 mg did not cause any changes in cholesterol, triglycerides or HDL cholesterol from pretreatment levels[26]. Farish and colleagues[27] likewise found that subcutaneous pellets of estradiol 50 mg and testosterone 100 mg had no effect on HDL fractions but testosterone appeared to slightly enhance the LDL cholesterol-lowering effect of estradiol. Following 2 years of treatment with an intramuscular combined estrogen–androgen depot preparation, Sherwin and associates[28] reported that combined replacement therapy did not adversely affect the lipoprotein cholesterol profile in these women compared with patients treated with parenteral estrogen alone and surgically menopausal women who were untreated. Other evidence suggests that the route of administration modulates the response to hormone therapy. For example, percutaneous and vaginal administration of estradiol do not cause the increases in triglycerides and very low-density lipoprotein (VLDL) observed during oral therapy[29]. Thus, it seems likely that parenteral routes of administration of combined estrogen–androgen drugs in the postmenopause may not cause the detrimental effect on HDL seen with oral preparations, as parenteral routes of administration bypass the so-called 'hepatic first-pass effect'.

It also seems clear that the cardioprotective effects of estrogen are only partially mediated through changes in lipids and lipoproteins. Indeed, it has been estimated that only 25–50% of cardiovascular risk reduction provided by estrogen replacement therapy can be predicted by lipoproteins[30]. Examples of non-lipoprotein-mediated actions are reduced atherosclerotic plaque formation unrelated to HDL cholesterol levels[31] and estrogen-induced vasodilatation[32]. In this regard, it is both interesting and potentially important that treatment of ovariectomized cynomolgus monkeys with oral estrogens improved indothelium-mediated vasodilatation of their atherosclerotic coronary arteries, and the addition of oral methyltestosterone did not alter this response[33]. These findings demonstrate that combined estrogen–androgen replacement therapy does not negate all cardiovascular benefits of estrogen alone.

Symptoms of virilization

Empirical data from controlled studies on the incidence of hirsutism in postmenopausal women treated with combined estrogen–androgen preparations could not be located. However, our own extensive clinical experience suggests that approximately 20% of women who receive 150 mg testosterone enanthate intramuscularly every 4 weeks along with estrogen will develop mild hirsutism manifested by an increased growth of hair on the chin and/or upper lip. When the dose is reduced to 75 mg testosterone enanthate per month, less than 5% of women have an increased hair growth. Moreover, hair growth decreases or usually stops entirely when the patient is switched to treatment with estrogen alone. There is little doubt that, in women, hirsutism is a dose-dependent side-effect of exogenous testosterone. Its development would depend also on the amount of estrogen given in combination, as both sex steroids influence the production of SHBG which, in turn, determines the concentration of free, or biologically available, testosterone.

Effects on endometrial histology

Of course, the postmenopausal uterus must be protected from excessive estrogenic stimulation during estrogen replacement therapy. The relevant question, therefore, is whether the addition of androgen to an estrogen replacement regimen should be co-administered with more or less progestin than would be used to prevent endometrial hyperplasia with estrogen alone. In a study that compared the effect of oral estrogen alone with an oral combined estrogen–androgen preparation on endometrial histology, similar changes in estrogen-stimulated proliferative growth occurred in both groups after 6 months of treatment[22]. The majority of women developed a moderately proliferative endometrial histology pattern and no woman displayed hyperplastic changes. Others have found endometrial hyperplasia both in women treated with estrogen alone and in those given a combined preparation[34]. It would seem, therefore, that the addition of testosterone neither facilitates nor antagonizes the stimulatory effect of estrogens on the endometrium. This suggests that a progestational agent should be added to the hormone regimen when a combined estrogen–androgen preparation is used.

CONCLUSION

On the basis of available data, it is now possible to conclude that the addition of testosterone to an estrogen replacement regimen for the treatment of postmenopausal women increases energy level, sense of well-being, and sexual desire and interest over and above treatment with estrogen alone. However, it is important to remember that human sexual behavior is extremely complex and that hormones are one among a multitude of factors that underlie this behavior. Menopause occurs during midlife, which can bring with it changes and stresses such as the need to take care of one's own aging parents and young adult children. Decreased libido is also a symptom of a major depressive episode. It is important, therefore, to exclude other possible contributing factors to a sexual dysfunction before recommending treatment with an estrogen–androgen combined drug.

A second indication for combined therapy is the persistence of a low energy level, fatigue and loss of well-being in a woman who has had a reasonable trial of treatment with estrogen alone. These symptoms are especially frequent in women who experience a premature or surgical menopause where the decrease in testosterone is more abrupt. Along with decreases in libido, these symptoms are more common than previously thought and may seriously impair a woman's quality of life, which combined therapy might restore.

The dose of testosterone used for combined estrogen–testosterone replacement therapy should induce physiological levels of plasma testosterone similar to the range of values in young, ovulating women, to preclude virilizing side-effects. Finally, testosterone should only be administered to women who are also receiving estrogen replacement therapy; when given alone to a postmenopausal woman unopposed by estrogen, the possibility of an adverse androgenic effect on plasma lipids would be increased.

ACKNOWLEDGEMENTS

The preparation of this manuscript was supported by a grant from the Medical Research Council of Canada (no. MA–11623) awarded to B. B. Sherwin.

References

1. Longcope C. Adrenal and gonadal androgen secretion in normal females. *Clin Endocrinol Metab* 1986;15:213–28

2. Longcope C, Franz C, Morello C, *et al.* Steroid and gonadotropin levels in women during their perimenopausal years. *Maturitas* 1986;8:189–96

3. Nisula BC, Rodbard D. Transport of steroid hormones. Binding endogenous steroids to both testosterone-binding globulin in human plasma. *J Clin Endocrinol Metab* 1981;53:58–68
4. McEwen BS. The brain as a target organ of endocrine hormones. In Kreiger DT, Hughes JS, eds. *Neuroendocrinology*. Sutherland, MA: Sinauer Association, 1980:33–42
5. Mendelson S, McEwen BS. Testosterone increases the concentration of (H^3 8-hydroxy-2-propylamine) tethelin binding at 5-HT$_3$A receptors in the medial preoptic nucleus of the castrated male rat. *Eur J Pharmacol* 1990;181:329–31
6. Everitt BJ, Herbert J. The effects of implanting testosterone propionate in the central nervous system on the sexual behavior of the female rhesus monkey. *Brain Res* 1975;86:109–20
7. Leiblum S, Bachmann G, Kemmann E, et al. Vaginal atrophy in the postmenopausal woman: the importance of sexual activity and hormones. *J Am Med Assoc* 1983;249:2195–8
8. McCoy N, Davidson J. A longitudinal study of the effects of menopause on sexuality. *Maturitas* 1985;7:203–10
9. Flöter A, Nathorst-Böös J, Carlstrom K, et al. Androgen status and sexual life in perimenopausal women. *Menopause* 1997;4:95–100
10. Dennerstein L, Smith AMS, Morse CA, et al. Sexuality and the menopause. *J Psychosom Obstet Gynaecol* 1994;15:59–66
11. Hallstrom T. Sexuality in the climacteric. *Clin Obstet Gynecol* 1977;4:227–39
12. Dennerstein L, Dudley EC, Hopper JL, et al. Sexuality, hormones and the menopausal transition. *Maturitas* 1977;26:83–93
13. Longcope C. Metabolism clearance and blood production rates of estrogen in postmenopausal women. *Am J Obstet Gynecol* 1981;111:779–85
14. Burger HG, Hailles J, Menelaus M, et al. The management of persistent menopausal symptoms with oestradiol testosterone implants: clinical, lipid and hormonal results. *Maturitas* 1984;6:351–8
15. Burger HG, Hailles J, Nelson J, et al. Effects of combined implants of estradiol and testosterone on libido in postmenopausal women. *Lancet* 1987;294:936–7
16. Davis SR, McClaud P, Strauss BJG, et al. Testosterone enhances estradiol's effects on postmenopausal bone density and sexuality. *Maturitas* 1995;21:227–36
17. Sherwin BB, Gelfand MM. Differential symptom response to parenteral estrogen and/or androgen administration in the surgical menopause. *Am J Obstet Gynecol* 1985;151:153–60
18. Sherwin BB, Gelfand MM. The role of androgen in the maintenance of sexual functioning in oophorectomized women. *Psychosom Med* 1987;49:397–409
19. Sherwin BB, Gelfand MM, Brender W. Androgen enhances sexual motivation in females: a prospective cross-over study of sex steroid administration in the surgical menopause. *Psychosom Med* 1985;7:339–51
20. Bancroft J, Wu FCW. Changes in erectile responsiveness during androgen replacement therapy. *Arch Sex Behav* 1983;12:59–66
21. Watts NB, Notelovitz M, Timmons MC, et al. Comparison of oral estrogens and estrogens plus androgen on bone mineral density, menopausal symptoms, and lipid–lipoprotein profiles in surgical menopausal women. *Obstet Gynecol* 1995;85:529–37
22. Raisz LG, Wiita B, Artis A, et al. Comparison of estrogen alone and estrogen plus androgen on biochemical markers of bone formation and resorption in postmenopausal women. *J Clin Endocrinol Metab* 1996;81:37–43
23. Grady D, Rubin SM, Petitti DB, et al. Hormone therapy to prevent disease and prolong life in postmenopausal women. *Ann Intern Med* 1992;117:1016–37
24. The Writing Group for the PEPI Trial. Effects of estrogen or estrogen/progestin regimens on heart disease risk factors in postmenopausal women. *J Am Med Assoc* 1995;273:199–208
25. Hickok LR, Toomey C, Speroff L. A comparison of esterified estrogens with and without methyltestosterone: effects on endometrial histology and serum lipoproteins in postmenopausal women. *Obstet. Gynecol* 1993;82:919–24
26. Teran AZ, Gambrell RD Jr. Androgens in clinical practices. In Speroff L, ed. *Androgens in the Menopause*. New York: McGraw-Hill, 1988:14–22
27. Farish E, Fletcher CD, Hart DM, et al. The effect of hormone implants on serum lipoproteins and steroid hormones in bilaterally oophorectomized women. *Acta Endocrinol* 1984;106:116–23
28. Sherwin BB, Gelfand MM, Schucher R, et al. Postmenopausal estrogen and androgen replacement and lipoprotein lipid concentrations. *Am J Obstet Gynecol* 1987;156:414–19
29. Mischell DR Jr, Moore RE, Roy S, et al. Clinical performance and endocrine profiles with contraceptive vaginal rings containing a combination of estradiol and d-norgestrel. *Am J Obstet Gynecol* 1978;130:155–61
30. Bush TL, Barrett-Connor E, Cowan LD, et al. Cardiovascular mortality and noncontraceptive use of estrogen in women: results from the Lipid Research Clinics Program follow-up study. *Circulation* 1987;75:1102–9
31. Adams MR, Clarkson TB, Koritnik DR, et al. Contraceptive steroids and coronary artery

32. Sarrel P. Ovarian hormones and the circulation. *Maturitas* 1990;590:287–98
33. Honoré EH, Williams JK, Adams MR, *et al.* Methyltestosterone does not diminish the beneficial effects of estrogen replacement therapy on coronary artery reactivity in cynomolgus monkeys. *Menopause* 1996;3:20–6
34. Gelfand MM, Ferenczy A, Bergeron C. Endometrial response to estrogen–androgen stimulation. In Hammond CB, Haseltine FB, Seniff I, eds. *Menopause Evaluation Treatment and Health Concerns.* New York: Alan R Liss, 1989:29–40

atherosclerosis of cynomolgus macaques. *Fertil Steril* 1987;47:1010–18

28

Andropause

A. Vermeulen and V. A. Giagulli

Whereas in women, at around age 50, the menopause, characterized by ovarian exhaustion of oocytes and arrest of cyclical ovarian hormonal secretion, signs the irreversible arrest of fertility and causes a state of estrogen deficiency, in the male, spermatogenesis persists until very old age. Children have been fathered by men well over 90 years old[1], and aging is not accompanied by a sudden decrease in plasma sex hormone levels. Hence, the male equivalent of the menopause, the andropause, does not exist in *strictu sensu*.

Nevertheless, both exocrine (spermatogenesis) and endocrine (testosterone secretion) functions decrease slowly and progressively with age.

AGE-RELATED CHANGES IN SERUM TESTOSTERONE LEVELS

In healthy young men, 20–30 years old, normal testosterone levels vary between 11 and 40 nmol/l. In normal males, testosterone circulates in plasma, about 60% bound to sex hormone binding globulin (SHBG), about 40% bound to albumin and about 2% as free testosterone[2,3]. Owing to the high association constant of SHBG for testosterone, SHBG-bound testosterone is not directly bioavailable, although SHBG appears to bind to receptors on the membrane of certain cells, activating cyclic adenosine monophosphate (cAMP)[4]. Only free testosterone and (part of) albumin-bound testosterone are directly available to the cells. Owing to the high plasma concentration of albumin with respect to the concentration of testosterone, the ratio of albumin-bound testosterone to free testosterone is independent of the free testosterone concentration and only determined by the albumin concentration[5]. At normal albumin concentration, the albumin-bound testosterone corresponds to about 20 times the level of free testosterone. The latter, therefore, is a reliable parameter of the bioavailable testosterone.

In young healthy males, free testosterone varies between 0.20 and 0.70 nmol/l. Cross-sectional[6] and longitudinal studies[7,8], involving large groups of healthy ambulant subjects, show that, between age 25 and 75 years, mean total testosterone levels decrease by about 30–40% (Figure 1), whereas the free testosterone decreases by 50–60% (Figure 2). Total

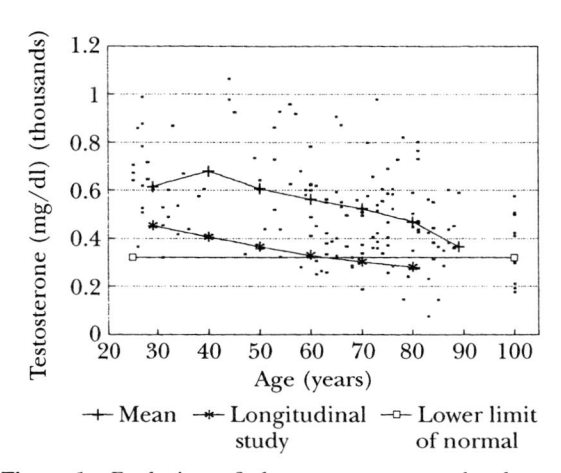

Figure 1 Evolution of plasma testosterone levels as function of age in men. From references 7 and 9

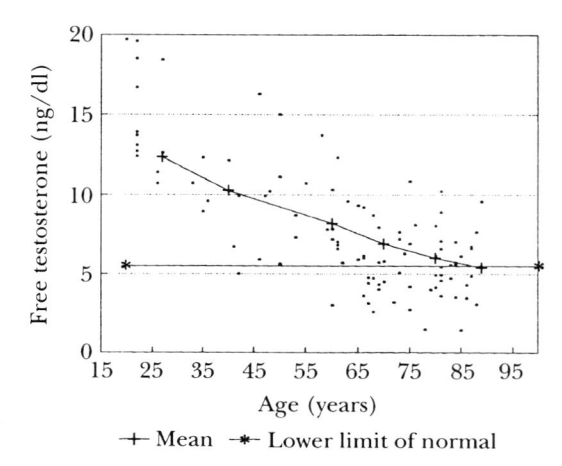

Figure 2 Evolution of free testosterone levels as function of age in men

testosterone levels, however, stay relatively stable until age 50–55 years and decrease thereafter at a rate of about 0.6–0.8% per year. The more important and earlier decline in free testosterone levels is the consequence of the age-associated increase in SHBG levels[3] which probably finds its origin in the age-associated decrease in growth hormone and insulin-like growth factor-I (IGF-I) levels[9–11]. At any age, there exists a wide interindividual variation in testosterone levels such that, even at age 75, some males have testosterone levels which fall within the normal range for young adults, while others have frankly hypogonadal values.

As to the frequency of hypogonadal values (< 11 nmol/l) of testosterone, in a study involving 300 healthy men, we observed subnormal values in one case in the age group 20–40 years ($n = 105$), in 8% of cases in the age group 40–60 years ($n = 68$) but in 22% in the age group 60–80 years ($n = 87$). In the age group over 80 years ($n = 40$), one-third had testosterone levels in the hypogonadal range[6]. As expected, the frequency was slightly higher when free testosterone levels were considered[12]. On the other hand, 20% of men over 80 years old had testosterone levels greater than 20 nmol/l, the mid-normal value for young men. The androgen deficiency of elderly men is generally moderate and has been coined PADAM or partial androgen deficiency of the aging male.

The wide interindividual variations in free testosterone levels in healthy males of any age are determined by a series of physiological factors. In addition, many acute or chronic diseases may accelerate the age-associated decrease in free testosterone levels.

Physiological factors affecting plasma testosterone levels

Genetics appears to play an important role in the interindividual variability of testosterone levels. Meikle and colleagues[13,14], on the basis of the variability of testosterone levels in homozygous and heterozygous twins, concluded that 63% of the variability of testosterone levels and 30% of the variability of SHBG levels was attributable to genetics. In accordance with this view is the observation that, in the same subject, testosterone levels show little variation over time[15].

Nevertheless, *seasonal influences* have been shown to influence testosterone levels, peak values being generally observed in the autumn[16,17], whereas *circadian* variations, with the highest values in the early morning and nadir values in the late afternoon, should not play a role in the variability of testosterone levels when plasma samples are taken between 8.00 and 11.00. As testosterone is secreted in a *pulsatile* manner with, according to Veldhuis and colleagues[18], a mean amplitude of 920 ng/dl in young healthy men, it is advised to pool 2–3 plasma samples taken with an interval of 20 min to minimize this variability.

Plasma insulin is an important determinant of SHBG and, hence, of total testosterone levels. Plymate and co-workers[19] as well as Singh and associates[20] in *in vitro* studies, showed an inhibitory effect of insulin/IGF-I on SHBG synthesis by human hepatoma cells. Clinical studies[9,21–23] showed an inverse correlation between insulin levels on the one hand and SHBG and testosterone levels on the other hand (Figure 3). Although it has been suggested that low SHBG and total testosterone levels are a risk factor for non-insulin dependent diabetes mellitus (NIDDM)[24], low SHBG and total testosterone levels seem to be rather the consequence than the cause of relative insulin resistance (Figure 4), preceding overt glucose intolerance.

The negative effect of *body mass index* (BMI) on SHBG (and testosterone levels) is probably mediated by the increased insulin levels[25].

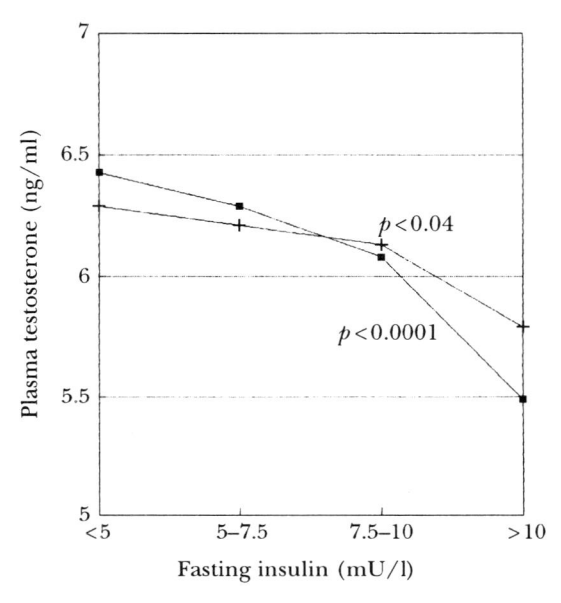

Figure 3 Insulin levels and testosterone. BMI, body mass index. From reference 23

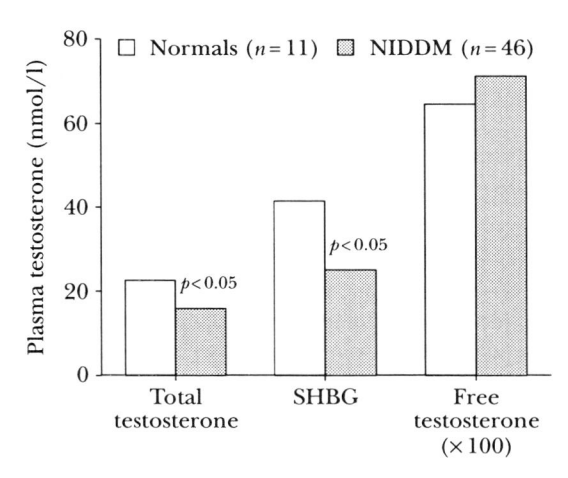

Figure 4 Plasma testosterone levels in men with non-insulin dependent diabetes mellitus (NIDDM) aged 57 ± 2.1 years. SHBG, sex hormone binding globulin. From reference 51

Whereas in moderate obesity (BMI < 40), only total testosterone levels are decreased, in morbid obesity (BMI > 40), also free testosterone levels are decreased, pointing towards alterations in the neuroendocrine regulation of testosterone secretion[25], with a decrease of the luteinizing hormone (LH) pulse amplitude.

The inverse correlation between *growth hormone and IGF-I levels*, respectively, and plasma SHBG and testosterone levels has already been mentioned. Growth hormone treatment of adults with isolated growth hormone deficiency causes a decrease of SHBG and total testosterone levels[9], independently of any increase in insulin levels. Similar results were seen after continuous growth hormone infusion in moderately obese middle-aged men[26].

Thyroid hormone levels are also important determinants of SHBG levels and, in hyperthyroidism, SHBG and testosterone levels are significantly, up to 3–5 times, increased[2,27]. However, also minor changes in thyroid hormone levels, within the normal range in apparently healthy men, without clinical signs of dysthyroidism, may influence SHBG levels[28]. Free testosterone levels, however, are not affected.

Diet also might influence SHBG and, indirectly, testosterone levels. Adlercreutz[29] reported that a western-type diet, rich in fat and animal protein, is accompanied by decreased SHBG and increased bioavailable testosterone levels, whereas Key and colleagues[30] reported higher SHBG and lower free testosterone levels in vegans than in omnivores (Figure 5). Belanger and co-workers[31] reported similar results, but these were not corrected for body mass index, whereas Reed and associates[32] observed that switching subjects from a very low-fat diet (< 20 g/day) to an isocaloric high-fat diet (> 100 g/day), caused a decrease in SHBG. However, as the latter diet was low in carbohydrates and proteins, the specific role of the fat content of the diet cannot be evaluated. Field and colleagues[33] observed an inverse correlation between SHBG levels and fiber intake but not with fat or calorie intake. Surprisingly, Schultz and associates[34] found no effect on free testosterone or SHBG levels after a 6-week consumption of fiber-rich bread.

Discordant results were reported my Meikle and co-workers[35], who observed that use of a high fat-containing meal resulted in a reduction of testosterone and free testosterone levels, and they suggest that fatty acids might modulate testosterone production.

The mechanism of the influence of the diet is unknown, but it might be hypothesized that at least part of the changes in SHBG levels is mediated through insulin, the plasma levels of which are low in vegetarians; possibly also phytoestrogens, present in large amounts in vegetarian and fiber-rich diets, might play a role.

It should be recalled, however, that changes in SHBG binding capacity should not affect free testosterone levels as this requires an additional effect at the hypothalamo–pituitary feedback system.

Fasting temporarily affects testosterone production through a decreased gonadotropin secretion[36].

Several authors[9,33,37,38] reported that *smokers* have 5–15% higher testosterone levels than non-smokers.

Alcohol abuse as well as *drug use* accentuates the age-associated decrease of testosterone levels[39–41].

Stress, finally, whether physical or psychological, as well as strenuous physical exercise depresses testosterone levels (Figure 6)[42,43].

Influence of disease on plasma testosterone levels

In addition to physiological factors, *acute and chronic diseases* accentuate and accelerate the age-associated decline in free testosterone levels. It is not the purpose of this review to discuss all diseases that may affect the testosterone levels. A recent review was published by Turner and Wass[44]. Any severe illness may produce hypogonadotropic hypogonadism[45], and the degree of hypogonadism is related to the severity of the disease[46]. Among the chronic diseases are chronic obstructive airway disease[47], diabetes mellitus[48–51], coronary artery disease[52], chronic renal insufficiency[53], chronic liver disease[54], acquired immunodeficiency syndrome (AIDS)[55] and rheumatoid arthritis[56].

Elderly persons frequently use a cocktail of *medications* (antihypertensives, neuroleptics, hypnotics, H2 antihistaminics, ketoconazol) which may also accentuate the decline in testosterone levels. Glucocorticoids also cause a marked depression of testosterone levels[57,58].

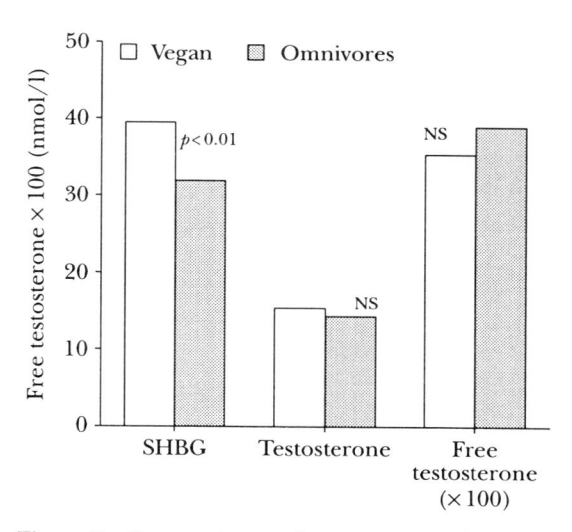

Figure 5 Comparison of testosterone levels in vegans and omnivores. SHBG, sex hormone binding globulin; NS, not significant. From reference 30

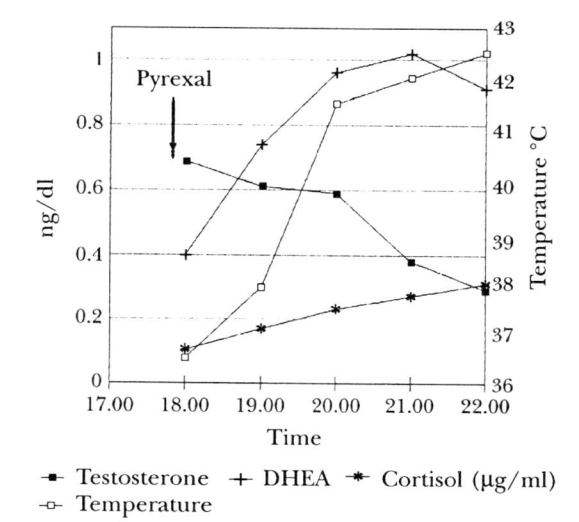

Figure 6 Influence of acute stress (pyrogen) on plasma androgen and cortisol levels. DHEA, dehydroepiandrosterone

In conclusion, it is evident that many factors may influence plasma testosterone levels in healthy men of any age, and that the variability of these levels in healthy males is largely attributable to a complex interplay of genetic, seasonal, social, environmental and economic factors.

Physiopathology of altered Leydig cell function in elderly men

It is now evident that the age-associated decrease of plasma testosterone levels has both a testicular and hypothalamo–pituitary origin. A wealth of data confirm the age-associated *alterations at the testicular level*: diminished response to human chorionic gonadotropin[59–62], the consequence of a decreased number of Leydig cells[63–65], and the decreased testicular perfusion[66,67] inducing a decreased oxygen supply with alterations in testicular steroid biosynthesis[68,69]. These testicular lesions explain the (modest) increase, observed in many elderly men (see reference 70 for review), of both immunoreactive and bioactive LH[71–73].

In many elderly men, the LH levels are not increased, notwithstanding decreased testosterone levels, indicating *alterations in the neuroendocrine control of gonadal function*. This is accompanied by a blunted circadian variation of the testosterone levels in elderly men[37,71,74,75] and a decreased amplitude of LH pulses, with preserved LH pulse frequency[76,77]. As the response of the pituitary gonadotrophs to physiological doses of gonadotropin releasing hormone (GnRH) is maintained[72], this decreased amplitude suggests that the bolus of GnRH, intermittently released in the portal circulation, is reduced. There appears to exist a linear correlation between LH pulse amplitude and plasma testosterone levels[76,77]. In elderly men, the hypothalamo–pituitary–gonadal axis is more sensitive to the negative feedback by sex hormones than in young men[78–80], and the opioid tone, restraining the GnRH pulse generator, is decreased in elderly men, receptor blockade by antiopioids failing to increase LH pulse frequency or amplitude, in distinction from the effect in young men[81].

CLINICAL RELEVANCE OF DECREASE IN ANDROGEN LEVELS IN ELDERLY MEN

Aging in men is generally accompanied by decreases in energy, muscle mass and strength, increases in body fat and osteopenia, lower blood cell counts and hemoglobin levels, generalized weakness, skin atrophy, decreases in virility, sexual pilosity, libido and sexual drive, increased frequency of impotence, increased sweating, forgetfulness, insomnia and irritability and a decrease of general well-being. It is striking that a number of these changes resemble features of androgen deficiency in younger men, and it is tempting to believe that at least some of these signs and symptoms are related to the age-associated decline in androgen levels. Therefore, one would expect a significant relationship between androgen levels and clinical signs and symptoms.

At best, the existence of a relationship between symptoms and plasma testosterone levels is doubtful, as no systematic studies on this issue have been performed. The etiology of the symptomatology accompanying the aging process is multifactorial, and the age-associated changes in the endocrine system do not concern only the gonadal system, but also growth hormone and IGF-I levels as well as adrenal androgen secretion, which decrease dramatically with age, whereas the age-associated gradual decline of all the other physiological functions contributes to the clinical picture of the aging male. Hence, the relative roles of hypoandrogenism, of the aging process itself and of the sequellae of intercurrent disease may be extremely difficult to unravel. The absence of significant correlations between subnormal testosterone levels and clinical symptoms is not necessarily in contradiction with the possible role of androgens in the symptomatology. Notwithstanding a widespread belief to the contrary, a similar situation exists also in the menopause, as no correlation has been observed between estrogen levels and the menopausal symptoms[82], and there is no universal set of symptoms, not even hot flushes, associated with the menopause, that all women cognitively share[83]. Improvement of subjective or even objective symptoms, such as an increase in muscle mass upon androgen therapy, does not prove the causal role of the androgens either, as this does not necessarily imply that the corrected symptom was due to the pre-existent androgen deficiency.

Among possible consequences of hypoandrogenism of the aging male, decreases in libido and sexual activity, increased frequency of impotence, and decreases in muscle mass, strength and energy as well as osteopenia are the most frequently mentioned.

Aging, libido, sexual activity and fertility

Other clinical symptoms of aging are *declining libido, sexual activity and fertility*.

Aging and ejaculate

Studies on the relationship between aging and quality of the ejaculate generally show a decrease in the ejaculatory volume, but a normal or even increased sperm count with, however, decreased motility and a decrease in the percentage of spermatozoa with normal morphology[84–86]. The decreased ejaculatory frequency, which leads to a higher sperm output and a lower motility[87], masks the decrease in spermatogenesis, the morphological basis of which is a reduction in the number of Sertoli cells[88], reflected biochemically by a decrease in plasma inhibin and an increase in follicle stimulating hormone (FSH) levels[89]. The role of the decreased testosterone levels in the reduced ejaculatory volume is unknown, but no relationship was observed by Rolf and colleagues[85].

In *in vitro* studies, the fertilizing capacity of sperm from elderly men was similar to that of young men[90,91], and Nieschlag and co-workers[92] observed that the reproductive function of grandfathers was not reduced. In view of the small number of semen samples from men over 60 years examined, moreover generally obtained from donors or elderly men having a wish for a child, not necessarily representative of the general elderly population, the data on sperm quality and fertilizing capacity of elderly men should be interpreted cautiously.

Aging, libido and plasma testosterone

Although, after castration, libido may persist for some time, it is evident that testosterone is required for normal sexual drive. Indeed, testosterone administration to men with subnormal testosterone levels stimulates sexual interest and activity[93] and, in these patients, a dose response was observed between testosterone levels and frequency of sexual thoughts and ejaculations[94,95], whereas Tsitouras and colleagues[96] reported that elderly men with higher testosterone levels were likely to be more sexually active than men with lower testosterone levels.

Aging is accompanied by decreases both of testosterone levels and of sexual drive[97,98]. Verwoerdt and co-workers[99] reported that only 15% of men over 60 years deny any sexual interest, and 80% remain sexually active. The correlation between testosterone levels and libido, however, is rather poor[100–102], and the testosterone concentration required to sustain sexual interest appears to be rather low[102] as androgen replacement therapy at a dose maintaining testosterone levels at half the baseline value was sufficient to sustain normal sexual function[103]. Similarly, Udry and associates[104,105] believe that healthy adults have substantially higher androgen levels than required for normal sexual behavior. This suggests that the influence of androgens on sexual activity is subject to a ceiling effect[105]. Nevertheless, Anderson and colleagues[106] observed that increasing testosterone levels to supraphysiological levels may increase sexual activity.

Bancroft[107] hypothesized that the threshold concentration required to sustain sexual activity would increase with age: plasma concentrations within the normal range for young adults may not be sufficient for adequate sexual function in elderly men. Consistent with this hypothesis is the observation that sleep erections, which are androgen-sensitive, are impaired in elderly men with testosterone levels within the normal range[102].

Aging, erectile function and impotence

Coital frequency declines almost linearly with age, from a mean maximal frequency, at around age 20–24, of about four times a week, to once a week at age 55–60, three times a month at age 70 and 1.7 times a month between age 75 and 79 years[108].

Frequency of coital impotence increases dramatically with age, from 8% at age 55 to 57% at age 75–79[109]. Although potency and nocturnal penile tumescence require adequate testosterone levels, most cases of impotence in the elderly have a non-hormonal cause, although hormonal alterations may play a subsidiary role in many cases of impotence[110,111]. Among the endocrinopathies, diabetes mellitus and hyperprolactinemia are a frequent cause of early impotence, usually accompanied by low testosterone levels. Among the non-hormonal factors, overall health status of both partners, medications (psychotropics, antihypertensives, H2 antihistaminics), stress and depressive states are the most important. Moreover, the level of sexual activity in old age is strongly related to sexual activity at a younger age[97,112].

Whereas the correlation between impotence of elderly men and plasma testosterone is rather poor, there exists a rather close correlation between nocturnal penile tumescence and testosterone levels. Schiavi[102] reported a significant correlation between biotestosterone and frequency of nocturnal penile tumescence, while sleep-related erections are restored by testosterone[93,113].

As to the *influence of age of the male partner on the fecundity of the couple*, this is essentially determined by the increasing frequency of impotence, the fertilizing capacity of sperm remaining apparently intact.

It should be mentioned that increasing paternal age has been associated with a variety of *autosomal dominant diseases* such as Marfan syndrome, polyposis coli and polycystic kidney disease. Friedman[114] estimates the risk at 1 pro mille at age 30–44, but 37 pro mille at age over 45, and he estimates that one-third of children with autosomal dominant mutations were fathered by men over age 40 years. Hence, it is recommended that men should have their children before the age of 45.

Atherosclerosis and cardiovascular disease

Among the age-associated diseases, atherosclerosis and cardiovascular diseases play an important role. Cardiovascular disease and cardiovascular mortality are more frequent in men than in women, and it is generally believed that the androgens are responsible for this increased risk, as they are considered to increase low density lipoprotein (LDL) cholesterol and decrease high density lipoprotein (HDL) cholesterol, important risk factors for cardiovascular disease. Indeed, at puberty, in parallel with the increase in testosterone levels, LDL cholesterol levels increase and HDL cholesterol levels decrease in boys whereas, in adults, blocking testosterone secretion with GnRH[115–117] leads to an increase in HDL cholesterol, an effect which is neutralized by co-administration of testosterone enanthate 100 mg every 2 weeks for 20 weeks[116]. Nevertheless, in most[118–120] but not all[121,122] cross-sectional studies in healthy adult males, a positive correlation between endogenous free testosterone levels and HDL cholesterol and a negative correlation with triglycerides was observed, correlations which persisted after correction for the other classical risk factors for cardiovascular disease. Whereas in some studies only total testosterone was considered, in several studies the same inverse correlation was observed between free testosterone and HDL cholesterol[118,119,123].

Epidemiological studies, moreover, show a positive correlation between endogenous testosterone levels and insulin sensitivity[124–126], whereas low testosterone levels are significantly related to the incidence of non-insulin dependent diabetes with its increased frequency of atherosclerosis[127]. This positive correlation, however, is only observed within the physiological male concentration range of testosterone[115,116]. Administration of testosterone to surgically or chemically castrated males, or to female-to-male trans-sexuals[128], induces a decrease in HDL cholesterol levels, whereas hyperandrogenic women also have an atherogenic lipid profile. This leads to the hypothesis that the atherogenic effects of testosterone are expressed when testosterone levels increase from normal female (or postgonadectomy) levels to 4–5 nmol/l, whereas, within the physiological male range, the insulin sensitizing effect would predominate. At supraphysiological levels, testosterone again induces a decrease in HDL cholesterol[103,129,130].

In conclusion, the age-associated hypotestosteronemia appears to constitute a risk factor for coronary atherosclerosis, an effect possibly mediated via a decrease in insulin sensitivity which might contribute to the development of an atherogenic lipid profile in elderly men. None the less, low testosterone levels appear not to be associated with an increased risk of cardiovascular death[131–133], suggesting that testosterone might have direct vascular effects which are independent of its effects on the plasma lipid profile.

Androgens, muscle mass, osteopenia

Both androgen levels and bone mass decrease with age, and several authors[134,135] reported a positive correlation between androgen levels and bone mass in elderly men. It is difficult, however, to evaluate the role of the decline in testosterone levels independently of the effect of aging itself. Cross-sectional studies have shown persistence of a weak correlation between androgen levels and bone mass at some skeletal sites after adjustment for age and body mass index (see reference 135 for review). Hypogonadism is reported to be a risk factor for hip fracture[137,138]. Behre and colleagues[139] as well as Finkelstein and co-workers[140] report favorable effects of testosterone substitution on bone mineral density (BMD) in males with hypogonadism. However, data are too limited to allow firm conclusions at this present time.

As for muscle mass, the age-associated decrease is probably multifactorial[141], contributing factors including relative physical inactivity, decreased activity of the growth hormone–IGF-I axis and decline in testosterone levels. The relative importance of these factors has not been clearly established, but testosterone treatment increases the lean body and muscle mass and the muscle strength of elderly men with low plasma testosterone levels[142–144].

ANDROGEN SUPPLEMENTATION IN ELDERLY MALES

The age-associated decrease in plasma testosterone levels, with more than 20% of men over 60 years old having plasma levels in the hypogonadal range[6], raises the problem of the necessity or desirability of androgen substitution in elderly males. Indeed, there is increasing evidence that at least some of the signs and symptoms of aging may be reversed by testosterone supplementation[141], profound hypogonadism responding best, whereas the evidence suggests that men with borderline low levels of testosterone are rather poor responders.

It seems evident that elderly men with androgen levels within the normal range *a priori* do not require androgen supplementation. In the absence of a reliable parameter of androgen activity, however, it remains difficult to determine the normal range of plasma testosterone levels in elderly men! It has already been mentioned that, as far as stimulation of sexual activity is concerned, androgen levels within the normal range for young adults may be insufficient to sustain erection in elderly men! In this connection, it is of interest to mention that Ono and colleagues[145] reported that the concentration of androgen receptors in pubic skin fibroblasts was reduced in elderly men, suggesting a decreased sensitivity to androgens.

The generally accepted lower limit of normal plasma testosterone concentration, 11 nmol/l, is based on values obtained in young adults, levels below this limit being observed in only 1% of healthy men aged 20–40 years but in over 20% of males over 65 years[6]. A more appropriate parameter is free testosterone, a parameter of the biologically active testosterone.

In the absence of clinical signs of androgen deficiency, and taking into account the paucity of data on the consequences of relative hypoandrogenism and the risks and benefits of androgen supplementation, it is certainly not advised to propose androgen supplementation on the basis of testosterone levels at or just below the lower limit for young adults. *Androgen supplementation should only be considered in the presence of androgen levels below the lower normal limit (11 nmol/l total testosterone or 0.20 nmol/l free testosterone) together with unequivocal signs and symptoms of androgen deficiency, in the absence of other factors known to decrease androgen levels.* Indeed, as already mentioned, many other hormonal and non-hormonal factors related to the aging process may play a role in the symptomatology.

As for the objective signs of relative androgen deficiency, a decrease of muscle mass and strength with a concomitant increase in central body fat, and osteoporosis, which may be asymptomatic or may lead to subjective complaints, can most easily be objectivated.

Decreased libido and sexual desire, loss of memory, difficulty in concentration, forgetfulness, insomnia, irritability, depressed mood and decreased sense of well-being are subjective feelings or impressions, more difficult to evaluate and to differentiate from hormone-independent aging. The recently reported data on the possible influence of decreased dehydroepiandrosterone sulfate levels on the symptoms of aging men add to the difficulty of evaluating the role of subnormal testosterone levels in the symptomatology of elderly men[146].

Risks and benefits of androgen supplementation

The decision to treat will finally depend upon the balance between possible benefits and risks. Unfortunately, few controlled studies, generally involving a small number of subjects only, have assessed this balance.

As to the benefits, all studies report improvements to the sense of general well-being, libido and muscle strength with an increase in lean body mass and a decrease in body fat[142–144,147–149]. Tenover[142,144], moreover, reports an improvement in spatial cognition, whereas Behre and colleagues[139] report an increased BMD in treated hypogonadal men, regardless of age. Also, Finkelstein and associates[140] reported favorable effects of testosterone on BMD in hypogonadal men.

As expected, effects on impotence were disappointing. As to the biochemical parameters, a generally moderate increase in hematocrit as well as an improvement of insulin sensitivity is frequently observed, whereas the effects on the biochemical indices of bone turnover (hydroxyproline, osteocalcin, alkaline phosphatase) have been inconsistent[12].

With regard to the risks of androgen replacement therapy in elderly men, the possible atherogenic *effects on plasma lipids* of androgens have been the subject of major concern. Indeed, androgen supplementation is prescribed to aged men, in whom alterations of lipid metabolism are very frequent. As already mentioned, there appears to exist a relatively low ceiling value of plasma testosterone, above which testosterone would not further unfavorably influence lipid metabolism, but rather improve the lipid profile. Increasing plasma testosterone female to male levels induces a clear-cut atherogenic lipid profile, but increasing testosterone levels from mildly hypogonadal to levels within the normal male range improves insulin sensitivity and the lipid profile[126,150–153]. The favorable effects of the androgens on the lipid profile are only seen if the androgen is aromatizable[153,154], treatment with non-aromatizable androgens, such as methyltestosterone, or simultaneous administration of an aromatase inhibitor, such as spironolactone, significantly decreasing HDL cholesterol levels[153]. A similar atherogenic effect is seen when supraphysiological doses of androgen are administered, for example for contraceptive purposes[103,129,130,155].

It should be repeated that, whereas several studies show that physiological doses of testosterone do not induce an atherogenic lipid profile, none addresses the effects on cardiovascular morbidity or mortality.

As to the effects of androgens on the cardiovascular system not related to the atherogenic lipid profile, both favorable and unfavorable effects have been reported. Occasionally, *thrombotic complications* have been reported after androgen treatment[156,157] but, on the other hand, also low testosterone levels have been associated with an increased thrombotic risk[137]. Testosterone, administered to female-to-male trans-sexuals *increases endothelin* (a potent vasoconstrictor) levels, while the antiandrogen, cyproterone acetate, together with ethinylestradiol, decreased endothelin levels[159]. In monkeys, testosterone significantly *inhibits prostacyclin and increases thromboxane B2*[160], which stimulates platelet aggregation. Adams and colleagues[161] observed that testosterone administration to female cynomolgus monkeys increased atherosclerotic plaque formation but, on the other hand, reversed the atherosclerosis-related impairment of endothelium-dependent vasodilatatory response to acetylcholine.

On the favorable side can be mentioned the *fibrinolytic effects*[162] and the *inverse correlation between testosterone and plasminogen activation inhibitor type I* (PAI-I)[163]. However, it is not evident whether replacement therapy with physiological doses of testosterone affects these different factors.

Another possible side-effect of androgen substitution, even in physiological doses, is *polycythemia*. A moderate increase in hematocrit in elderly males is probably beneficial, but Hajjar and associates[149] observed that, out of 45 elderly, hypogonadal males receiving 200 mg of testosterone enanthate or cypionate every 2 weeks, 11 (24%) developed polycythemia sufficient to require phlebotomy or temporary withholding of testosterone, one-third of which occurred less than 1 year after starting treatment. Sih and co-workers[148] reported a similar frequent development of polycythemia. It is well known that testosterone stimulates erythropoietin production by the kidney.

Androgens may favor *obstructive sleep apnea*[164]. Therefore, chronic obstructive pulmonary disease, especially in overweight subjects or heavy smokers, is a relative contraindication to androgen therapy.

Gynecomastia, related to the conversion of testosterone to estradiol in peripheral tissues, mainly fat tissue which is relatively increased in elderly men, is a not infrequent, medically innocent side-effect in elderly men, more frequent in the obese.

Although testosterone causes some *sodium and water retention*[165], this effect usually does not cause a problem, except in patients with heart decompensation, hypertension or renal insufficiency.

Hepatoxicity is very rare and most frequently seen after use of 17-alkylated anabolic steroids.

Of greater concern are the possible *effects on the prostate*, which is an androgen-dependent organ. Stimulation of *benign prostatic hyperplasia* (BPH) does not seem to represent a major problem as, to date, all studies failed to observe an important growth of the prostate[166] and no relationship between plasma levels and BPH tissue levels of testosterone, dihydrotestosterone or estradiol has been reported. Indeed, tissue levels are determined more by the enzyme activity in the tissue itself, rather than by surrounding plasma androgen levels[167]. Prostatic specific antigen (PSA) levels, a parameter of androgen stimulation of the prostatic tissue, increase moderately during short-term treatment but, after stopping treatment, the values return to pretreatment levels[141,144,149]. Nevertheless, larger, long-term studies are required to confirm definitively these reassuring results.

Clinical *prostatic carcinoma* undoubtedly is an androgen-sensitive tumor[168]: hence, *presence of a clinical prostatic carcinoma is an absolute contraindication to testosterone supplementation.*

A major problem is the high frequency (> 50% of males over 70 years) of *subclinical carcinoma*, only detectable by prostate biopsy but undetectable by biochemical or clinical procedures. Whereas only a small percentage of these subclinical carcinomas will, eventually, further develop to a clinical carcinoma, it is not known whether testosterone treatment would stimulate the progression of subclinical carcinoma and, although to date no data are available indicating that testosterone substitution will activate subclinical carcinoma[169–171], all studies to date concern only a small number of elderly males treated for a relatively short period of time. Anyway, *before starting testosterone supplementation, careful exclusion of the presence of a prostatic carcinoma by rectal examination and testing of PSA levels, when required supplemented by echography, followed by 6-monthly controls, is mandatory.*

Aims of replacement therapy

In young healthy men, testosterone levels vary between 11 and 35 nmol/l and show a circadian variation with an amplitude of ± 35%, highest levels being reached in the early morning and nadir values in the evening around 18.00–20.00.

Testosterone supplementation should aim at alleviating the symptoms related to the relative androgen deficiency, if possible by achieving plasma testosterone levels that mimic the levels of their nycthemeral variations as found in young adults. Even transient suprapysiological concentrations should be avoided as they may be responsible for many of the side-effects. As the hypothalamo–pituitary–testicular axis is very sensitive to negative feedback, and even more so in elderly males[78,79], it is important to ascertain that the dose administered increases the testosterone levels within the physiological range and does not just suppress LH secretion with, as a consequence, just a replacement of endogenous testosterone production by exogenous testosterone administered.

Modalities of androgen substitution

Testosterone administered orally is completely inactivated through the liver. The only *orally active testosterone derivate* suitable for substitution therapy is testosterone undecanoate which partially escapes hepatic inactivation, being partially taken up via the lymph. The usual dose in elderly men is 40–80 mg, two or three times a day; as the absorption is rather variable from person to person, the dose should be determined on the basis of plasma testosterone levels obtained[172]. Intramuscularly administered long-chain *testosterone esters* are the most frequently used galenic form. Generally, 200 mg of testosterone enanthate or cypionate is injected every 2–3 weeks; this yields suprapysiological levels the first 2–3 days after injection followed by a steady decline to subphysiological levels just before the next injection; these fluctuations are certainly not physiological[173], and are unpleasant for the patient.

Preliminary studies with intramuscular injection of testosterone undecanoate suggest that this would yield physiological levels during about 8 weeks; other new preparations under experimentation are testosterone buciclate which would act over 3–4 months and biodegradable testosterone microspheres[174]. A recent development are patches for *transdermal testosterone* administration[175]. One type is applied daily at 22.00 on the shaved scrotal skin and produces plasma testosterone levels in the physiological range for 6–8 h, with a subsequent decline during the following hours; dihydrotestosterone levels, however, are unphysiologically high. Recently, a permeation-enhanced non-scrotal patch has become available; it produces normal testosterone and dihydrotestosterone levels for 8–12 h following nightly application, and the plasma pattern mimics the physiological circadian variations[176]. However, the patch frequently causes local irritation. Subcutaneous testosterone pellets (6 × 100 mg every 6 months yield physiological testosterone levels for 4–6 months, but are not widely used. In about 5% of the patients, the pellet is rejected by the organism[177].

Other galenic forms are under development.

CONCLUSIONS

Summarizing, although the andropause *in strictu sensu* does not exist, fertility persisting in elderly men, the progressive decrease of testosterone secretion contributes to a series of symptoms of aging in males. This is all the more evident in a subgroup of males with subnormal testosterone levels, the importance of which increases sharply after age 60. Testosterone supplementation should only be considered in men with subnormal free testosterone levels and clinical signs suggestive for hypoandrogenism, and treatment should only be initiated after exclusion of all possible causes of secondary hypogonadism. Moreover, all men over 40 years should have a digital rectal examination and a determination of PSA levels to exclude prostatic carcinoma.

Clinical prostatic carcinoma is an absolute contraindication for testosterone replacement therapy. Impotence in elderly men is rarely an indication for androgen therapy.

Patients under treatment should be followed on a 6-monthly basis with rectal examination and PSA and hematocrit determinations. Any increase of PSA requires complementary investigations to exclude prostatic carcinoma.

Most subjects on testosterone supplementation will experience an improvement of general well-being and mood and increases of muscle mass, strength and energy. As, to date, only a few, small-scale and relatively short-term studies concerning the effects of androgen substitution in elderly men have been completed, more large-scale, long-term, well-controlled studies are required before final assessment of the risk/benefit ratio of androgen supplementation in elderly men will be possible.

References

1. Silber SJ. Effects of age on male fertility. *Semin Reprod Endocrinol* 1991;9:241–8
2. Vermeulen A, Stoica T, Verdonck L. The apparent free testosterone concentration, an index of androgenicity. *J Clin Endocrinol Metab* 1971;33:759–67
3. Vermeulen A, Rubens R, Verdonck L. Testosterone secretion and metabolism in male senescence. *J Clin Endocrinol Metab* 1972;39:730–40
4. Rosner W, Hryb DJ, Kahn MS, *et al.* Sex hormone binding globulin (SHBG) anatomy and physiology of a new regulatory system. *J Steroid Biochem Mol Biol* 1991;40:813–20
5. Vermeulen A, Verdonck L. Studies of the binding of testosterone to human plasma. *Steroids* 1968;11:609–35
6. Vermeulen A. Discussion. In Oddens B, Vermeulen A, eds. *Androgens and the Aging Male.* Carnforth, UK: Parthenon Publishing, 1996:202
7. Pearson USD, Blackman MR, Metter EJ, *et al.* Effect of age and cigarette smoking on longitudinal changes in androgens and SHBG in healthy males. Presented at the *77th Annual Meeting of the Endocrinology Society*, Washington, June 1995:abstr 129
8. Morley JE, Kaiser FE, Perry HM, *et al.* Longitudinal changes in testosterone, SHBG, LH and FSH in healthy older males. Presented at the *10th International Congress of Endocrinology*, San Francisco, June 1996:abstr 174
9. Vermeulen A, Kaufman JM, Giagulli VA. Influence of some biological indices on sex hormone binding globulin and androgen levels in aging and obese males. *J Clin Endocrinol Metab* 1996;81:1821–6
10. Erfurth EM, Hagmart LE, Säär M, *et al.* Serum levels of insulin-like growth factor I and insulin-like growth factor binding protein 1 correlate with free testosterone and sex hormone binding globulin in healthy young and middle aged men. *Clin Endocrinol* 1996;44:654–64
11. Pfeilschifter J, Scheidt-Nave C, Leidig-Bruckner G, *et al.* Relationship between circulating insulin-like growth factor components and sex hormones in a population based sample of 50–80 year old men and women. *J Clin Endocrinol Metab* 1996;81:2534–40
12. Kaufman JM, Vermeulen A. Declining gonadal function in elderly men. *Baillière's Clin Endocrinol Metab* 1997;11:289–309
13. Meikle HW, Bishop DT, Stringham JD, *et al.* Quantitating of genetic and non genetic factors that determine sex steroid variation in normal male twins. *Metabolism* 1986;35:1090–5
14. Meikle AW, Stringham JD, Bishop J, *et al.* Quantitation of genetic and non genetic factors influencing androgen production and clearance rates in men. *J Clin Endocrinol Metab* 1988;67:104–9
15. Vermeulen A, Verdonck L. Representativeness of a single point plasma testosterone level for the long term hormonal milieu in men. *J Clin Endocrinol Metab* 1992;74:939–42
16. Reinberg A, Lagoguey M, Chauffournier MM, *et al.* Circannual and circadian rhythms in plasma testosterone in five healthy, young Parisian males. *Acta Endocrinol* 1975;80:723–43
17. Smals AGH, Kloppenburg PWC, Benraad TJ. Circannual cycles in plasma testosterone levels in man. *J Clin Endocrinol Metab* 1976;42:479–82
18. Veldhuis JP, King JC, Urban RJ, *et al.* Operating characteristics of the male hypothalamo–pituitary–gonadal axis. Pulsatile release of testosterone and follicle stimulating hormone and their temporal coupling with luteinizing hormone. *J Clin Endocrinol Metab* 1987;65:929–47
19. Plymate SR, Matej LA, Jones RE, *et al.* Inhibition of sex hormone binding globulin production in the human hepatoma cell-line. *J Clin Endocrinol Metab* 1988;67:460–4
20. Singh A, Hamilton FD, Koistinen V. Effect of insulin like growth factor type I (IGF-I) and insulin, on the secretion of sex hormone binding globulin and IGF-I binding protein by human hepatoma cells. *J Endocrinol* 1990;124:R1–3

21. Haffner JM, Katz MS, Stern MP, et al. The relationship of sex hormones to hyperinsulinemia and hyperglycemia. *Metabolism* 1988;7:686–8
22. Haffner SM, Valdez RM, Mykkanen L, et al. Decreased testosterone and dehydroepiandrosterone sulfate concentrations are associated with increased insulin and glucose concentration in non diabetic men. *Metabolism* 1994;43:599–603
23. Simon D, Charles MA, Nahoul K, et al. Androgen therapy improves insulin sensitivity in healthy men with low plasma total testosterone. *Diabetes* 1996;45(Suppl 2):232A
24. Lindstedt G, Lunberg PA, Lapidus L, et al. Sex hormone binding globulin concentration, an independent risk factor for the development of NIDDM. *Diabetes* 1991;40:123–8
25. Giagulli VA, Kaufman JM, Vermeulen A. Pathogenesis of decreased androgen levels in obese men. *J Clin Endocrinol Metab* 1994;79:997–1000
26. Oscarsson J, Lindstedt G, Lundberg PA, et al. Continuous subcutaneous infusion of low dose growth hormone decreases serum sex-hormone binding globulin and testosterone in moderately obese middle-aged men. *Clin Endocrinol* 1996;44:23–9
27. Dray F, Sebaoun J, Mowszowisz I. Facteurs influençants le taux de la testostérone plasmatique chez l'homme: rôle des hormones thyroidiennes. *C R Acad Sci (Paris)* 1967;364:2578–84
28. Faber J, Perrild H, Johansen JS. Bone Gla protein and sex hormone binding globulin in non toxic goiter: parameters of metabolic status at the tissue level. *J Clin Endocrinol Metab* 1990;70:49–55
29. Adlercreutz H. Western diet and Western diseases: some hormonal and biochemical mechanisms and associations. *Scand J Clin Lab Invest* 1990;201(Suppl): S3–23
30. Key T, Roe L, Thorogood M, et al. Testosterone, sex hormone binding globulin, calculated free testosterone and estradiol in male vegetarians and omnivores. *Br Med J* 1990;64:111–19
31. Belanger A, Locong A, Noel CJ, et al. Influence of diet on plasma steroids and plasma steroid hormone binding globulin levels in adult males. *J Steroid Biochem* 1989;32:829–33
32. Reed MJ, Cheng RW, Simmonds M, et al. Dietary lipids: an additional regulator of plasma levels of sex hormone binding globulin. *J Clin Endocrinol Metab* 1987;64:1083–5
33. Field AE, Colditz CA, Willett WC, et al. The relation of smoking, age, relative weight and dietary intake to serum adrenal steroids, sex hormones and sex hormone binding globulin in middle aged men. *J Clin Endocrinol Metab* 1994;79:1310–16
34. Schultz TD, Bonorden WR, Seaman WR. Effect of short time flax seed consumption on lignan and sex hormone metabolism in man. *Nutr Res* 1991; 11:1089–100
35. Meikle AW, Stringham JD, Woodward MG, et al. Effect of fat containing meal on sex hormones in men. *Metabolism* 1990;39:943–6
36. Cameron JM, Weltzin TE, Conaha C, et al. Slowing of pulsatile luteinizing hormone secretion after forty-eight hours of fasting. *J Clin Endocrinol Metab* 1991;73:35–41
37. Deslypere JP, Vermeulen A. Leydic cell function, in normal men: effect of age, life style, residence, diet and activity. *J Clin Endocrinol Metab* 1984;59:593–600
38. Dai WS, Gutai SP, Kuller LH, et al. Cigarette smoking and serum sex hormones in man. *Am J Epidemiol* 1988;128:796–808
39. Cicero TJ. Alcohol induced defects in the hypothalamo–pituitary–luteinizing hormone action in the male. *Alcoholism* 1982;6:207–15
40. Irwin M, Dreyfus E, Baird D, et al. Testosterone in chronic alcoholic disease. *Bri J Addiction* 1988; 83:449–53
41. Ida Y, Tsyjitrama S, Nakamura K, et al. Effect of acute and repeated alcohol ingestion on hypothalamo–pituitary–gonadal functioning in normal males. *Drug Alcohol Depend* 1992;31: 57–64
42. Bernton E, Hoover D, Galloway R, et al. Adaptation to chronic stress in military trainees: adrenal androgens, testosterone, glucocorticoids, IGF-I and immune function. *Ann NY Acad Sci* 1995;774:217–31
43. Nilsson P, Möller L, Solstad K. Adverse effects of psychosocial stress on gonadal function and insulin levels in middle aged males. *J Int Med* 1995;237:479–86
44. Turner HE, Wass JAH. Gonadal function in chronic illness. *Clin Endocrinol* 1997;47: 379–401
45. Woolf PD, Hamill RW, McDonald JV, et al. Transient hypogonadotropic hypogonadism caused by critical illness. *J Clin Endocrinol Metab* 1985;60: 444–50
46. Spratt DI, Cox P, Orav J, et al. Reproductive axis suppression in acute illness is related to disease severity. *J Clin Endocrinol Metab* 1993;76:1548–54
47. Semple P d'A, Beastall GH, Watson WS, et al. Hypothalamic–pituitary dysfunction in respiratory hypoxia. *Thorax* 1987;36:605–9
48. Semple CG, Gray CE, Beastall GH. Androgen levels in men with diabetes mellitus. *Diabetic Med* 1988;5:122–5
49. Barrett-Connor E. Lower endogenous androgen levels and dyslipidemia in men with non-insulin-dependent-diabetes mellitus. *Ann Intern Med* 1992;117:807–11

50. Chang TC, Tung CC, Hsiao YL. Hormonal changes in elderly men with non-insulin-dependent diabetes mellitus and the hormonal relationships to abdominal obesity. *Gerontology* 1994;40:260–7
51. Andersson B, Vermeulen A, Marin P, *et al.* Testosterone concentration in women and men with NIDDM. *Diabetes Care* 1994;17:405–11
52. Phillips GB, Pinkernell BJ, Jing TY. The association of hypotestosteronemia with coronary heart disease. *Atheroscl Thromb* 1994;14:710–6
53. Handelsman DJ, Dong Q. Hypothalamo–pituitary–gonadal axis in chronic renal failure. *Endocrinol Metab Clin North Am* 1993;22:145–61
54. Baker HWG, Burger HCG, de Kretser DM, *et al.* A study of the endocrine manifestations of hepatic cirrhosis. *Q J Med* 1976;45:145–7
55. Dobs AS, Dempsey MA, Ladenson PW, *et al.* Endocrine disorders in men affected with human immunodeficiency virus. *Am J Med* 1988;84:611–16
56. Gordon D, Beastall GH, Thomson JA, *et al.* Prolonged hypogonadism in male patients with rheumatoid arthritis during flares in disease activity. *Br J Rheumatol* 1988;27:440–4
57. Doerr P, Pirke KM. Cortisol induced suppression of plasma testosterone in normal adult males. *J Clin Endocrinol Metab* 1976;43:622–9
58. MacAdams MP, White RH, Chipps BG. Reduction of serum testosterone levels during chronic glucocorticoid therapy. *Ann Intern Med* 1986;104:648–51
59. Longcope C. The effect of human chorionic gonadotropin on plasma steroid levels in young and old men. *Steroids* 1973;21:583–90
60. Nieschlag E, Kley KM, Wiegelman W, *et al.* Lebensalter und endokrine Funktion des erwachsenen Mannes. *Deutsch Med Wschr* 1973;98:1281–4
61. Nankin HR, Lin T, Murono EP, *et al.* The aging Leydig cell. III Gonadotropin stimulation in man. *J Androl* 1981;2:181–9
62. Rubens R, Dhont M, Vermeulen A. Further studies on Leydig cell function in old age. *J Clin Endocrinol Metab* 1984;39:40–5
63. Sniffen RC. The testes.I. The normal testis. *Arch Pathol* 1950;50:259–84
64. Harbitz TB. Morphometric studies of Leydig cells in elderly men with special reference to the histology of the prostate. *Acta Pathol Microbiol Scand* 1973;81:301–13
65. Neaves B, Johnson L, Porter JC, *et al.* Leydig cell numbers, daily sperm production and gonadotropin levels in aging men. *J Clin Endocrinol Metab* 1984;49:269–76
66. Sasano N, Ichijo S. Vascular pattern of the human testis with special reference to senile changes. *Tokutu J Exp Med* 1969;99:269–76

67. Suoranta H. Changes in small vessels of the adult testes in relation to age and some pathological conditions. *Virchow's Arch A: Pathol Anat Histopathol* 1971;352:765–81
68. Pirke KM, Sintermann R, Vogt HJ. Testosterone and testosterone precursors in the spermatic vein and in the testicular tissue of old men. *Gerontology* 1980;26:221–30
69. Vermeulen A, Deslypere JP. Intratesticular unconjugated steroids in elderly men. *J Steroid Biochem* 1986;24:1079–83
70. Tsitouras PD, Bulat T. The aging male reproductive system. *Endocrinol Metab Clin North Am* 1995;24:297–315
71. Tenover JS, Matsumoto AM, Clifton DK, *et al.* Age related alteration in the circadian rhythms of pulsatile luteinizing hormone and testosterone secretion in healthy men. *J Gerontol* 1988;43:M163–9
72. Kaufman JA, Giri M, Deslypere JP, *et al.* Influence of age on the responsiveness of the gonadotrophs to luteinizing hormone releasing hormone in males. *J Clin Endocrinol Metab* 1991;72:1255–60
73. Matzkin H, Braf Z, Nava D. Does age influence the reactivity of follicle stimulating hormone in men? *Age Aging* 1991;20:199–205
74. Bremner WJ, Vitiello M, Prinz PN. Loss of circadian rhythmicity in blood testosterone levels with aging in normal men. *J Clin Endocrinol Metab* 1983;56:1278–81
75. Plymate JR, Tenover JS, Bremner WJ, *et al.* Circadian variation in testosterone sex hormone binding globulin bound testosterone in healthy young and elderly men. *J Androl* 1989;10:366–71
76. Veldhuis JD, Urban RJ, Lizarreld G, *et al.* Attenuation of luteinizing hormone secretory burst amplitude as a proximate basis for the hypoandrogenism of healthy aging in men. *J Clin Endocrinol Metab* 1992;75:707–13
77. Vermeulen A, Kaufman JM, Deslypere JP, *et al.* Attenuated LH pulse amplitude but normal LH pulse frequency and its relation to plasma androgens in hypogonadism of obese men. *J Clin Endocrinol Metab* 1993;76:1140–6
78. Winters SJ, Sherins RJ, Troen P. The gonadotropin suppressive activity of androgen is increased in elderly men. *Metabolism* 1984;33:1052–9
79. Deslypere JP, Kaufman JM, Vermeulen A. Influence of age on pulsatile luteinizing hormone release and responsiveness of the gonadotrophs to sex hormone feedback in men. *J Clin Endocrinol Metab* 1987;64:68–73
80. Winters SJ, Atkinson L. Serum LH concentrations in hypogonadal men during transdermal testosterone replacement therapy through

scrotal skin: further evidence that aging enhances testosterone negative feedback. *Clin Endocrinol* 1997;47:317–22
81. Vermeulen A, Deslypere JP, Kaufman JM. Influence of antiopioids on luteinizing hormone pulsatility in aging men. *J Clin Endocrinol Metab* 1989;68:68–7
82. Whitehead M. The Pieter Van Keep Memorial Lecture. In Berg G, Hammar M, eds. *The Modern Management of the Menopause. Proceedings of the VIIth International Congress of the Menopause.* Carnforth, UK: Parthenon Publishing, 1993: 1–13
83. Flint M. Menopause. The global view. In Berg G, Hammer M, eds. *The Modern Management of the Menopause. Proceedings of the VIIth International Congress of the Menopause.* Carnforth, UK: Parthenon Publishing, 1993: 17–22
84. Schwarz D, Mayaux MJ, Spira A, *et al.* Semen characteristics as a function of age in 833 fertile men. *Fertil Steril* 1983;39:530–5
85. Rolf CD, Behre HM, Nieschlag E. Reproductive parameters of older compared to younger men of infertile couples. *Int J Androl* 1996;19: 135–42
86. Lemcke B, Behre HM, Nieschlag E. Frequently subnormal semen profiles of normal volunteers recruited over 17 years. *Int J Androl* 1997;20: 144–52
87. Cooper TG, Keck C, Oberdieck U, *et al.* Effects of multiple ejaculations after extended periods of sexual abstinence on total, motile and normal sperm numbers as well as on accessory gland secretions from healthy normal and oligospermic men. *Hum Reprod* 1993;8:1251–8
88. Johnston L. Spermatogenesis and aging in the human. *J Androl* 1986;7:331–4
89. Illingworth PJ, Groome NP, Byrd W, *et al.* Inhibin B: a likely candidate for the physiologically important form of inhibin in men. *J Clin Endocrinol Metab* 1996;81:1321–5
90. Guanes PP, Gallardo E, Levy M, *et al.* Effect of age on sperm fertilizing potential: oocyte donation as a model. In *Human Reproduction* Vol. 11. *12th Annual Meeting,* ESHRE, Maastricht, June 1996:abstr 112, p52
91. Johnston RC, Kovacs GT, Lording DH, *et al.* Correlation of semen variables and pregnancy rates for donor insemination: a 15 year retrospective. *Fertil Steril* 1994;61:355–9
92. Nieschlag E, Lammers U, Freischem CW, *et al.* Reproductive functions in young fathers and grandfathers. *J Clin Endocrinol Metab* 1982;55: 676–81
93. Kwan M, Greenleaf WJ, Mann J, *et al.* The nature of androgen action on male sexuality. A combined laboratory/self report study on hypogonadal men. *J Clin Endocrinol Metab* 1983;57: 557–62
94. Davidson JM, Camargo C, Smith ER. Effects of androgens on sexual behaviour in hypogonadal men. *J Clin Endocrinol Metab* 1979;48:955–8
95. O'Carroll R, Bancroft J. Testosterone therapy for low sexual interest and erectile dysfunction in men: a controlled study. *Br J Psychiatry* 1984; 145:146–51
96. Tsitouras PD, Martin CE, Harman SM. Relation of serum testosterone to sexual activity in healthy elderly men. *J Gerontol* 1982;37:288–93
97. Pfeiffer E. Sexuality in the aging individual. *Arch Sex Behav* 1974;22:481
98. McKinlay JD, Feldman HA. Age related variation in sexual activity and interest in normal men: results of the Massachusetts male aging study. In Rossi AS, ed. *Sexuality Across the Life Course.* University of Chicago Press, 1994:261–86
99. Verwoerdt A, Pfeiffer E, Wangh AS. Sexual behaviour in senescence. *Geriatrics* 1969;24: 137–54
100. Davidson JM, Chen JJ, Crapo L, *et al.* Hormonal changes and sexual function in aging men. *J Clin Endocrinol Metab* 1983;57:71–7
101. Bagatell CJ, Knopp RH, Bremner WJ. Physiological levels of estradiol stimulate plasma high density lipoprotein-2-cholesterol levels in normal men. *J Clin Endocrinol Metab* 1991;73:1360–9
102. Schiavi RC. Androgens and sexual function in men. In: Oddens B, Vermeulen A, eds. *Androgens and the Aging Male.* Carnforth, UK: Parthenon Publishing, 1996;111–28
103. Bagatell CJ, Heiman JR, Matsumoto AM, *et al.* Metabolic and behavioral effects of high dose exogenous testosterone in healthy men. *J Clin Endocrinol Metab* 1994;79:561–7
104. Udry JR, Belly JOG, Morris NM, *et al.* Serum androgenic hormones motivate normal behavior in adolescent boys. *Fertil Steril* 1985;43: 136–41
105. Udry JR, Talbert LM, Morris NM. Biosocial foundation for adolescent female sexuality. *Demography* 1986;23:217–30
106. Anderson RA, Bancroft J, Wu FCW. The effects of exogenous testosterone on sexuality and mood of normal men. *J Clin Endocrinol Metab* 1992;75:1503–7
107. Bancroft J. Androgens, sexuality and the aging male. In: Labrie F, Proulx L, eds. *Endocrinology.* Amsterdam:Elsevier, 1984:913–16
108. Masters WH. Sex and aging – expectations and reality. *Hosp Pract* 1986;15:175–98
109. Martin CE. Factors affecting sexual functioning in 60–79 year old married males. *Arch Sex Behav* 1981;10:399

110. Morley JE. Impotence. *Am J Med* 1986;80: 897–906
111. Dobs AS, Burnett AL, Fagan PJ, *et al.* Serum testosterone levels of men with erectile dysfunction presenting to a general urology clinic. *J Androl* 1995; Suppl:56, abstr 120
112. Martin CE. Marital and sexual factors in relation to age, disease and longevity. In: Wirdt RD, Winokur G, Ruff M, eds. *Life History Research in Psychopathology*, Vol.4. Minneapolis: University of Minnesota Press, 1975:326
113. Bancroft J, Wu FCW. Changes in erectile responsiveness during androgen replacement therapy. *Arch Sex Behav* 1983;12:59–66
114. Friedman JM. Genetic disease in the offspring of older fathers. *Obstet Gynecol* 1981;5:745–9
115. Goldberg RB, Rabin AN, Alexander AN, *et al.* Suppression of plasma testosterone leads to an increase in serum total and high density lipoprotein cholesterol and Apo A$_1$ and B. *J Clin Endocrinol Metab* 1985;60:203–7
116. Moorjani S, Dupont A, Labrie F, *et al.* Increase in plasma high density lipoprotein concentration following complete androgen blockade in men with prostatic carcinoma. *Metabolism* 1987; 36:244–50
117. Bagatell CJ, Knopp RH, Vale WW, *et al.* Physiologic levels of testosterone suppress HDL-cholesterol levels in normal men. *Ann Intern Med* 1992;116:967–73
118. Heller RF, Wheeler MJ, Micallef J, *et al.* Relationships of high density lipoproteincholesterol with total and free testosterone and sex hormone binding globulin. *Acta Endocrinol* 1983;104:253–60
119. Hamalainen E, Adlercreutz H, Ehnhorn C, *et al.* Relationships of serum lipoproteins and apoproteins for the binding capacity of sex hormone binding globulin (SHBG) in healthy Finnish men. *Metabolism* 1986;35:535–54
120. Bagatell CJ, Bremner WJ. Androgens and progestogen effects on plasma lipids. *Progr Cardiovasc Dis* 1995;38:255–72
121. Semmens J, Rouse I, Berlin LJ, *et al.* Relationship of plasma HDL cholesterol to testosterone, estradiol and sex hormone binding globulin levels in men and women. *Metabolism* 1983;32: 428–31
122. Handa K, Ishii H, Kono S, *et al.* Behavioral correlates of plasma sex hormones and their relationships with plasma lipids and lipoproteins in Japanese men. *Atherosclerosis* 1997; 130:37–44
123. Haffner SM, Mykkanen L, Valdez RA, *et al.* Relationship of sex hormones to lipids and lipoproteins in non-diabetic men. *J Clin Endocrinol Metab* 1993;77:1610–15
124. Haffner SM. Andrgens in relation to cardiovascular disease and insulin resistance in ageing men. In: Oddens B, Vermeulen A, eds. *Androgens and the Aging Male*. Carnforth, UK: Parthenon Publishing, 1996:65–83
125. Simon D, Preziosi P, Barrett-Connor E, *et al.* The influence of aging on plasma sex hormones in men: the TELECOM study. *Am J Epidemiol* 1992; 135:783–91
126. Simon D, Nahoul K, Charles MA. Sex hormones, aging, ethnicity and insulin sensitivity: an overview of the TELECOM study. In Oddens B, Vermeulen A, eds. *Androgens and the Aging Male*. Carnforth, UK: Parthenon Publishing 1996:85–102
127. Haffner SM, Shaten JS, Stern MP, *et al.* Low levels of sex hormone binding globulin and testosterone predict the development of non-insulin dependent diabetes mellitus. *Am J Epidemiol* 1996;143:889–97
128. Asscheman H, Gooren LJG, Megens JAJ, *et al.* Serum testosterone is the major determinant of male–female differences in serum levels of high-density lipoprotein-cholesterol and HDL-2 cholesterol. *Metabolism* 1994;43:935–9
129. Wu FCW, Farley TMM, Peregourdov A, *et al.* and the World Health Organization Task Force for the Regulation of Male Fertility. Effects of testosterone enanthate in normal men. Experience from a multicenter contraceptive efficacy study. *Fertil Steril* 1996;65: 626–36
130. Anderson RA, Wallace BM, Wu FCW. Effects of testosterone enanthate on serum lipoproteins in man. *Contraception* 1995;52:115–19
131. Cauley SA, Gutai JP, Kuller LH, *et al.* Usefulness of sex steroid hormone levels in predicting coronary artery disease in men. *Am J Cardiol* 1987; 60:771–7
132. Barrett-Connor E, Khaw KS. Endogenous sex hormone levels and cardiovascular disease in men: a prospective population based study. *Circulation* 1988;78:539–43
133. Haffner SM, Moss SE, Klein BEK, *et al.* Sex hormones and DHEA SO$_4$ in relation to ischemic heart disease in diabetic subjects: the WESDR study. *Diabetes Care* 1996;19:1045–50
134. Foresta C, Ruzza G, Mioni R, *et al.* Osteoporosis and decline of gonadal function in the elderly males. *Horm Res* 1984;19:18–24
135. Murphy S, Khaw KT, Cassidy A, *et al.* Sex hormones and bone mineral density in elderly men. *J Bone Miner Res* 1993;20:133–40
136. Kaufman JM. Androgens, bone metabolism and osteoporosis. In Oddens B, Vermeulen A, eds. *Androgens and the Aging Male*. Carnforth, UK: Parthenon Publishing, 1996:39–60
137. Stanley HL, Schmitt BP, Poses RM, *et al.* Does hypogonadism contribute to the occurrence of a minimal trauma hip fracture in men? *J Am Geriatr Soc* 1991;39:766–71

138. Jackson JA, Rigg MW, Spiekerman AM. Testosterone deficiency as a risk factor for hip fractures in men. A case control study. Am J Med Sci 1992;304:4–8
139. Behre HM, Kliesch AS, Leifke E, et al. Long term effects of testosterone therapy on bone mineral density in hypogonadal men. J Clin Endocrinol Metab 1997;82:2386–90
140. Finkelstein JS, Klibanski A, Nees RM, et al. Increase in bone mineral density during treatment of men with idiopathic hypogonadotropic hypogonadism. J Clin Endocrinol Metab 1989;69:776–83
141. Tenover JS. Androgen administration to aging men. Endocrinol Metab Clin North Am 1994;23:877–92
142. Tenover JS. Effect of testosterone supplementation to the aging male. J Clin Endocrinol Metab 1992;72:1092–8
143. Morley ME, Perry MM, Kaiser SE, et al. Effects of testosterone replacement therapy in old hypogonadal males: a preliminary study. J Am Geriatr Soc 1993;41:149–52
144. Tenover JS. Effect of androgen supplementation in the aging male. In Oddens B, Vermeulen A, eds. Androgens and the Aging Male. Carnforth, UK: Parthenon Publishing, 1996:191–221
145. Ono K, Haji M, Nawata H, et al. Age-related changes in glucocorticoid and androgen receptors of cultured human skin fibroblasts. Gerontology 1988;34:128–33
146. Berr C, Lafont S, Debuire B, et al. Relationships of dehydroepiandrosterone sulfate in the elderly with functional, psychological and mental status and short term mortality: a French community based study. Proc Natl Acad Sci 1996;93:13410–15
147. Marin P, Holmang S, Gustafson C, et al. Androgen treatment of abdominally obese men. Obesity Res 1993;1:245–51
148. Sih R, Morley JE, Kaiser FE, et al. Testosterone replacement in older hypogonadal men: a 12 month randomized controlled study. J Clin Endocrinol Metab 1997;82:1661–7
149. Hajjar RR, Kaiser FE, Morley JE. Outcomes of long term testosterone replacement therapy in old hypogonadal males: a preliminary study. J Am Geriatr Soc 1997;43:149–52
150. Conway AJ, Boylan LM, Howe C, et al. Randomized clinical trial of testosterone replacement therapy in hypogonadal men. Int J Androl 1988;11:247–64
151. Marin P, Holmang S, Jönsson L, et al. The effects of testosterone treatment on body composition and metabolism in middle aged men. Int J Obesity 1992;16:991–7
152. Marin P, Lönn L, Anderson B, et al. Assimilation of triglycerides in subcutaneous and intraabdominal adipose tissues in vivo in men: effects of testosterone. J Clin Endocrinol Metab 1996;81:1018–22
153. Friedl KE, Hannan CS, Jones RE, et al. High density lipoprotein-cholesterol is not decreased if an aromatizable androgen is administered. Metabolism 1990;39:69–74
154. Zmuda JN, Fahrenbach ML, Youkin BT, et al. The effect of testosterone aromatization on high density lipoprotein cholesterol level and post heparin lipolytic activity. Metabolism 1993;42:446–50
155. Bashin S, Storer TW, Berman N, et al. The effects of supraphysiological doses of testosterone on muscle size and strength in normal men. N Engl J Med 1996;335:1–7
156. Shiozowa Z, Yamada H, Mabuchi C, et al. Superior sagittal sinus thrombosis associated with androgen therapy. Ann Neurol 1982;12:57–88
157. Nagelberg JB, Lae L, Loriaux DL, et al. Cardiovascular accident associated with testosterone therapy in a 20 year old hypogonadal man (letter). N Engl J Med 1986;314:649–50
158. Bonithon-Kopp C, Scarabin PY, Bara I, et al. Relationship between sex hormones and haemostatic factors in healthy middle aged men. Atherosclerosis 1988;71:71–6
159. Polderman KH, Stehouwer CDA, Van de Kamp GJ, et al. Influence of sex hormones on plasma on plasma endothelin levels. Ann Intern Med 1993;118:429–32
160. Ajayi AA. Testosterone increases human platelet thromboxane A2 receptor density and aggregation responses. Circulation 1995;91:2742–7
161. Adams MR, Williams JK, Kaplan JR. Effects of androgens on coronary artery atherosclerosis related impairment of vascular responsiveness. Arterioscler Thromb Vasc Biol 1995;15:562–70
162. Fearnley CR, Chakrabarti R. Increase of blood fibrinolytic activity by testosterone. Lancet 1962;2:128–32
163. Beer NA, Jakubowicz DS, Matt DW, et al. Oral dehydroepiandrosterone administration reduces plasma levels of plasminogen activator type I and tissue plasminogen activator antigen in men. Am J Med Sci 1996;311:205–10
164. Matsumoto AM, Sandblom RE, Schoene RE, et al. Testosterone replacement in hypogonadal men. Clin Endocrinol 1985;22:713–21
165. Wilson JD. Androgen abuse by athletes. Endocr Rev 1988;9:203–8
166. Wallace EM, Pye SD, Wild ST, et al. Prostate specific antigen and prostate gland size in men receiving exogenous testosterone for male contraception. Int J Androl 1993;16:35–40
167. Krieg M, Tunn S. Androgens and human benign prostatic hyperplasia (BPH). In Nieschlag

E, Behre HM, eds. *Testosterone, Action, Deficiency, Substitution.* Berlin: Springer-Verlag, 1990: 219–44

168. Goldenberg SL, Bruchowsy N, Gleave ME, *et al.* Intermittent androgen suppression in the treatment of prostate cancer. *Urology* 1995;45:839–45

169. Jackson JA, Waxman J, Spiekerman M. Prostatic implications of testosterone replacement therapy. *Arch Intern Med* 1989;149:2364–6

170. Schröder FH. Androgens and carcinoma of the prostate. In Nieschlag E, Behre HM, eds. *Testosterone, Action, Deficiency, Substitution.* Berlin: Springer-Verlag, 1990:245–60

171. Schröder FM. The prostate and androgens: the risk of supplementation. In Oddens B, Vermeulen A, eds. *Androgens and the Aging Male.* Carnforth, UK: Parthenon Publishing, 1996: 223–32

172. Gooren LJG. Androgen levels and sexual function in testosterone treated hypogonadal men. *Arch Sex Behav* 1987;16:463–76

173. Snyder P, Lawrence DA. Treatment of hypogonadism with testosterone-enanthate. *J Clin Endocrinol Metab* 1980;51:1335–6

174. Bashin S, Bremner W. Emerging issues in androgen replacement therapy. *J Clin Endocrinol Metab* 1997;82:3–8

175. Cunningham CR, Cordero E, Thornby JL. Testosterone replacement with transdermal therapeutic systems. *J Am Med Assoc* 1989;261:2525–30

176. Meikle AW, Mazer NA, Noellmer JF, *et al.* Enhanced transdermal delivery of testosterone across nonscrotal skin produces physiological concentrations of testosterone and its metabolites in hypogonadal men. *J Clin Endocrinol Metab* 1992;74:623–8

177. Handelsman DJ. Pharmacology of testosterone pellet implants In Nieschlag E, Behre HM, eds. *Testosterone, Action, Deficiency, Substitution.* Berlin: Springer-Verlag, 1990:136–54

Index

abortion, incidence of and maternal age, 68
abstinence, use by age, 70
activin, action of, 2
adenocarcinoma, links with endometrial hyperplasia, 113
age,
    biological cf. anagraphic, 51
    bone mineral density changes and, 7
    effect on bladder, 39
    fertility decline with, 67, 95
    incontinence and, 41
    Leydig cell function in elderly men, 293
    rheumatoid arthritis and age at menopause, 61
    testosterone levels change in men with, 279
alcohol,
    effects on testosterone levels in men, 282
    osteoporosis and high level intake, 161
aluminium and osteoporosis, 159
Alzheimer's disease,
    diagnostic criteria for, 183
    estrogen effects on brain and, 184
    estrogens and, 178
    gender difference in incidence, 172
    prevention of and estrogens, 183–8
    reduced risk of and HRT, 186
    response of cognition to estrogen in, 185
    risk factors for, 184
amenorrhea and HRT, 115
androgen replacement therapy,
    role in aging males, 279–90
    role in female androgen deficiency syndrome, 52
androgens,
    changing levels at menopause, 4
    clinical relevance of decrease in men with age, 283
    combined estrogen–androgen HRT preparations, 271–5
    decrease in levels with age in men, 279–82
    production in women, 271
    role in rheumatoid arthritis, 61
    supplementation of in aging males, 286
        aims of, 288
        benefits of, 287
        methods of, 289
        risks of, 287
andropause, 279–90
angiogenesis, inhibition by phytoestrogens, 86
anovulatory cycles during menopausal transition, 4
antioxidant activity of phytoestrogens, 87

aromatase inhibition by phytoestrogens, 85
arthritis,
    menopause and, 59–63
    see also carpal tunnel syndrome; osteoarthritis; rheumatoid arthritis; systemic lupus erythematosus
assisted reproduction,
    ovum donation for premature menopause, 93–8
    success rates of ovum donation cf. regular IVF, 94
atherosclerosis,
    in aging men, 285
    in carotid artery, 180
    reduction in and estrogen, 215
attitude, role of negative in depression at menopause, 16

barrier contraception,
    see also by method
    use by age, 70
bilateral oophorectomy, as an indication for HRT use after hysterectomy, 259
bisphosphonates,
    as an alternative to progestogens, 253
    use in osteoporosis treatment, 128
bladder,
    effect of aging on, 39
    see also urinary problems, 41
bleeding,
    patterns of on HRT, 115, 116
    prevention and treatment of, 243
    problems with progestogens, 242
bone cells, effect of estrogens on osteoclasts and osteoblasts, 123
bone loss,
    accelerated after discontinuation of HRT, 137
    biochemical markers of, 152
    in diabetes mellitus, 234
bone markers,
    clinical value in osteoporosis, 143–55
    of formation,
        bone-specific alkaline phosphatase, 145
        osteocalcin, 144
        procollagen type I carboxy-terminal propeptide, 146
    of resorption,
        C-telopeptide degradation products, 149
        N-telopeptide degradation products, 148
        pyridinolines, 147

prediction of fractures from, 153
bone mass,
    effect of HRT on, 125
    need for long-term estrogen to improve, 128
bone metabolism, role of lysine in, 161
bone mineral density,
    changes in after discontinuation of HRT, 138
    effects of estradiol–norethisterone on, 126
    effects of HRT on, 125
    in diabetes mellitus, 233
    optimization by dietary changes, 161
    skeletal response prediction to therapies, 151
    timing of HRT for optimal, 135–40
    variations with age, 7
bone remodeling, mechanism of, 123
bone resorption,
    markers for, 143–55
    role of estrogen in, 122, 124
bone structure, 121
bone turnover,
    at menopausal transition, 7
    markers of, use in monitoring therapy, 129
bone-specific alkaline phosphatase, 145
boron and osteoporosis, 162
brain,
    as a target for estrogen, 169
    blood flow in and estrogens, 177–81
    effects of estrogens on, 184
breast cancer,
    combined oral contraceptives and increased risk of, 74
    detection rates, 193
    development of and estrogen, 201
    effect of pregnancy on prognosis, 201
    epidemiology of, 81
    estrogen use after, 199–206
    incidence bias in studies of HRT, 195
    mortality from and HRT, 193–6
    possible effects of progestogens on, 245
    premature menopause after treatment for, 199
    progestogen-only menopausal treatment in, 206
    risk factors for, 200
    risk of and HRT, 202
    survival and estrogen replacement therapy, 204
    use of HRT after, 204
    use of HRT in premature menopause after, 199
breast cell,
    estrogen effects on, 200
    progestogen effects on, 200
breast cell internal signaling system, 200

C-telopeptide degradation products, 149
cadmium and osteoporosis, 159
caffeine and fracture risk, 160
calcitonin, skeletal response to, 151
calcitonin use in osteoporosis treatment, 129
calcitriol use in osteoporosis treatment, 129
calcium and osteoporosis, 163
cancer,
    diet and, 82
    incidence of and vegetable-rich diets, 88
    see also under breast cancer; endometrial cancer; ovarian cancer; prostate cancer
carbohydrate metabolism,
    effects of estrogen on, 232
    effects of menopause on, 231
    effects of opposed HRT on, 233
cardioprotective effects of estrogen, 211–18
cardiovascular disease,
    combined oral contraceptives and increased risk of, 73
    effects of estrogen in women with previous disease, 222
    effects of estrogen–testosterone regimens on, 273
    estrogen use in women with, 213
    ever-use of hormones and risk, 212
    in aging men, 285
    mechanisms of cardioprotection by estrogen, 224
    risk factors for at menopausal transition, 8
    risk factors for in women, 225
    see also coronary heart disease
cardiovascular protection of HRT, 264
carotid artery,
    atherosclerosis of, 180
    wall thickness at menopause, 22
carpal tunnel syndrome, effect of HRT on, 63
cerebral blood flow,
    and estrogens, 177–81
    measurement of, 178
    physiology of, 178
    progestogens and, 181
    pulsatility index measurement, 179
    SPECT scan, 179
    vascular morphology and, 180
cerebrovascular disease, epidemiology of, 177
cholesterol,
    effect of estrogen on in coronary artery disease in monkeys, 217
    hyperlipidemia as a risk factor for cardiovascular disease, 225
    levels at menopausal transition, 8
    see also high-density lipoprotein; low-density lipoprotein
cognitive function,
    estrogen effects on, 185
    influence of estrogen on, 170

INDEX

collagen,
    effect of HRT on, 20
    effect of sex steroids on levels in skin, 21
    role in skin, 19
condom,
    female, 71
    use by age, 70
contraception,
    in women over forty, 67–77
    masking of menopause by hormonal methods, 76
    methods available to older women, 70
    need for in perimenopause whilst taking HRT, 77
    see also under specific methods
    when to stop, 76
copper and osteoporosis, 163
coronary heart disease,
    epidemiology, 211
    estrogen and primary prevention of, 211
    risk in diabetes mellitus, 236
coronary risk factors in women, 225
counseling for ovum donation, 97

dehydroepiandrosterone and rheumatoid arthritis, 61
delivery systems,
    advantages of, 102
    intramuscular injections, 105
    menopausal vaginal rings, 105
    new methods for HRT delivery, 101–8
    subdermal, 104
    transdermal, 102
dementia, *see under* Alzheimer's disease
Depo-Provera, 75
depression,
    changes after hysterectomy, 262
    decreased estrogen levels postmenopause and, 171
    incidence in menopausal transition, 6
    is there a specific menopausal syndrome, 14
    menopausal transition and, 13
    predictors for, 16
dermis, *see* skin
diabetes mellitus,
    as a risk factor for cardiovascular disease, 225
    complications of and HRT, 233
    coronary heart disease risk in, 236
    diabetic dyslipidemia, 235
    diabetic osteopenia, 234
    HRT and, 231–7
    hypertension risk in, 235
    increased risk of osteoporosis in, 233
    potential usefulness of HRT in, 237
    testosterone levels in, 281
diaphragm, use by age, 70
diet,
    cancer and, 82
    changes in to optimize bone mineral density, 161
    modern Western and osteoporosis, 160
    vegetable-rich diets and cancer incidence, 88
DNA topoisomerase inhibition by phytoestrogens, 86
dopamine, role in mood, 172
douche, use by age, 70
droloxifene, 253
drug abuse, effects on testosterone levels in men, 282
dysfunctional uterine bleeding,
    estrogen secretion and, 7
    hypothalamic–pituitary–ovarian axis alterations in, 4
dyslipidemia, diabetic, 235

employment as a buffer to depression at menopause, 16
endometrial cancer,
    combined oral contraceptives and reduced risk, 111
    epidemiology of, 81
    estrogen and increased risk, 111
    protective effect of combined oral contraceptives against, 75
    relative risk of and combined estrogen and progestin use, 112
    relative risk of and estrogen use, 111
endometrium,
    bleeding patterns, 115
    effect of progestogens on, 242
    effects of estrogen–testosterone regimens on, 275
    hyperplasia of, 113–15
        incidence, 114
        links with adenocarcinoma, 113
        links with endometrial cancer, 113
        links with HRT, 115
        links with long-cycle HRT regimens, 117
    receptivity and success rates in assisted reproduction cycles, 95
    thickness measurement by transvaginal sonography, 118
β-endorphin, effect of sex steroids on, 170
epidermis, *see* skin
erectile function in aging men, 284
estradiol,
    hot flushes and levels of, 7

levels after hysterectomy with bilateral oophorectomy, 258
levels in older cf. younger women, 3
transdermal delivery of, 103
estrogen,
Alzheimer's disease and, 172, 178
prevention and, 183–8
antioxidant activity, 216
atherosclerosis reduction and, 215
cardioprotective effects of, 211–18
mechanisms, 224
cerebral blood flow and, 177–81
cf. other osteoporosis treatments, 128
combined with progestin and endometrial cancer risk, 112
continence mechanism and, 41
decrease in and decreased cognitive function, 171
effect in women with previous cardiovascular disease, 222
effect of deficiency on bladder, 39–45
effect on bone, 121
effect on bone resorption rate, 124
effect on brain, 184
effect on breast cancer incidence, 193
effect on breast cell, 200
effect on carbohydrate metabolism, 232
effect on cognition in Alzheimer's disease, 185
effect on cognitive function, 185
effect on inflammation in gingiva, 28
effect on lipid profile, 215
effect on mood, 185
effect on osteoblasts, 123
effect on osteoclasts, 123
effect on vascular endothelium, 224
effect on wound healing, 27
hemodynamic effects, 216
in plants, 83
influence on cognitive function, 170
levels at menopausal transition, 5
links with endometrial cancer, 111
mechanism of action on bone cells, 122
monitoring of therapy with, 129
neurotransmitters and, 169–73
osteoporosis therapy with, 121–31
primary prevention of coronary heart disease, 211
problems associated with long-term therapy, 128
role in arousal, 55
role in breast cancer development, 201
role in granulation in wound healing, 32
role in matrix formation and remodeling in wound healing, 32
role in mood, 14
role in osteoarthritis, 59
role in systemic lupus erythematosus, 62
role in treatment of incontinence, 42
see also phytoestrogens
short-term memory and, 171
short-term studies of therapy for optimal bone mineral density, 135
synthesis and menopause, 122
targeting of brain by, 169
transdermal, 102
unopposed and endometrial cancer risk, 111
use after breast cancer, 199–206
use in women with postmenopausal women with cardiovascular disease, 213
vaginal atrophy and, 106
estrogen receptors,
in bone, 122
in brain, 169
in lower urinary tract, 40
in skin, 27
ethical issues and ovum donation, 96
exercise,
osteoporosis and, 159
protective effect against cardiovascular disease, 225

female androgen deficiency syndrome, 52
femininity, changing perception of and sexuality at menopause, 51–54
fertility,
decline with age, 67, 95
in aging men, 284
flavonoids, 83
flushes, *see* hot flushes
folic acid and osteoporosis, 164
follicle stimulating hormone (FSH),
hot flushes and levels of, 7
levels after hysterectomy with bilateral oophorectomy, 258
levels in older cf. younger women, 3
levels in perimenopausal cycles, 68
production of by pituitary, 1
follicular development during menopausal transition, 4
fractures,
caffeine and increased risk of, 161
effects of HRT on, 127
prediction of from biochemical markers, 153

genitourinary changes at menopause, 39–45
gingival inflammation and estrogens, 28
glucose, effects of estrogen on fasting levels, 232
glycosaminoglycans,
effect of estrogens on, 21

role in skin, 19
gonadotropin releasing hormone, pituitary regulation by, 1

high-density lipoprotein (HDL) cholesterol,
    effect of estrogen on, 215
    effect of estrogen plus progestin, 224
    levels at menopausal transition, 8
    levels in aging men, 285
    levels in diabetic dyslipidemia, 235
    raised by estrogen alone, 224
hormone replacement therapy (HRT),
    advantages of delivery systems, 102
    after coronary artery thrombosis, 221–7
    Alzheimer's disease risk and, 186
    androgen supplements in aging males, 286–90
    bleeding patterns and, 115
    breast cancer mortality and, 193–6
    breast cancer risk and, 202
    cardiovascular protection by, 264
    combined estrogen–androgen preparations, 271–5
    compliance with after hysterectomy, 265
    continuous combined regimens, 243
    contraception requirements whilst taking, 77
    diabetes complications and, 233
    discontinuation and accelerated bone loss, 137
    discontinuation rates, 130
    effect on bone balance, 124
    effect on bone mass, 125
    effect on bone mineral density, 126
    effect on carbohydrate metabolism, 233
    effect on collagen, 20, 22
    effect on fractures, 127
    effect on rheumatoid arthritis, 62
    effect on skin changes at menopause, 19–23
    effect on wound healing, 27–34
    endometrial hyperplasia and, 115
    estradiol-releasing rings, 106
    estrogen-only,
        breast cancer survival and, 204
        deep vein thrombosis risk and, 223
        monitoring of, 129
        problems associated with, 128
        pulmonary embolism risk and, 223
    future developments in, 173
    guidelines to improve compliance, 267
    immediate benefits of after hysterectomy, 260
    indications for use after hysterectomy, 259
    intramuscular injections, 105
    intrauterine systems, 107
    lack of compliance, 130
    late start, 137
    levonorgestrel-releasing intrauterine system, 107
    lifelong use, 101
    limitations in osteoporosis treatment, 139
    long-cycle regimens, risk of endometrial hyperplasia and, 117
    long-term benefits of after hysterectomy, 264
    menopausal vaginal rings, 105
    need for improved delivery for acceptance, 101
    need for trials in diabetic women, 237
    neural effects of, 172
    new delivery systems for, 101–8
    new treatment regimens, 125
    osteoporosis prevention and, 8
    osteoporosis protection by, 264
    prediction of skeletal response, 151
    progestogen dose used and bleeding problems, 243
    quarterly regimens, 243
    reasons for poor compliance, 266
    risk of coronary events and, 221
    role in carpal tunnel syndrome, 63
    role in osteoarthritis, 60
    role in systemic lupus erythematosus, 63
    subdermal implants, 104
    timing of for optimal bone mineral density, 135–40
    transdermal delivery systems,
        percutaneous estrogen gels, 102
        skin patches, 102
    use after breast cancer, 204
    use after hysterectomy, 257–68
    use at menopausal transition, 9
    use in postmenopausal women with cardiovascular disease, 213
    use in premature menopause after breast cancer, 199
hormones,
    dynamics in menopause, 2
    effect on skin collagen content, 21
    effects on breast tissues, 200
    ever-use and cardiovascular risk, 212
    influence on lower urinary tract, 40
    normal physiological dynamics in reproduction, 1
    rheumatoid arthritis and, 61
    role in genitourinary system, 39
    role in mood postmenopause, 13
    role in osteoarthritis, 59
    role in reduced fertility with increased age, 68
    see also individual hormones
hot flushes,
    estradiol levels and, 7
    estrogen deficiency and neural control of, 171
    FSH levels and, 7
    incidence in menopausal transition, 6

17β-hydroxysteroid dehydrogenase inhibition by phytoestrogens, 85
hyperlipidemia as a risk factor for cardiovascular disease, 225
hypertension,
 as a risk factor for cardiovascular disease, 225
 increased risk in diabetes mellitus, 235
 pregnancy-induced, increased incidence in ovum donation, 96
hypothalamic–pituitary–ovarian axis,
 altered sensitivity during menopausal transition, 4
 normal physiology of, 1
hysterectomy,
 as an alternative to progestogens, 252
 changes in sexuality after, 262
 compliance with HRT after, 265
  guidelines to improve, 267
  reasons for poor, 266
 HRT after, 257–68
  immediate benefits, 260
 psychological morbidity after, 262
 with bilateral oophorectomy, endocrine changes after, 258
 with ovarian conservation, endocrine changes after, 257

impotence in aging men, 284
incontinence,
 estrogens and mechanism of, 41
 incidence of, 41
 role of estrogens in treatment, 42–44
 stress cf. urge, 42
infections, recurrent urinary, 44
inhibin,
 levels in older cf. younger women, 3
 production by ovary, 1
insulin,
 effects of estrogen on, 232
 resistance and progestogens, 251
 testosterone levels and, 280
intrauterine device,
 levonorgestrel-releasing intrauterine system, 72, 107, 244
 suitability for older women, 71
 use by age, 70
involutional melancholia, 13
irregular menstruation at menopausal transition, 7
isoflavonoids, 83
 biological properties of, 84

lead and osteoporosis, 159
levonorgestrel-releasing intrauterine system, 107
 adverse effects with, 249
 suitability for older women, 72
 use in HRT, 244
Leydig cell function in elderly men, 293
libido, loss of, 54
lignans, 83
 biological properties of, 84
lipid metabolism,
 effect of estrogen on, 215
 effect of estrogen–testosterone regimens on, 273
 effect of oral contraception on at menopausal transition, 8
 effect of progestogens on, 250
low-density lipoprotein (LDL) cholesterol,
 effect of estrogen on, 215
 levels at menopausal transition, 8
 levels in aging men, 285
 levels in diabetic dyslipidemia, 235
 lowering by estrogen, 224
luteinizing hormone production of by pituitary, 1
lysine, role in bone metabolism, 161

magnesium and osteoporosis, 163
management at menopausal transition, 9
manganese and osteoporosis, 163
memory reduction in and decreased estrogen levels postmenopause, 171
menopausal symptoms, incidence after hysterectomy, 261
menopausal syndrome, as a depressive syndrome, 14
menopausal transition,
 anovulatory cycles during, 4
 bone turnover at, 7
 cardiovascular risks at, 8
 changes in sexuality at, 50
 female sexual identity during, 50
 hormonal dynamics in, 2
 hormonal levels during, 5
 management of, 9
 symptoms at, 6
 wound healing at, 27
menopause, premature see under premature menopause
mineralocorticoid activity and progestogens, 245
Monash assay, 2
mood,
 estrogen and, 14
 estrogen effects on, 185
 psychosocial factors affecting, 15
 role of hormones in postmenopause, 13
mood disorders, decreased estrogen levels postmenopause and, 171
moral issues and ovum donation, 96
mucus changes in menopausal transition, 5

myocardial infarction, combined oral
    contraceptives and increased risk of, 73

N-telopeptide degradation products, 148
natural methods of fertility regulation, 73
nervousness, incidence in menopausal transition, 6
neuropeptide Y, effect of sex steroids on, 171
neurotransmitters and estrogen, 169–73
norepinephrine, role in mood, 172
norethisterone enanthate, 75
Norplant, 76
nutrition,
    deficiencies caused by modern Western diet,
        160–1
    see also diet

obesity and menopausal osteoarthritis, 60
oocyte quality changes with age, 67
oral contraception,
    combined,
        non-contraceptive health benefits of, 74
        risk of arterial disease and, 73
        risk of breast cancer and, 74
        risk of venous thromboembolism and, 74
    effect on lipid concentrations at menopausal
        transition, 8
    progestogen-only, 75
    use by age, 70
osteoarthritis,
    generalized, sex hormone binding globulin
        levels in, 60
    hormonal factors in, 59
    obesity and, 60
    role of HRT in, 60
osteoblasts, effect of estrogen on, 123
osteocalcin, 144
osteoclasts, effect of estrogen on, 123
osteopenia,
    androgen levels in men and, 286
    diabetic, 234
osteoporosis,
    alcohol intake and risk of, 161
    bisphosphonate therapy, 128
    calcitonin therapy, 129
    calcitriol therapy, 129
    clinical value of bone markers in, 143–55
    diet and, 159–65
    estrogen treatment for, 121–31
        cf. other treatments, 128
    follow-up of therapy, 150
    HRT for prevention, 8
    incidence,
        and skin transparency, 20
        increasing, 159

    increased risk in diabetes mellitus, 233
    induction by high sucrose diet in hamsters, 160
    minerals useful against, 162–4
    nutritional supplements for, 162
    phosphorus intake and risk of, 161
    protection against by HRT, 264
    reasons for increased incidence, 159
    risk determination, 143
    skin thickness as an indicator for, 23
    sodium intake and risk of, 161
    suggested diet for, 162
    timing of HRT for optimal protection, 135–40
    vitamins useful against, 164–5
ovarian cancer,
    epidemiology of, 82
    protective effect of combined oral
        contraceptives against, 75
ovarian failure, as an indication for HRT use after
    hysterectomy, 259
ovariectomy, effect on granulation in wound
    healing in mice, 31
ovary, inhibin production by, 1
ovum donation,
    counseling for, 97
    donors for, 97
    future developments, 98
    history of, 93
    moral and ethical issues of, 96
    postpartum hemorrhage after, 96
    pregnancy-induced hypertension and, 96
    procedure for, 94
    self-donation before chemo- or radiotherapy, 98
    success rates cf. regular IVF, 94

Parkinson's disease, gender difference in
    incidence, 172
perimenopause, see menopausal transition
pessary use by age, 70
phosphorus, high intake and osteoporosis, 161
phytoestrogens,
    angiogenesis inhibition by, 86
    antioxidant activity of, 87
    aromatase inhibition by, 85
    cancer and, 81–8
    DNA topoisomerase inhibition by, 86
    estrogenic activity of, 84
    flavonoids, 83
    17β-hydroxysteroid dehydrogenase inhibition
        by, 85
    isoflavonoids, 83
        biological properties of, 84
    lignans, 83
        biological properties of, 84
    menstrual cycle and, 85

tumorigenesis inhibition by, 87
tyrosine-specific protein kinase inhibition by, 86
pituitary, gonadotropin production by, 1
pregnancy,
    effect on prognosis after breast cancer, 201
    in older women, 68
    risks in older women, 68
pregnanediol, levels at menopausal transition, 5
premature menopause,
    after treatment for breast cancer, 199
    causes, 93
    incidence, 93
    ovum donation for, 93–8
premature ovarian failure as an indication for HRT use after hysterectomy, 259
procollagen type I carboxy-terminal propeptide, 146
progesterone vaginal gel, 249
progesterone-releasing intrauterine system, 244
progestogen, effect on breast cell, 200
progestogen-only contraception,
    injectables, 75
    pills, 75
progestogens,
    adverse effects of, 241
    alternatives to, 252
    antimineralocorticoid forms of, 250
    breast cancer risk and, 202
    cerebral blood flow and, 181
    chemical classification, 242
    clinical management of intolerance, 253
    effects on neurotransmitters, 246
    insulin resistance and, 251
    intolerance to, treatment of, 241–54
    metabolic side-effects of, 241, 250
    minimum doses, 248
    physical effects of, 241
        on skin, 245
    psychological effects of, 241, 245
    subcutaneous injection of, 249
    transdermal, 249
    treatment of adverse metabolic effects of, 251
    treatment of adverse physical and psychological effects of, 247
    use in breast cancer against menopausal symptoms, 206
    vascular effects, 251
prostate cancer, epidemiology of, 82
psychopathology at menopause, 13
psychosocial factors affecting mood, 15
pulmonary embolism, risk of and HRT, 223
pulsatility index, measurement of for cerebral blood flow, 179
pyridinolines, 147

pyridoxine and osteoporosis, 164

quarterly regimens of HRT, 243, 248

raloxifene, 253
rheumatoid arthritis,
    age at menopause and, 61
    effect of HRT on, 62
    role of androgens in, 61
    role of dehydroepiandrosterone in, 61

safe period, use by age, 70
selective estrogen-receptor modulators, 253
self-perception,
    changes in mental, 53
    changes in sensory, 52
serotonin,
    effects of progestogens on, 246
    effects of testosterone on, 272
sex hormone binding globulin, levels in women with osteoarthritis, 60
sexual activity, 69
sexuality,
    and need for contraception, 69
    arousal difficulties, 54
    changes after hysterectomy, 262
    changes at menopausal transition, 50
    clinical implications for gynecologist, 53
    couple relationship and, 56
    cybernetic model of, 54
    female sexual function, 54
    importance for gynecologists to understand, 50
    in aging men, 284
    libido loss, 54
    menopause and, 49–56
    perception of femininity and, 51
    problems with at menopause, 49
        choice of doctor, 49
        diagnosis, 49
    sensory self-perception changes and, 52
    testosterone and in postmenopause, 272
skin,
    anatomy of, 19
    androgenic effects of progestogens on, 245
    as a window on menopausal transition, 53
    changes in,
        and sexuality, 51
        at menopause, 20
        thickness at menopause, 21
    estrogen receptors in, 27
    thickness of as a measure of carotid wall thickness, 22
    thickness of as a measure of osteoporosis, 23
    transparent skin and osteoporosis incidence, 20

sleeplessness incidence in menopausal transition, 6
smoking as a risk factor for cardiovascular disease, 225
social support as a buffer to depression at menopause, 16
sodium, high intake and osteoporosis, 161
sponge, use by age, 70
sterilization,
    female,
        incidence, 72
        use by age, 70
    male,
        cancer risk and, 72
        use by age, 70
stress, effects on testosterone levels in men, 282
strontium and osteoporosis, 163
systemic lupus erythematosus,
    effect of HRT on, 63
    role of estrogen in, 62

testosterone,
    age-related changes in men, 279
    aging and libido and, 284
    changes after hysterectomy, 262
    changing levels at menopause, 4
    clinical relevance of decrease in men with age, 283
    disease and levels, 282
    effects of stress on, 282
    effects on central nervous system, 272
    effects on serotonin system, 272
    erectile function and, 284
    impotence and, 284
    levels after hysterectomy with bilateral oophorectomy, 259
    levels in diabetes mellitus, 281
    physiological factors affecting, 280
    production in women, 271
    sexuality in postmenopause and, 272
thrombosis,
    coronary artery, HRT use after, 221–7
    deep vein, risk of and HRT, 223
    venous, 74
thrombotic stroke, combined oral contraceptives and increased risk of, 73
tibolone as an alternative to progestogens, 252
transvaginal sonography, *see under* ultrasound
triglyceride levels at menopausal transition, 8

tumorigenesis inhibition by phytoestrogens, 87
tyrosine-specific protein kinase inhibition by phytoestrogens, 86

ultrasound,
    Doppler measurement of cerebral blood flow, 179
    transvaginal sonography, endometrial thickness measurement by, 118
urinary problems,
    at menopause, 39–45
    continence and estrogens, 41
    epidemiology, 41
    estrogen treatment for incontinence, 42
        stress, 43
        urge, 44
    estrogen treatment for recurrent urinary infections, 44
urinary tract,
    embryology of lower, 40
    sex steroids influence on, 40

vaginal atrophy, estrogen creams and cure of, 106
vascular endothelium, effects of estrogen on, 224
vasectomy, *see under* sterilization, male
venous thromboembolism, combined oral contraceptives and increased risk of, 74
very low-density lipoprotein (VLDL) cholesterol levels in diabetic dyslipidemia, 235
virilization, estrogen–testosterone regimens and, 274
vitamin B6 and osteoporosis, 164
vitamin C and osteoporosis, 164
vitamin D and osteoporosis, 164
vitamin K and osteoporosis, 164

withdrawal, use by age, 70
wound healing,
    changes in at menopause, 27–34
    effect of estrogens on, 27
    granulation phase, 31
    inflammatory phase of and estrogens, 28
    matrix formation and remodeling, 32
    process of, 28–34
    proliferative phase of and estrogens, 30

zinc and osteoporosis, 164